HYSTEROSCOPY

Alvin M. Siegler, M.D., D.Sc.

Clinical Professor, Department of Obstetrics and Gynecology,
State University of New York, Downstate Medical Center, Brooklyn, New York

Hans J. Lindemann, M.D.

Medical Director and Head, Department of Obstetrics and Gynecology,
Elisabeth Krankenhaus, Hamburg, West Germany

With 94 contributors

HYSTEROSCOPY

PRINCIPLES AND PRACTICE

J. B. LIPPINCOTT

Philadelphia

London   St. Louis
Mexico City   São Paulo
New York   Sydney

Acquisitions Editor: Lisa A. Biello
Sponsoring Editor: Richard Winters
Manuscript Editor: Martha Hicks-Courant
Indexer: Julie Schwager
Art Director: Maria S. Karkucinski
Designer: Arlene Putterman
Production Supervisor: N. Carolyn Kerr
Production Assistant: S. M. Gassaway
Compositor: Progressive Typographers
Printer: Princeton Polychrome Press
Binder: Haddon Craftsmen

The authors and publisher have exerted every effort to ensure that drug selection and dosage set forth in this text are in accord with current recommendations and practice at the time of publication. However, in view of ongoing research, changes in government regulations, and the constant flow of information relating to drug therapy and drug reactions, the reader is urged to check the package insert for each drug for any change in indications and dosage and for added warnings and precautions. This is particularly important when the recommended agent is a new or infrequently employed drug.

1 3 5 6 4 2

Library of Congress Cataloging in Publication Data
Main entry under title:

Hysteroscopy: principles and practice.

  Bibliography: p.
  Includes index.
  1. Hysteroscopy. I. Siegler, Alvin M. II. Lindemann,
Hans J. [DNLM: 1. Endoscopy—Congresses. 2. Uterus—
Congresses. 3. Uterine diseases—Diagnosis—Congresses.
4. Uterine diseases—Therapy—Congresses. WP 400 H999
1982]
RG304.5.H97H97 1984   618.1′407545   83-767
ISBN 0-397-50613-9

Contributors ☐

ASGHAR AFSARI, M.D.
Human Reproductive Resources
Infertility and Reproductive Research and
    Diagnostic Services
West Bloomfield, Michigan

JEAN M. ANTOINE, M.D.
Department of Obstetrics and Gynecology
Hôpital Tenon
Paris, France

ALFONSO ARIAS, M.D.
Foreign Assistant
Instituto Dexeus
Facultad de Medicina
Universidad Autónoma de Barcelona
Barcelona, Spain

SANDRA ARONBERG, M.D.
Department of Obstetrics and Gynecology
Cedars-Sinai Hospital
Los Angeles, California

MICHAEL S. BAGGISH, M.D.
Director
Department of Obstetrics and Gynecology
Mt. Sinai Hospital;
Professor
Department of Obstetrics and Gynecology
University of Connecticut School of Medicine
Hartford, Connecticut

WILHELM BRAENDLE, M.D.
Professor
Department of Obstetrics and Gynecology
Division of Experimental and Clinical
    Endocrinology
University of Hamburg
Hamburg, West Germany

FRANCESCO BRANCONI, M.D.
Department of Obstetrics and Gynecology
University of Florence
Florence, Italy

DORIS C. BROOKER, M.D.
Assistant Professor
Department of Obstetrics and Gynecology
University of Minnesota Medical School
Minneapolis, Minnesota

PHILIP G. BROOKS, M.D.
Associate Clinical Professor
Department of Obstetrics and Gynecology
University of Southern California School of
    Medicine
Los Angeles, California

JAN O. BRUNDIN, M.D., Ph.D.
Associate Professor
Department of Obstetrics and Gynecology
Karolinska Institute
Danderyd, Sweden

MILAN BUROS, M.D.
Head
Anesthesiology Department
Elisabeth Krankenhaus
Hamburg, West Germany

ELISABETTA CHELO, M.D.
Department of Obstetrics and Gynecology
University of Florence
Florence, Italy

INA CHOLST, M.D.
Department of Obstetrics and Gynecology
Yale University School of Medicine
New Haven, Connecticut

ANDRE CHOURAQUI, M.D.
Department of Anesthesiology
Hôpital Tenon
Paris, France

CHUNG KUN-CHIN, M.D.
Associate Professor
Department of Obstetrics and Gynecology
Chung Shan Medical College
Taichung, Taiwan

ETTORE CITTADINI, M.D.
Professor
Institute of Endocrinology and Physiopathology
   of Reproduction
Obstetric and Gynecological Clinic
University of Palermo
Palermo, Italy

MAURIZIO COLAFRANCESCHI, M.D.
Anatomy Pathology Institute
University of Florence
Florence, Italy

JAY M. COOPER, M.D.
Obstetrics and Gynecology Consultants, Inc.
Phoenix Baptist Hospital and Medical Center
Phoenix, Arizona

STEPHEN L. CORSON, M.D.
Department of Obstetrics and Gynecology
Pennsylvania Hospital
University of Pennsylvania School of Medicine
Philadelphia, Pennsylvania

ALAN H. DeCHERNEY, M.D.
Associate Professor
Department of Obstetrics and Gynecology
Director of Reproductive Endocrinology Division
Yale University School of Medicine
New Haven, Connecticut

JORIS F.D.E. DeMAEYER, M.D.
O. Lieve Vrouw U. Troost
Antwerp, Belgium

CHRISTIAN DEUTSCHMANN, M.D.
Department of Obstetrics and Gynecology
Elisabeth Krankenhaus
Hamburg, West Germany

SANTIAGO DEXEUS, M.D., F.I.A.C.
Associate Professor
Instituto Dexeus;
Head
Department of Obstetrics and Gynecology
Universidad Autónoma de Barcelona
Barcelona, Spain

MICHAEL DOLFF, M.D.
Universitätsfrauenklinik Düsseldorf
Düsseldorf, West Germany

ROBERT A. ERB, Ph.D.
Institute Fellow
Franklin Research Center
Division of the Franklin Institute
Philadelphia, Pennsylvania

YOSHIHIKO FUKUDA, M.D.
Department of Obstetrics and Gynecology
Osaka Medical College
Osaka, Japan

ADOLF GALLINAT, M.D.
Department of Obstetrics and Gynecology
Elisabeth Krankenhaus
Hamburg, West Germany

MARC GAMERRE, M.D.
Hôpital de la Conception
Clinique Obstétricale et Gynécologique
Marseille, France

RONALD E. GEORGE, B.Eng., M.Sc., Ph.D.
Director
Academic Computing Services
University of Calgary
Calgary, Alberta, Canada

DOMENICO GULLO, M.D.
Institute of Endocrinology and Physiopathology
   of Reproduction
Obstetric and Gynecological Clinic
University of Palermo
Palermo, Italy

JACQUES E. HAMOU, M.D.
Department of Obstetrics and Gynecology
Hôpital Tenon
Paris, France

MANUEL HILGARTH, M.D., F.I.A.C.
Department of Gynecology
University of Freiburg
Freiburg, West Germany

HANS-JOACHIM HINDENBURG, M.D.
Department of Obstetrics and Gynecology
Auguste Viktoria Krankenhaus
Berlin, West Germany

RICHARD HOUCK, M.D.
Obstetrics and Gynecology Consultants, Inc.
Phoenix Baptist Hospital and Medical Center
Phoenix, Arizona

INGEMAR S. JOELSSON, M.D.
Professor
Department of Obstetrics and Gynecology
Umeå University School of Medicine
Umeå, Sweden

BODO KARACZ, M.D.
Hamburg, West Germany

RICHARD K. KLEPPINGER, M.D.
Director
Department of Obstetrics and Gynecology
Reading Hospital and Medical Center
Reading, Pennsylvania

RICHARD A. KOPHER, M.D.
Reproductive Endocrinologist
Group Health, Inc.
St. Louis Park, Minnesota

RAMON LABASTIDA, M.D.
Chief
Endoscopic Section
Instituto Dexeus
Facultad de Medicina
Universidad Autónoma de Barcelona
Barcelona, Spain

ARTHUR LEADER, M.D.
Assistant Professor
Division of Obstetrics and Gynecology
University of Calgary
Calgary, Alberta, Canada

FRANKLIN D. LOFFER, M.D.
Chief
Division of Endoscopy
Department of Obstetrics and Gynecology
Maricopa County General Hospital
Phoenix, Arizona

PATRICIA S. LOFFER, R.N.
Gynecological Associates, Ltd.
Phoenix, Arizona

FRIEDHELM LÜBKE, M.D.
Professor
Department of Gynecology
Freie Universität Berlin
Berlin, West Germany

ROLF PETER LUEKEN, M.D.
Senior Registrar
Department of Obstetrics and Gynecology
Elisabeth Krankenhaus
Hamburg, West Germany

GENEVIEVE MAILLARD, M.D.
Department of Anesthesiology
Hôpital Tenon
Paris, France

VALENTIN MARLESCHKI, M.D.
Chief
Private Gynecological Clinic
Tuttlingen, West Germany

RENE MARTY, M.D.
Hôpitaux de Paris
Université XIII
Paris, France

LUCA MENCAGLIA, M.D.
Department of Obstetrics and Gynecology
University of Florence
Florence, Italy

COL. KUNIO MIYAZAWA, M.D.
Assistant Chief
Department of Obstetrics and Gynecology;
Chief
Gynecologic Oncology Service
Tripler Army Medical Center
Honolulu, Hawaii

FREDERICK NAFTOLIN, M.D., Ph.D.
Professor and Chairman
Department of Obstetrics and Gynecology
Yale University School of Medicine
New Haven, Connecticut

THEODORE C. NAGEL, M.D.
Associate Professor
Department of Obstetrics and Gynecology
University of Minnesota Medical School
Minneapolis, Minnesota

ROBERTO NANNINI, M.D.
Department of Obstetrics and Gynecology
University of Florence
Florence, Italy

ROBERT S. NEUWIRTH, M.D.
Babcock Professor
Department of Obstetrics and Gynecology
College of Physicians and Surgeons
Columbia University
New York, New York

KIMIYASU OHKAWA, M.D.
Professor and Director
Department of Obstetrics and Gynecology
Nippon Medical School
Tokyo, Japan

RYOKI OHKAWA, M.D.
Associate Professor
Department of Obstetrics and Gynecology
Nippon Medical School
Tokyo, Japan

TAKASHI OKAGAKI, M.D.
Professor
Department of Obstetrics and Gynecology
University of Minnesota Medical School
Minneapolis, Minnesota

GERLINDE PARTECKE, M.D.
Anesthesiology Department
Elisabeth Krankenhaus
Hamburg, West Germany

ANTONIO PERINO, M.D.
Institute of Endocrinology and Physiopathology
    of Reproduction
Obstetric and Gynecological Clinic
University of Palermo
Palermo, Italy

RAFAEL L. PINEDA, M.D.
Servicio de Ginecología
Hospital de Emergencias Dr. Clemente Alvarez
Rosario, Argentina

LOTHAR W. POPP, M.D.
Head
Department of Obstetrics and Gynecology
Elisabeth Krankenhaus
Hamburg, West Germany

ROBERT PORTO, M.D.
Hôpital de la Conception
Clinique Obstétricale et Gynécologique
Marseille, France

RODOLFO G. QUIÑONES, M.D.
Professor
Department of Obstetrics and Gynecology
Facultad Nacional de Medicina U.N.A.M.;
Medical Advisor
Subdirección Médica ISSS
Mexico City, Mexico

THEODORE P. REED, III, M.D.
Associate Clinical Professor
Jefferson Medical College
Thomas Jefferson University
Philadelphia, Pennsylvania

HANS-HARALD RIEDEL, M.D.
Department of Obstetrics and Gynecology
Michaelis Midwifery School

University of Kiel
Kiel, West Germany

JACQUES E. RIOUX, M.D., M.P.H.
Professor
Department of Obstetrics and Gynecology
Centre Hospitalier de l'Université Laval
Quebec, Canada

MAXWELL ROLAND, M.D.
Honorary Gynecologist
Department of Obstetrics and Gynecology
Booth Memorial Medical Center
Flushing, New York

HANS ROLL, M.D.
Akademisches Lehrkrankenhaus
Tuttlingen, West Germany

JACQUES SALAT-BAROUX, M.D.
Professor
Department of Obstetrics and Gynecology
Hôpital Tenon
Paris, France

LUCIANO SAVINO, M.D.
Department of Obstetrics and Gynecology
University of Florence
Florence, Italy

GIANFRANCO SCARSELLI, M.D.
Department of Obstetrics and Gynecology
University of Florence
Florence, Italy

SIEGFRIED SCHULZ, D.V.M.
Theoretical Surgery
Veterinary School
University of Marburg
Marburg, West Germany

ALBRECHT SCHULZ-CLASSEN, M.D.
Department of Obstetrics and Gynecology
University of Hamburg
Hamburg, West Germany

KARL W. SCHWEPPE, M.D.
Department of Obstetrics and Gynecology
Westfälischen Wilhelms Universität
Münster, West Germany

JOHN J. SCIARRA, M.D., Ph.D.
Professor and Chairman
Department of Obstetrics and Gynecology
Northwestern University School of Medicine
Chicago, Illinois

H. ASCHER SELLNER, M.D.
Assistant
Clinical Obstetrics and Gynecology
Columbia University
New York, New York

KURT SEMM, M.D., D.V.M.
Professor
Department of Obstetrics and Gynecology
Michaelis Midwifery School
University of Kiel
Kiel, West Germany

HENRI SERMENT, M.D.
Professor
Department of Obstetrics and Gynecology
Hôpital de la Conception
Marseille, France

HANS-EGON STEGNER, M.D.
Department of Obstetrics and Gynecology
Division of Histopathology
University of Hamburg
Hamburg, West Germany

OSAMU SUGIMOTO, M.D.
Chairman and Professor
Department of Obstetrics and Gynecology
Osaka Medical College
Osaka, Japan

MARK W. SURREY, M.D.
Assistant Professor
Department of Obstetrics and Gynecology
University of California in Los Angeles
School of Medicine
Los Angeles, California

GIANLUCA TADDEI, M.D.
Anatomy Pathology Institute
University of Florence
Florence, Italy

GEORGE E. TAGATZ, M.D.
Professor
Department of Obstetrics and Gynecology
University of Minnesota Medical School
Minneapolis, Minnesota

CARLO TANTINI, M.D.
Department of Obstetrics and Gynecology
University of Florence
Florence, Italy

PATRICK J. TAYLOR, M.B.
Professor
Division of Obstetrics and Gynecology

University of Calgary
Calgary, Alberta, Canada

DUANE E. TOWNSEND, M.D.
Department of Obstetrics and Gynecology
Cedars-Sinai Medical Center
Los Angeles, California

ROBERTO I. TOZZINI, M.D.
Associate Professor
Department of Gynecology
Rosario Medical School
National University of Rosario
Rosario, Argentina

TAKAHISA USHIROYAMA, M.D.
Department of Obstetrics and Gynecology
Osaka Medical College
Osaka, Japan

SERGE UZAN, M.D.
Department of Obstetrics and Gynecology
Hôpital Tenon
Paris, France

RAFAEL F. VALLE, M.D.
Associate Professor
Department of Obstetrics and Gynecology
Northwestern University School of Medicine
Prentice Women's Hospital and Maternity Center
Chicago, Illinois

HARRY VAN DER PAS, M.D.
Department of Gynecology
St. Elisabeth Hospital
Turnhout, Belgium

BRUNO J. VAN HERENDAEL, M.D.
Department of Gynecology
A.Z. Jan Palfijn O.C.M.W. Merksem
Merksem, Belgium

PIERRE VERGES, M.D.
Department of Bacteriology
Hôpital Tenon
Paris, France

HORST WAGNER, M.D.
Professor
Department of Obstetrics and Gynecology
Westfälischen Wilhelms Universität
Münster, West Germany

KEES WAMSTEKER, M.D., Ph.D.
Department of Obstetrics and Gynecology
Mariastichting
Haarlem, Holland

Preface □

Hysteroscopy is an endoscopic procedure utilizing a fiberoptic telescope and a method to distend the uterine cavity for examination.

Early attempts to inspect the uterine cavity were thwarted because of inability to obtain sustained adequate expansion of the uterus, concern about infection of the peritoneal cavity through the tubes by liquid or gaseous media, and endometrial bleeding during manipulation. Theoretically, development of a reliable and reproducible hysteroscopic procedure should improve the diagnostic accuracy of gynecologists, permitting them to treat many uterine diseases more effectively than before. Techniques for hysteroscopy have been employed sporadically for many years with limited acceptance, but recent reports claiming more successful and diverse applications have renewed interest in the procedure.

Hysteroscopy: Principles and Practice is based on the proceedings of the First World Congress of Hysteroscopy held in Miami, Florida, in January of 1982. The chapters are based on the contributions made by the experts at this meeting, with editorial modifications to provide guidance for beginners and descriptions of advanced refinements in technique for those with more experience. The fundamentals involved have been carefully described in the first section of this book to furnish the gynecologist with some guidelines. Although experience is the best teacher, a review of indications, instruments, anesthesia, and hazards involved in hysteroscopy is essential.

Certainly the logic of looking into the uterine cavity for the cause of abnormal bleeding seems irrefutable. Perhaps the time has come for the curet to be used selectively rather than simply as a tool to scrape the entire uterine cavity haphazardly in hopes of finding the cause of bleeding. It is an acknowledged fact that curettage misses about 25% of the endometrial surface, and in too many instances, a repeated curettage fails to disclose an endometrial polyp, a submucous myoma, or even an early localized endometrial adenocarcinoma. For specialists in infertility and physicians dealing with gynecologic oncology, hysteroscopy holds special promise for the establishment of a more precise diagnosis. Furthermore, in selected instances, therapeutic measures can be performed under hysteroscopic control. Some of these procedures are described by experts in hysteroscopy, who note the advantages and limitations of the operations.

The quest for a simple, safe, effective procedure for sterilization continues, and several authors detail new experiences with the hysteroscope used to guide an occlusive device into the uterotubal ostia. Hysteroscopy may be used in early pregnancy to examine the embryo, permit performance of selected biopsies of the trophoblast, and facilitate removal of an intrauterine contraceptive device, allowing a pregnancy to continue. The practical value of hysteroscopy as an office procedure is documented by many investigators. Combinations of hysteroscopy with ultrasound and a new microcolpohysteroscope are described.

Illustrations have been used throughout the text to show the hysteroscopic appearances of all the intrauterine lesions discussed as well as methods for their differential diagnosis and removal.

Is the hysteroscope still an instrument looking for an indication? The editors, as well as the experts who have contributed their excellent research and discussions, firmly believe that no gynecologist can be considered thoroughly trained without having had access to this technique of endoscopy.

ALVIN M. SIEGLER, M.D., D.SC.
HANS J. LINDEMANN, M.D.

Acknowledgments □

We wish to thank all the contributors for their active participation in the historic First World Congress of Hysteroscopy, for their splendid help in developing this book, and for their kindness in responding to the pressures of the editors. Many of the contributors describe different instruments and techniques and give different indications for hysteroscopy. Contradictory beliefs concerning several aspects of hysteroscopy are expressed throughout the book, but the editors believe that these remarks are essential so that the total international picture of current practices can be reviewed.

We also express our sincerest appreciation to Dr. Leon Chesley for the conscientious application of his literary talents toward improving the quality of this book. Without his keen insights and ability to clarify the essence of each manuscript, the editors could not have fulfilled their objective of writing a complete guide to the current applications of hysteroscopy. The staff of the American Association of Gynecologic Laparoscopists, especially Miss Linda Bojorquez, deserve special mention for their care and concern during the repeated retyping of the edited manuscripts. Finally, this book would not have been possible without the driving force, organizational skills, and guidance of Dr. Jordan M. Phillips, Chairman of the Board of the American Association of Gynecologic Laparoscopists.

We hope that this text will serve as a reference for the gynecologist who practices hysteroscopy and as a stimulus and incentive for those who contemplate a beginning in hysteroscopy, so that in the end, the carefully executed procedure will appreciably improve the care of our patients.

Addresses Presented at the First World Congress of Hysteroscopy □

Gynecologists from 23 countries are meeting to compare notes about their extensive experiences with hysteroscopy. This intrauterine endoscopic technique is efficient, safe, and relatively simple. The remarkable increase in its use during the last few years has assured its importance in gynecology. Its application for investigating causes of female sterility or abnormal uterine bleeding should become routine. With hysteroscopy, the examiner is able to see the interior of the uterine cavity in detail. Carbon dioxide gas or liquid solutions can be used to distend the uterine cavity, the medium employed depending upon the indication for the hysteroscopy and the preference of the gynecologist.

After 130 years, transuterine sterilization still is in a state of research, but present trials with plastic substances may disclose a successful, reliable, and simple method for outpatient sterilization. New contact and microcolpohysteroscopes may become valuable additions to the instruments used in hysteroscopy. The continued progress of every endoscopic method depends on further development of telescopic and technical instruments, light sources, and photodocumentation. We should like to take this opportunity to thank all of the firms involved with this task for their excellent teamwork with the doctors, all of which contributes to the well-being of the patient. My thanks also to the American Association of Gynecologic Laparoscopists, its Chairman, Dr. Jordan M. Phillips, and the Chairman of the Scientific Program Committee, Dr. Alvin M. Siegler, who arranged for this meeting.

HANS J. LINDEMANN, M.D.
Honorary President
First World Congress of Hysteroscopy

As it enters its second decade, the American Association of Gynecologic Laparoscopists can look back with some pride to advances made in laparoscopy and microsurgery as a direct result of a congress such as this. But the AAGL is a forward-looking organization, and as we look into the near future, we see hysteroscopy at a crossroads. Remember, only a few years ago, hysteroscopy was termed a "procedure in search of an indication."

What are the indications for hysteroscopy? What are the therapeutic procedures that legit-imately should be pursued with this modality? Is there a place for office hysteroscopy? What is the status of hysteroscopic sterilization?

These and many other basic questions will be raised at this congress, and some answers may also be forthcoming. Perhaps more questions will be raised than answered, but in any case, this collection of manuscripts from the world's experts will have a major impetus in making hysteroscopy a well-utilized routine gynecologic procedure.

STEPHEN L. CORSON, M.D.
President
American Association of Gynecologic
Laparoscopists, 1982

It is with a feeling of pleasure and deep appreciation that I cordially welcome you to this important meeting. The overwhelmingly positive responses by the invited guests were most gratifying and indeed facilitated the fulfillment of my responsibility. I wish to thank all of you for your support, which ensures the superior quality of this convention. This meeting is a testimony to international interest in hysteroscopy and a tribute to an esteemed colleague in this field, our Honorary President, Dr. Hans-Joachim Lindemann. I thank Dr. Jordan Phillips for lending us his remarkable organizational talents and for his vision in sensing the need for such a congress. I am grateful to my colleagues in the American Association of Gynecologic Laparoscopists who have afforded me the benefits of their expertise. Finally, I would like to thank the office staff of AAGL for their diligent and careful attention to every detail. May this be a productive meeting and one that shall be remembered for its contribution to improving the diagnosis and management of many uterine diseases.

ALVIN M. SIEGLER, M.D., D.SC.
Chairman
Scientific Program Committee
First World Congress of Hysteroscopy

Contents ☐

HYSTEROSCOPY

The Uterus Throughout the Ages ■ Introduction

Hans J. Lindemann

When I was invited to speak on the occasion of the First World Congress of Hysteroscopy, it seemed appropriate to choose the uterus as my theme. I shall reflect on some philosophic aspects. Various questions spring to mind. What is the uterus and what purpose does it have? Answers are found only within a wider context of creation by examination of the role of the uterus in the history of human life and reproduction.

The first references to the existence of this organ appear in the philosophic writings of the ancient world. The Old Testament tells us that God created man in His own image. Having created *Homo sapiens,* He thought it unfair that man should walk this earth without a partner of the opposite sex. So God caused the first man, whom we know as Adam, to fall into a deep sleep. From Adam, He took a rib and fashioned from it the first woman, known to us as Eve. Henceforth, man had a permanent companion, in good times and in bad. Woman's primary role was to serve the needs of love and procreation. So when God created Woman, the uterus itself came into being.

An alternative, and no less interesting, version of man's creation is recorded in ancient Greek mythology. Accordingly, the first human beings were bisexual with two heads, four arms, four legs, and both male and female genitalia. These spherically shaped creatures, also known as *androgynes,* were too powerful for the gods. When they wanted to move quickly, they could propel themselves forward like a wheel, rolling swiftly toward their goal on the tips of their four arms and legs (Fig. 1). The Olympian gods were alarmed. To lessen the power of these creatures and at the same time increase their numbers, Zeus split them in two. The offspring were either male or female. Most were ordinary men and women with normal sexuality. The two halves had a natural longing to be reunited, and from this developed the love between man and woman. Hence modern man's incessant search for his ideal partner, or "other half," as we still say. Some became homosexual, whereas others chose a life of celibacy, a tradition that persists in monasticism today.

According to Hellenic tradition, the creation of a separate man (*andro*) and woman (*gyne*) brought into being the uterus, which became an integral part of Greek culture. From the age of Hippocrates onwards, references to this organ are found in the writings of philosophers. Many famous thinkers, including Plato, Aristotle, Galen, and Paracelsus, were also practicing physicians.

The oldest representations of the female body occur in prehistoric models, cave drawings, and carved reliefs found in eastern Spain (Fig. 2). These representations, which date

1

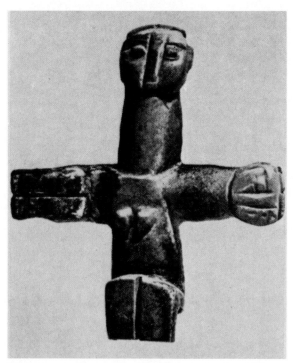

FIG. 1. Androgynes propelled themselves like a wheel.

from about 20,000 B.C., reveal an understanding of the function and structure of the genitals that seems irrational. Many prehistoric tribes regarded the uterus as a living being in its own right. This was also a common view in European folk medicine, particularly in Greece. When the uterus failed to perform its function properly, it was regarded by some as a type of wild beast roaming through the woman's body and endangering her life. If, for example, a woman failed to conceive, fear and serious illness were thought to result. The uterus was an organ that attracted moisture, like the bladder, and liquid was thought essential for its proper functioning. Physical exertion and sexual abstinence were considered to dry out the uterus, making it lighter. Consequently it was thought to roam about in search of moisture. Its wanderings took it to the liver, stomach, lungs, and thyroid gland and eventually to the head. Symptoms of illness associated with these movements became known as *hysteria.* This term, with which we are all familiar, comes

from the Greek word *hystera,* meaning womb or uterus. From the beginning of civilization, people have regarded the "hystera" as the root of all evil, and rightly so, according to Galen. Physicians of antiquity attributed all kinds of ailments to a uterine cause, even those that logically could not possibly have anything to do with the uterus. By affinity, symptoms were allegedly transmitted through the body. Even fever was said to be caused in this way. This theory of Plato profoundly influenced the Hippocratic teachings on hysteria.

As a therapy for hysteria (which was very widespread), Greek physicians of the Hippocratic School recommended coitus. This "remedy" had been practiced among primitive peoples and remained standard treatment until the late Middle Ages. The uterus thereby received an adequate supply of moisture, causing it to stay in its proper place. The people of the Pacific island of Bali even today believe that the uterus needs to be placated with a constant diet of semen. This must surely be one of the most simple and natural remedies in all of medical science. Is there, I wonder, a lesson for us here? It was not unknown for a young woman married to an aging husband to take advantage of this situation. Coitus was recommended by physicians of antiquity as a remedy for amenorrhea, dysmenorrhea, leukorrhea, and hysteria. In a witty epigram, the poet Martial described a young woman who cunningly persuaded her impotent older husband to delegate his marital duties to younger men because she was suffering from hysteria. I rather doubt that modern husbands would consent so amicably to such an arrangement.

Another therapy consisted of bleeding the uterus by placing cupping glasses on the breast. In the Middle Ages, cupping was thought to be the only way of drawing blood from the uterus. Theoretically, the uterus and breast were linked by blood vessels that played a part in nourishing the fetus.

From ancient times until the Middle Ages, the shape of the uterus was compared to that of a toad. The uterine corpus, cervix, tubes, and ligaments combined resembled the body of this animal. The toad motif recurred constantly in

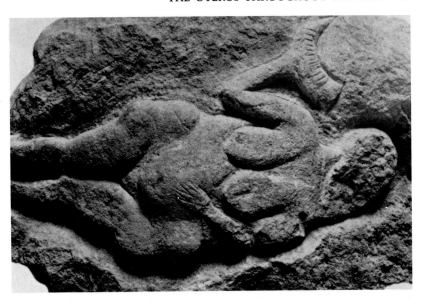

FIG. 2. Cave drawing seen in carved relief.

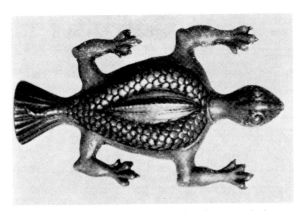

FIG. 3. The toad motif was a fertility symbol.

relation to infertility (Fig. 3). Cast in wax or metal, the form of a toad is still offered as a votive gift to bring fertility to the supplicant. Among certain peoples, the uterus was thought to be like a spiny animal or prickly ball, resembling the inverted uterus of a cow. As students of veterinary medicine know, the uterus of ruminants has many projections and lobes, giving it the appearance of a hedgehog. The most accurate portrayal of the uterus before the modern era dates from the 15th century, when Leonardo daVinci prepared a series of anatomic drawings for midwifery (Fig. 4).

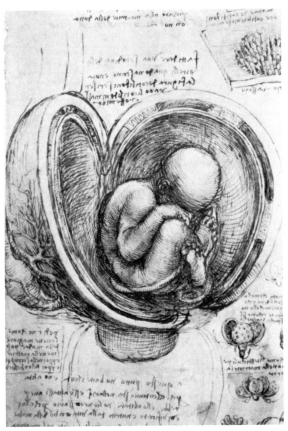

FIG. 4. Anatomic drawing of the uterus made by Leonardo da Vinci.

Sterility has been an important problem in gynecology throughout history. Even when nothing was known about the existence of spermatozoa or the ovum, it was broadly understood that the male ejaculate and secretion and menstruation in women were important for fertilization. Women were examined for fertility by the so-called smoke test. With the lower part of her body uncovered, the woman sat on a special chair with a perforated seat. Clothing was draped around the lower part of her body, sealing it completely from the surrounding air. Special herbs were burned underneath the seat of the chair. If the woman identified the herbs, she was deemed fertile. In another test, a peeled garlic bulb was placed in the vagina overnight. If the woman awoke the next morning with the taste of garlic, it meant that the system of ducts extending from the vagina to the breasts and mouth through the uterus, tubes, and blood vessels was patent, and the woman was judged fertile. The modern technique of tubal insufflation, the Rubin test, is not much different.

To ascertain the fertility of a male, a sample of urine was poured over certain types of grain such as barley or lentils. Germination after 7 days signified that the man was fertile. In another method, the ejaculate was placed in a vessel containing water. If the semen remained on the surface or dispersed in the water, the man was considered infertile. If it all sank to the bottom of the container, the man was considered fertile. An ancient tradition taught that fertility of males was improved by bleeding of the blood vessels behind the ears. The seminal passages were thought to extend from the brain to the testicles, so that if they became blocked, they could cause infertility. This indicates a premonition of the existence of the gonadotropic hormones.

The woman's ability to sustain a pregnancy was thought to be due to her body being filled with air, aided by a thin skin and a porous skull. The infant in the womb needed an ample and continuous supply of air. As the supply of food and air became inadequate, the baby felt "hemmed in," and labor began because of shrinkage of the uterus. The infant and the placenta were regarded as twins. The umbilical cord could be cut only after delivery of the placenta, which would otherwise remain behind.

A few words must be said about the modern understanding and medical knowledge of the uterus. This organ is situated between the bladder and the rectum. It is held in position by round ligaments anteriorly and the uterosacral ligaments posteriorly. These ligaments are elastic, so that the uterus can move in any direction within the pelvis. The uterus is a hollow, muscular organ approximately 7 cm to 9 cm long with a flat, slitlike cavity. It is roughly triangular, with lobe-shaped protrusions to which the tubes are connected. Safely protected by the fluids of the uterine cavity, the tiny, delicate spermatozoa make their way toward the tubes, in which they unite with the ovum to create a new life.

The pear-shaped uterus changes during puberty and in the menopause, and it is affected by processes within the organ. In pregnancy and childbirth, the womb expands to 500 times its usual size. The uterus may also be dramatically structurally and functionally altered by benign and malignant diseases.

Hysteroscopy, the oldest gynecologic endoscopic technique, has enabled us to study the anatomy of the uterine cavity and the endocervical canal and to observe the processes that take place within them. To illustrate its range and efficiency, I will describe a few of the physiologic changes relating to the menstrual cycle that may be seen through the hysteroscope. Normally, the myometrium is evenly lined with the endometrium. During the proliferative phase, the lining appears reddish yellow and looks like a "close-cropped carpet." At ovulation, it takes on a more yellowish hue. Occasionally, some diffuse discharge of blood is seen, and many women experience intermenstrual bleeding. Throughout the secretory phase, as the endometrium becomes swollen, its surface frequently produces cystlike eruptions and furrows. The color also changes to reddish purple. Soon afterward, desquamation or shedding results. Necrosis around the edges is seen together with small, curled fragments that have already been detached. The tissue is interspersed with areas of blood, though sometimes coagulation occurs and the blood clots. The endometrium initially breaks down in the fundus, and the process spreads to the sidewalls and then to the isthmus. When shedding is completed, regeneration of the mucous membrane begins. Bloodlike growths appear, interspersed with minor sporadic bleeding. This sequence is demonstrated by the pattern of myometrial contractions.

The blastocyst is implanted in the uterine cavity approximately 1 week after ovulation, where it is nourished as it develops into the embryo and fetus.

If we compare our present understanding of the uterus with the ideas of the ancients, it seems to me that the old thinking on the subject still has some merit, especially when we are faced by apparently inexplicable ailments or bodily functions in some way attributed to this organ. All ancient mythologies, whether derived from the Greeks, Romans, Hebrews, Egyptians, or peoples of India, tell us that the uterus has a significance far beyond its physical function in procreation. These views were inextricably bound with mystical conceptions.

The history of the uterus and woman's role in society is fascinating, and a great deal more could be said about it. Although modern science has brought us a long way in our understanding of the world, we are only just beginning to comprehend the great mystery of life. The ultimate question, why are we here, remains unanswered. Paracelsus called the uterus "the smallest microcosm" in which all human life is reproduced, contrasting it with the macrocosm or "great womb," where life in its totality is enacted. And the medieval humanist Buonaccioli said of this unique female organ, "Of all the miracles which the human body shows us, none is more marvelous and admirable than the womb of the woman, from whence man in all his wondrous complexity, is most ingeniously derived."

PRINCIPLES OF HYSTEROSCOPY   I

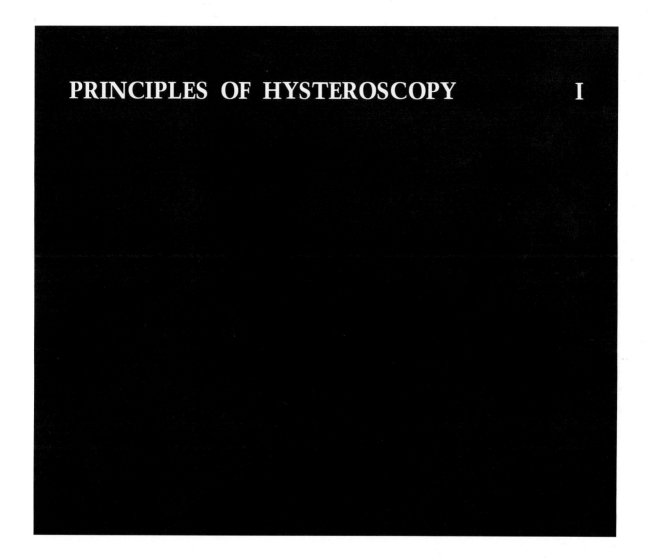

Although the hysteroscopic procedure has been available for over 100 years, inconsistent success with the operation and a presumed lack of good indications prevented its widespread application. Inadequate uterine distention, inferior optical systems, and disconcerting endometrial bleeding disappointed many observers.

The contributors to this section show the potential value of hysteroscopy in solving many gynecologic problems. Lindemann thoroughly traces its history and development during the past century, while Valle carefully describes its practical and potential diagnostic and therapeutic values. His paper is followed by an analysis of over 1000 operations performed by different authors who have used this endoscopic approach successfully. One of the most common indications is abnormal uterine bleeding. Hysteroscopy enables the physician to see into the uterine cavity, making a directed or target biopsy possible. Infertility and postabortal hypomenorrhea are also given as important indications.

The advantages and disadvantages of different media to distend the uterine cavity are described by Rioux. The intrauterine pressure developed during instillation of gaseous or liquid media is sufficient to have a hemostatic effect on the fragile endometrium, provided the physician is gentle and slow in manipulating the hysteroscope. The physiologic principles involving carbon dioxide are listed by Gallinat, who correctly cautions against the use of unmonitored systems of delivery of gas into the uterine cavity. Note that the rate of flow should never exceed 100 ml/min. Although most physicians in Europe seem to prefer carbon dioxide, those in the United States and Japan use liquid media more commonly. Physicians should use the technique that gives them the best results. Quiñones continues to advocate 5% dextrose for uterine distention because of its availability, low cost, and effectiveness. With his instrumental innovation, a continuous flow of fluid is ensured under constant pressure. Roll and Hilgarth did most of their 560 carbon dioxide hysteroscopic examinations under general anesthesia; prostaglandin E_2 was given intramuscularly 6 hr preoperatively to soften the cervix.

Experience with hysteroscopy increases the operator's skill and confidence in interpretation. The principles of this technique include a review of the history and previous hysterosalpingogram to alert the physician to search for specific defects and a preliminary pelvic examination to ascertain uterine position and size; then a tenaculum is placed on the anterior lip of the cervix for traction. The speculum should have an opening on one lateral aspect to enable greater manipulation of the hysteroscope. The patient's buttocks are elevated about 5 degrees, the medium for uterine distention and the fiberoptic light projector are adjusted, and their connections are fixed to the appropriate place on the sheath of the hysteroscope. The tip of the instrument is gently inserted into the cervical canal as the surgeon observes its entrance

through the ocular. As the cervix fills, its projections are clearly seen within the canal while it is dilated by gas or liquid. Usually some resistance is encountered just before the uterine cavity is entered.

The surgeon is then ready to explore systematically the fundus, both horns and ostia, and the lateral, anterior, and posterior walls of the uterine cavity. As the cavity distends, the endometrium appears pale yellow, tan, or pink with occasional hemorrhagic spots. Since the endometrial surfaces are fairly close together, the hysteroscope must be carefully rotated for exploration of the entire endometrial cavity. The procedure is relatively simple, since the uterine cavity is readily visible in a panoramic view. The horns and tubal ostia are seen by manipulating the scope very slightly. It is important to proceed slowly, initially observing the endocervical canal and following the dark opening of the lower uterine segment until the fundus comes into view. A normal cavity is easily identified, since it is distended with either liquid or gas. Most patients have minimal abdominal discomfort postoperatively. Instruments created over the past decade offer increased clarity of vision, a sheath reduced to 5 mm or less, and larger, rigid accessory instruments, so that therapeutic procedures under hysteroscopic control are now performed in a more definitive manner.

Microhysteroscopy, according to Hamou and Salat-Baroux, can be used in women who have abnormal cervical smears to examine the squamocolumnar junction *in vivo* at the cellular level with vital stains. This relatively common new instrument can magnify up to 150 times during contact. Because of its small size, it may be able to locate the transitional zone beyond the reach of the colposcope. Many procedures and multicenter studies must be done to confirm this hope before a definitive conclusion can be reached. Contact hysteroscopy has been advocated for many years by Marleschki, but his observations and interpretations have not been duplicated by other investigators. Of course, no distending medium is needed, but then panoramic vision is not possible. Vascular patterns are very important for proper diagnosis.

In a preliminary report of small series, Brooks and coauthors confirmed the usefulness of the Hamou hysteroscope for panoramic observation, and we look forward to their impressions on the microcolposcopic value of the instrument. It is reports of such investigators with experience in colposcopy and the new approach that will provide the quality control needed to ascertain the dimensions of this technologic innovation. Incidentally, this hysteroscope cannot be used effectively with high-molecular dextran as a medium for uterine distention, and it is not generally considered useful for therapeutic hysteroscopic procedures.

Hysterosonography is a technique for "looking inside" the uterine cavity indirectly with a rotating, intrauterine ultrasound probe in place of a hysteroscope. Popp and Lueken's excellent illustrations and description of the technique add yet another method to enable a more precise intrauterine examination. Scarselli and co-workers attempted to correlate some physiopathologic endometrial changes as seen by conventional ultrasound and panoramic hysteroscopy, while Ohkawa and Ohkawa compared histologic findings with cellular morphologic changes seen on *in vivo* staining. Both of these contributions must be judged as preliminary reports and need further evaluation before definitive conclusions can be reached on the accuracy of *in vivo* observations during hysteromicroscopy.

The large series of 4000 hysteroscopic examinations performed by Salat-Baroux and colleagues was done without any anesthesia except in 53 patients, 13 of them because of other associated operative procedures. These authors confirmed the safety of carbon dioxide hysteroscopy with a series of blood gas studies and the minimal chance of infection on the basis of clinical results and bacteriologic studies. It is strange that aerobic and anaerobic cultures revealed so few organisms, because the cervix is normally inhabited by numerous bacteria. They rinsed the hysteroscope with saline and 70% alcohol between patients, and few infections were found. Although this evidence seems convincing (7 infections in 4000 operations), perhaps autoclaving the sheath between patients or at least once a day is warranted. Maybe even this precaution will prove unnecessary as additional data are accumulated in other centers.

Karacz presented the results of 125 hysteroscopic office examinations, giving a realistic approach of the time and effort involved. Although we cannot agree that either a special room or a trained nurse or assistant is a prerequisite, certainly a sufficient number of patients with appropriate indications and reliable, reasonably priced instruments would increase the use of the hysteroscope in private practice.

Local paracervical nerve block, cervical dilatation, suction cups, carbon dioxide hysteroscopy, and high-molecular dextran are used during hysteroscopy, the methods being tailored to the patient's needs and the physician's experience. The most important ingredients for success are gentleness and patience to avoid provoking endometrial bleeding and spasm. Biopsy must accompany observation of suspicious areas. Therapeutic hysteroscopy requires additional experience and dexterity; these maneuvers should be adapted to the endoscopist's experience, particularly for the removal of submucous myomas, the division of thick connective tissue adhesions and uterine septae, and tubal sterilization.

One Hundred Years of Hysteroscopy: 1869–1969 ■

Hans J. Lindemann

Observation ranks with percussion, auscultation, and palpation as one of the principal methods of clinical examination. For this reason physicians sought a simple method to look into the cavities of the human body. Until the beginning of the 20th century, this possibility existed only for external orifices. Archigenes of Apameia already had a grasp of illumination procedures, "et hoc ad clarem lucem siat."[2] Subsequently anal and vaginal specula were developed, from simple tubes to more "complex" instruments for dilatation and observation. Various methods were devised, using systems of concave mirrors and lenses, to collect and focus light from natural and artificial sources and direct it into a cavity.

HISTORY OF ENDOSCOPY

The history of endoscopy really begins in the early years of the 19th century. In 1805 Bozzini (1773–1809) constructed a device, called a *light conductor*, that enabled him to inspect various passages and body cavities (Fig. 1-1).[7] This instrument consisted of a square, windowed tube. Candlelight was directed by a concave mirror through a narrow tube into the cavity. The results were not satisfactory. Bozzini recommended his device for the detection of small tumors and changes in the uterine cavity, for the diagnosis of causes of female sterility, and for internal examinations when complications occurred during pregnancy. He said that physicians should "look to the foetus." According to McCrea, the Viennese Academy of Medicine disapproved of Bozzini's unseemly interest in exploring the most inaccessible regions of the human body.[26] In 1864 Aubinais observed a baby's head emerge from the cervix with a tube he inserted into the vagina, and for this reason he has been described incorrectly as the first hysteroscopist.[3]

The first hysteroscopy (also called *metroscopy* or *uteroscopy*) was described in 1869 by Pantaleoni.[45] The patient was 60 years old with resistant uterine bleeding. A straight tube 12 mm in diameter, similar to the device Désormeaux used in 1865 to examine the urethra, was inserted into the uterine cavity (Fig. 1-2).[11] Polypoid endometrial growths were observed. Pantaleoni used reflected candlelight from a concave mirror to illuminate the uterine cavity.

ENDOSCOPY AT PRESENT

The present era in endoscopy began with Nitze, who demonstrated a cystoscope to the Royal Medical Board of Saxony and in 1879 published an account of the instrument (Fig.

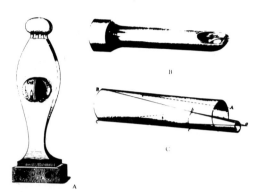

FIG. 1-1. Light conductor of Bozzini, 1805.

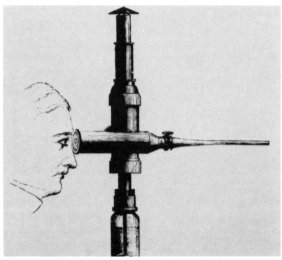

FIG. 1-2. First hysteroscopy with cystoscope of Désormeaux by Pantaleoni, 1869.

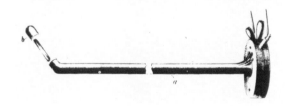

FIG. 1-3. First cystoscope by Nitze, 1877.

1-3).[36] Nitze inserted the illuminator and endoscope directly into the bladder. In collaboration with Leiter, a Viennese instrument maker, he added optical lenses. Both illumination and field of vision were increased.

To obtain a good view of the uterine cavity, it is necessary to maintain an adequate distance between the endoscopic lens and the endometrium. Early practitioners of uteroscopy proceeded without initially distending the uterus. The instruments were straight tubes of varying lengths and diameters. The light came from candles, kerosene lamps, or incandescent bulbs directed by a reflector to illuminate the area. This method did not produce satisfactory results. In 1880 Munde published an account of his experience with hysteroscopy and wrote, "If one compares the information derived in this way with that which can be obtained by using the tip of the index finger, the proverbial 'eye of the gynaecologist,' then it has to be said that this fleeting glimpse of the endometrium is of little clinical value."[35] The tube could not be moved easily within the uterine cavity, and the value of hysteroscopy remained limited.

The Nitze principle of endoscopy was not adopted for hysteroscopy. In 1893 Morris used a straight silver and brass tube 9 mm in diameter and 22 cm long.[34] An obturator inside the

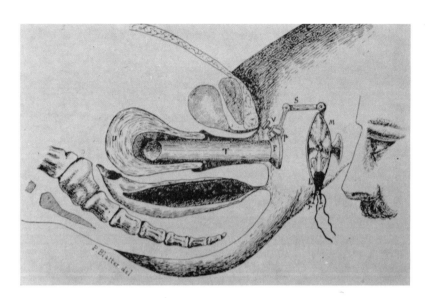

FIG. 1-4. First hysteroscope with a built-in lens to magnify the image. The illumination system is mounted externally, near the viewing end of the instrument.

tube was withdrawn once the instrument had been introduced into the uterine cavity, leaving the hollow tube to serve as an endoscope. Morris observed the tubal ostia and the endometrium. Bumm, using a head lamp with a reflector and the cystoscope, described endometrial changes, including granulations, ulcers, and polyps.[8] Bleeding and mucus frequently obstructed his vision. Blondel complained of similar difficulties, and, to alleviate these problems, a new type of hysteroscope was proposed by Beutner in 1898.[5,6] It was equipped with a water sprinkler system. Simultaneously, Duplay and Clado experimented with a hysteroscope equipped with a mandrin and an illuminator located near the eyepiece.[13] David constructed an endoscope modeled on Nitze's cystoscope with a built-in lens to magnify the image (Fig. 1-4).[10] The illuminating system was mounted externally, near the viewing end of the instrument. When the device was inserted into the uterine cavity, the physician was able to look directly toward the uterine fundus. David demonstrated that hysteroscopy was useful for diagnosis of uterine disorders.

Heineberg developed a water sprinkler system to rinse off the blood that often covered the lens and hindered vision.[18] Rubin insuf-

flated the uterine cavity with carbon dioxide instead of water.[50] The procedure was similar to tubal pertubation. The hysteroscope was a modified McCarthy cystourethroscope. The pointed end was rounded off to avoid trauma.

Seymour introduced a hysteroscope fitted with a suction tube that could drain mucus and blood from the uterine cavity.[58,59] In 1927 von Mikulicz-Radecki and Freund collaborated to produce a "curettoscope" with a rinsing system to wash away the blood that obstructed vision.[30,31] The view was angled toward the side with an optical magnification of 1:4. The instrument afforded a good view of the cavity and enabled the physician to perform directed endometrial biopsies.

In 1928 Gauss reported experiments with a similar instrument.[17] Anesthesia was used only in nulliparous women. Schroeder succeeded in developing an instrument with an excellent forward-viewing optical system, a significant advantage over earlier designs with side-mounted apertures.[53] It thus became possible to inspect larger areas of the cavity and to achieve three-dimensional views. The instrument had an external diameter of 10 mm. Examinations on multiparous women were done without need for anesthesia. A few drops of epinephrine (Adrenalin) solution were often added to the rinsing fluid to reduce the tendency of the endometrium to bleed.

Schroeder collected important data on the intrauterine pressure during hysteroscopy. He found that water instilled into the cavity from 650 mm above the patient resulted in an intrauterine pressure between 25 mm Hg and 30 mm Hg. When the height of the water column was increased to 950 mm, the pressure inside the uterus rose to 35 mm Hg. These pressures were sufficient to distend the uterine cavity. When the intrauterine pressure increased to more than 55 mm Hg, water flowed through the tubes into the peritoneal cavity. Schroeder performed hysterosalpingography using a radiopaque solution diluted to approximately the same viscosity as water to show these changes. Pressures of 35 mm Hg can distend the cavity sufficiently to ensure an adequate space between the endoscopic lens and the endometrium.

Encouraged by the work of Dickinson and of von Mikulicz-Radecki, Schroeder also attempted transuterine tubal sterilization.[12,30,31] Other pioneers of hysteroscopy during these years were Bank, Schack, and Segond.[4,51,54-57] Norment reported a new technique that called for a transparent rubber balloon mounted on the tip of the hysteroscope and illumination provided by an external light through a glass fiber conductor.[37-43] This system of illumination has become standard practice in hysteroscopy. The electric light bulb, previously mounted on the tip of the hysteroscope shaft, was replaced by the lens. When the instrument was inserted into the uterine cavity, the balloon was filled with air, and the resulting pressure against the endometrium was supposed to prevent the bleeding. Since this technique failed to solve the problem, Norment reverted to the traditional water-rinsing system.

Mohri and colleagues reported on the possibility of embryoscopy and presented a film showing embryos inside the uterus from the 8th to the 17th weeks of pregnancy.[32,33] They also introduced the first tubaloscope. Under favorable anatomic conditions, this slender instrument, 1.2 mm in diameter, was inserted into the tubal lumen. Illumination was poor, and the images appeared blurred.

Palmer proposed a hysteroscope with a diameter of 5 mm to obviate the need to dilate the cervical canal.[44] To distend the uterine cavity, he advised using the standard water-irrigation system. Silander devised a balloon made of transparent plastic fitted to the tip of the hysteroscope and filled with water.[60-62] Other early efforts to improve hysteroscopy were made by Burnett, Lyon, Esposito, and Schmidt-Matthiesen.[9,16,23,52] Englund and colleagues performed hysteroscopy after curettage. Since curettage failed to remove a substantial proportion of the endometrium, they recommended hysteroscopy for uterine bleeding resistant to therapy.[15] Marleschki made a special study of the blood circulation of the endometrium with an instrument 5 mm in diameter and $\times 12.5$ magnification placed in direct contact with the endometrium.[24,25] Agüero and associates performed hysteroscopy on 118 pregnant women between their 8th and 40th weeks of gestation, believing that in complicated cases a hysteroscopic examination was of great diagnostic value.[1]

A new era in hysteroscopy began with the introduction of viscous fluids as media for distending the uterine cavity. Menken reported on his experiments with Luviscol, a polyvinylpyrrolidone with a molecular weight of 200,000.[27-29] Media currently in use include dextran 70 (Hyskon) (Edström and Fernström), carbon dioxide gas (Lindemann and Porto and Gaujoux,) and a 5% glucose solution (Quiñones and colleagues).[14,19-22,46-49]

Improvements in instruments, light sources, and ancillary apparatus have facilitated the development of hysteroscopy (Table 1-1). Ultimately, a successful examination of the uterine cavity depends on the physician's skill. The endometrium remains highly sensitive, and blood and secretions can hinder vision during hysteroscopy. As far as the future role of hysteroscopy is concerned, a vigilant eye in the uterine cavity is better than numerous blind curets.

Table 1-1
HISTORICAL TIMETABLE: 1869–1969

INVESTIGATOR	YEAR	TECHNIQUE	INSTRUMENT DIAMETER	RESULTS	DISADVANTAGES
Pantaleoni (Great Britain)	1869	Désormeaux tube	10 mm	First uterine endoscopy; examination and therapy (silver nitrate)	Cervical dilatation; blood and mucus obstruct tubes
Blondel (France)	1893	Open-ended tube sliding a perforated outer tube (four sections reinforced by a collar at each end)	20 mm	Opportunity to inspect the uterine walls, which were separated and held apart by the perforated outer tube; work abandoned	Cervical dilatation; bleeding; heat emitted by light source
Morris (USA)	1894	"Endoscopic tubes" ?		Expressed little confidence in future of hysteroscopy	
Bumm (Germany)	1895			Expressed reservations about method and its safety	Bleeding; frequent tamponade ineffective; one case of salpingitis
Duplay and Clado (France)	1898	Open-ended tube; external light source, battery powered		Observation and therapy (silver nitrate)	Apparatus unwieldy and difficult to operate; frequent blockages caused by blood and mucus
David (France)	1907	Tube terminating in a window sliding within an open-ended outer tube; internal light source	10.5 mm, 12 mm, and 18 mm	Observation and cauterization of three models, one normal, one post-abortal, and one post-partal	Cervical dilatation; bleeding
Heineberg (USA)	1914	Internal light source; water-rinsing system			
Rubin (USA)	1925	Used a cystourethroscope; rinsed with saline solution; air injected with syringe; insufflation with carbon dioxide	15 mm	Observation; samples taken; coagulation	Inadequate distention; bleeding

(*Continued*)

Investigator (country)	Year	Technique	Diameter	Observations	Complications
Seymour (Great Britain)	1926	Sealed tube; internal light source; continuous evacuation by suction		Observation; samples taken	Cervical dilatation; no uterine distention
von Mikulicz-Radecki and Freund (Germany)	1927	Dual-circuit water-rinsing system			
Gauss (Germany)	1928	Pressurized water-rinsing system			Cervical dilatation; passage of fluid into abdominal cavity
Schroeder (Germany)	1934	Pressurized water-rinsing system	10 mm	Wider field of vision	
Schack (Germany)	1936	Pressurized water-rinsing system		50% failure rate	Cervical dilatation; passage of fluid into abdominal cavity
Segond (France)	1934	Pressurized water-rinsing system (elevated douche); water outlet larger than return intake (to avoid over distention); fore-oblique optical system with light source mounted on sliding rod inside tube	8 mm and 11 mm	Exploratory model and operative model; cornua of uterus not visible	Partial cervical dilatation, forcible insertion; inadequate distention; passage of several liters of fluid into abdominal cavity
Litwak (Germany)	1936			Postabortal study of the uterus; drawings made of various features observed	
Palmer (France)	1937	Modified version of Segond's hysteroscope (shortened and calibrated); water-rinsing system (elevated douche)	8 mm and 11 mm	Cornua of uterus rarely visible	Dilatation caused by fluid
Palmer (France)	1942	Performed cervicoscopy with a glass tube with a conical end, into which Segond's optical system was inserted	8 mm	Examination restricted to cervical canal	
Fourestier and colleagues (France)	1952	Application to endoscopy of quartz light transmission		Cold light source	Quartz rods very fragile

[16]

	Year	Diameter	Instrument	Purpose	Technique
Silander (Sweden)	1962	7 mm	Hysteroscope with small balloon derived from cardioscope of Carlens and Silander; balloon filled with serum or air	Observation only	Cervical dilatation (Hegar 8); anesthesia (optional); compression of endometrium by balloon
Burnett (USA)	1964		Norment's hysteroscope	Hysteroscopy as an aid to curettage	General anesthesia; cervical dilatation; flooding of peritoneal cavity
Lyon (USA)	1964	7 mm	Hysteroscope with small balloon (Silander type)		General anesthesia; cervical dilatation (Hegar 8); compression of endometrium
Schmidt-Matthiesen (W. Germany)	1966		Silander's hysteroscope		Compression of endometrium
Marleschki (E. Germany)	1966		Contact hysteroscope with a glass shield to keep mucus at a distance from lens		No distention of uterus
Esposito (Italy)	1965 to 1968	7 mm	Silander's hysteroscope with a modified balloon and more powerful illumination	Observation only	General anesthesia; cervical dilatation; compression of endometrium
Menken (W. Germany)	1968		Cold light hysteroscope, concave, with spring-loaded conical valve; injection with polyvinylpyrrolidone	No anesthesia and no dilatation	Passage of fluid into peritoneal cavity
Agüerrero and associates (Mexico)	1970		Cold light hysteroscope with small balloon	Observation only	General anesthesia; cervical dilatation; compression of endometrium
Edström and Fernström (Sweden)	1970	6 mm	Cold light hysteroscope		General or local anesthesia; cervical dilatation (Hegar 7); passage of injected liquid into peritoneal cavity
Porto and Gaujoux (France)	1971	4 mm and 8 mm	Pneumohysteroscopy (insufflation with carbon dioxide)	Observation; controlled biopsy; no cervical dilatation and no anesthesia	Design of insufflation apparatus must be perfected

Table 1-1 (*Continued*)

INVESTIGATOR	YEAR	TECHNIQUE	INSTRUMENT DIAMETER	RESULTS	DISADVANTAGES
Norment (USA)	1950 to 1956	Illumination by external light source; various methods: rubber balloon, transparent plastic balloon, water-rinsing system	9.5 mm	Observation; biopsy; sterilization by electrocoagulation; first photographs, showing that curettage leaves behind 25% of endometrium	Cervical dilatation; general anesthesia; flooding
Englund (Sweden) Ingleman-Sundberg	1952 1954	McCarthy's panendoscope; rinsing with saline solution at 37°C (elevated douche)		Study of metrorrhagia	Cervical dilatation; local or general anesthesia; one case of salpingitis and two cases of hyperthermia
Mohri and colleagues (Japan)	1954	Self-designed hysteroscope (no further information available)		Film	
Palmer (France)	1957	Segond's endoscope, reduced in diameter and fitted with a more powerful bulb	5 mm	No dilatation, only observation	Copius flooding of peritoneal cavity
Muller (France)	1956	Urethroscope with water-rinsing system (water evacuated by suction); cold light source through quartz tube (principle pioneered by Vulmiere and Forestier, 1952)	9 mm	Observation; openings of the uterine tubes not visible; color film	Cervical dilatation; general anesthesia; forcible insertion of outer tube; copious flooding of peritoneal cavity
Wulfsohn (Great Britain)	1959	Cystoscope; distention with small balloon filled with water	6 mm	Observation only	Cervical dilatation; general anesthesia
Gribb (USA)	1960	Norment's hysteroscope			Cervical dilatation; general anesthesia
Bánk (Hungary)	1960	Hysteroscope with small balloon (Wulfsohn type); method abandoned and a return to water rinsing but with manometer to regulate pressure	6 mm		Rubber formed folds that hampered vision; compression altered appearance of endometrium

REFERENCES

1. Agüero O, Aure M, López R: Hysteroscopy in pregnant patients—A new diagnostic tool. Am J Obstet Gynecol 94:925, 1966
2. Archigenes: cit. in Aumiller, Die Entwicklung der Endoskope. Inaugural dissertation, 1971
3. Aubinais EJ: De l'uteroscopie. J Sect Med Soc Acad Dept Loire Infer 39:71, 1863
4. Bánk EB: Erfahrungen mit der Metroskopie. Zentralbl Gynaekol 82:866, 1960
5. Beutner O: Über Hysteroskopie. Zentralbl Gynaekol 22:580, 1898
6. Blondel R: CR Soc d'Obstét, December 1907
7. Bozzini P: Der Lichtleiter oder Beschreibung einer einfachen Vorrichtung und ihrer Anwendung zur Erleuchtung innerer Höhlen und Zwischenräume des lebenden animalischen Körpers. Weimar, Landes—Industrie—Comptoir, 1807
8. Bumm E: Diskussion über Endometritis. In Chrobak R, Pfannenstiel J (eds): Verhandlungen der Deutschen Gesellschaft für Gynäkologie, 6th Kongress (Wien), p 524. Leipzig, Breitkopf und Hartel, 1895
9. Burnett JE Jr: Hysteroscopy-controlled curettage for endometrial polyps. Obstet Gynecol 24:621, 1964
10. David C: L'Endoscopie utérine (hystéroscopie). Applications au diagnostic et au traitement des affections intrautérines. Master's thesis, University of Paris, G Jacques, Paris, 1908
11. Désormeaux AJ: De l'endoscope et de ses Applications au Diagnostic et au Traitement des Affections de l'Uréthre et de la Verrie. Paris, Balliere, 1865
12. Dickinson RL: Simple sterilization of women by cautery stricture at the intrauterine tubal openings, compared with other methods. Surg Gynecol Obstet 23:203, 1916
13. Duplay S, Clado S: Traite d'Hysteroscopie. Rennes, Simon, 1898
14. Edström K, Fernström I: The diagnostic possibilities of a modified hysteroscopic technique. Acta Obstet Gynecol Scand 49:327, 1970
15. Englund, S, Ingelman-Sundberg A, Westin B: Hysteroscopy in diagnosis and treatment of uterine bleeding. Gynaecologia 143:217, 1957
16. Esposito A: Une exploration gynécologique trop negligée: l'hystéroscopie. Gynecol Pract 19:167, 1968
16a. Fourestier M, Gladu A, Vulmière J: Perfectionnements de l'endoscope médicale. Presse Med 60:1292, 1952
17. Gauss CL: Hysteroskopie. Arch Gynaekol 133:18, 1928
18. Heineberg A: Uterine endoscopy, an aid to precision in the diagnosis of intra-uterine disease. Surg Gynecol Obstet 18:513, 1914
19. Lindemann HJ: Eine neue Untersuchungsmethode für die Hysteroskopie. Endoscopy 4:194, 1971
20. Lindemann HJ: The use of CO_2 in the uterine cavity for hysteroscopy. Int J Fertil 17:221, 1972
21. Lindemann HJ: Pneumometra für die Hysteroskopie. Geburtshilfe Frauenheilkd 33:18, 1973
22. Lindemann HJ: Historical aspects of hysteroscopy. Fertil Steril 24:230, 1973
23. Lyon FA: Intrauterine visualization by means of a hysteroscope. Am J Obstet Gynecol 90:443, 1964
24. Marleschki V: Die moderne Zervikoskopie und Hysteroskopie. Zentralbl Gynaekol 88:20, 1966
25. Marleschki V: Hysteroskopische Feststellung der spontanen Perfusionsschwankungen am menschlichen Endometrium. Zentralbl Gynaekol 90:1094, 1968
26. McCrea LE: Clinical Cystoscopy, Vol I, p 5. Philadelphia, F A Davis, 1945
27. Menken FC: L'endocervicoscopie. Bull Soc Sci Med Grand Duche Luxemb 104:97, 1967
28. Menken FC: Endoscopic observations of endocrine processes and hormonal changes. In Simposio Esteroides Sexuales, p 24. Bogota, 1968
29. Menken FC: Fortschritte der gynäkologischen Endoskopie. In Demling L, Allenjann R (eds): Fortschritte der Endoskopie. Stuttgart, F K Schattauer, 1969
30. Mikulicz-Radecki F von, Freund A: Das Tubenhysteroskop und seine diagnostische Verwendung bei Sterilität, Sterilisierung und Tubenerkrankungen. Arch Gynaekol 123:68, 1927
31. Mikulicz-Radecki F von, Freund A: Ein neues Hysteroskop und seine praktische Anwendung in der Gynäkologie. Geburtshilfe Gynaekol 92:13, 1928
32. Mohri T, Mohri C: Hysteroscopy. World Gynecol Obstet 6:48, 1954
33. Mohri T, Mohri C, Yamadori F: The original production of the glassfibre hysteroscope and a study of the intrauterine observation of the human fetus, things attached to the fetus and the inner side of the uterus wall in late pregnancy and the beginning of delivery by means of hysteroscopy and its recording on the film. J Jpn Obstet Gynecol Soc 15:87, 1968
34. Morris RT: Endoscopic tubes for direct inspection of the interior of the bladder and uterus. Trans Am Assoc Obstet Gynecol 6:275, 1893
35. Munde PF: Minor Surgical Gynecology, p 99. New York, W Wood, 1880
36. Nitze M: Über eine neue Beleuchtungsmethode der Höhlen des menschlichen Körpers. Wien Med Presse 20:851, 1879
37. Norment WB: A study of the uterine canal by direct observation and uterogram. Am J Surg 60:56, 1943
38. Norment WB: Visualization and photography of the uterine canal in patients. North Carolina Med J 9:619, 1948
39. Norment WB: Improved instrument for diagnosis of pelvic lesions by hysterogram and water hysteroscope. North Carolina Med J 10:646, 1949
40. Norment WB: A diagnostic test for tumors of the uterine canal. Am J Surg 82:240, 1951
41. Norment WB: Hysteroscopy in diagnosis of pathological conditions, of uterine canal. JAMA 148:917, 1952

42. Norment WB: The hysteroscope. Am J Obstet Gynecol 71:426, 1956

43. Norment WB: Hysteroscopic examination in older women. Geriatrics 11:13, 1956

44. Palmer R: Un nouvel hystéroscope. Bull Fed Soc Gynecol Obstet Franc 9:300, 1957

45. Pantaleoni D: On endoscopic examination of the cavity of the womb. Med Press Circ 8:26, 1869

46. Porto R, Gaujoux J: Une nouvelle méthode d'hystéroscopie: Instrumentation et technique. J Gynecol Obstet Biol Reprod 1:691, 1972

47. Porto R, Gaujoux J, Serment H: Premiers resultats d'une nouvelle méthode d'hystéroscopie: Communication á la Sociéte Nationale de Gynécologie et d'Obstétrique de France (groupement de Marseille), June 20, 1972.

48. Quiñones RG: A symposium on advances in fiberoptic hysteroscopy. Contemp Obstet Gynecol 3:115, 1974

49. Quiñones RG, Alvarado DA, Aznar RR: Tubal catheterization: Applications of a new technique. Am J Obstet Gynecol 114:674, 1972

50. Rubin IC: Uterine endoscopy, endometroscopy with the aid of uterine insufflation. Am J Obstet Gynecol 10:313, 1925

51. Schack L: Unsere Erfahrungen mit der Hysteroskopie. Zentralbl Gynaekol 60:1810, 1936

52. Schmidt-Matthiesen H: Die Hysteroskopie als klinische Routinemethode. Geburtshilfe Frauenheilkd 26:1498, 1966

53. Schroeder C: Über den Ausbau und die Leistungen der Hysteroskopie. Arch Gynakol 156:407, 1934

54. Segond R: Hystéroscope. Bull Fed Soc Obstet Gynecol 23:709, 1934

55. Segond R: L'hystéroscopie. Gaz Med Franc 42:285, 1935

56. Segond R: Le diagnostic des métrorragies par l'hystéroscopie. Gaz Méd Franc 43:1031, 1936

57. Segond R: L'hystéroscopie, description des images critiques. Gaz Med Franc 44:271, 1937

58. Seymour HF: A method of endoscopic examination of the uterus with its indications. Proc R Soc Med 19:74, 1926

59. Seymour HF: Endoscopy of the uterus with a description of a hysteroscope. J Obstet Gynaecol Br Emp 33:52, 1926

60. Silander T: Hysteroscopy through a transparent rubber balloon. Surg Gynecol Obstet 114:125, 1962

61. Silander T: Hysteroscopy through a transparent rubber balloon in patients with carcinoma of the uterine endometrium. Acta Obstet Gynecol Scand 42:284, 1963

62. Silander T: Hysteroscopy through a transparent rubber balloon in patients with uterine bleeding. Acta Obstet Gynecol Scand 42:300, 1963

63. Wulfsohn NL: A hysteroscope. J Obstet Gynaecol Br Emp 65:657, 1959

Indications ■   2

Rafael F. Valle

Indications being established for hysteroscopy undoubtedly include potential applications. An application represents a potential use without proven benefit in a clinical study, whereas an indication implies clinical value because of previous findings. The number of patients or trials required to support such a study has not been elucidated. In this chapter, an indication is defined as the use of hysteroscopy in the diagnosis and treatment of gynecologic patients as documented by published reports of at least one investigator.

EARLY INDICATIONS

In 1869 hysteroscopy was used by Pantaleoni to diagnose and treat abnormal uterine bleeding.[19] No significant advances in the development of hysteroscopy occurred until 40 years later, when David introduced a contact hysteroscope to evaluate abnormal uterine bleeding and to search for retained placental tissue and uterine anomalies.[3]

Additional indications for hysteroscopy appeared between 1920 and 1930, with the introduction of low-viscosity fluids for uterine distention by Gauss, Schroeder, and Schack and of carbon dioxide gas insufflation by Rubin.[7,25-27]

In 1935, Ahumada and Gandolfo-Herrera specified the following indications for hysteroscopy (based on reports of these previous investigators): polyps, submucous leiomyomas, endometrial hyperplasia, endometrial adenocarcinoma, abnormal uterine bleeding, incomplete abortion, uterine anomalies, tubal catheterization, and ascertainment of the phase of the endometrium in the menstrual cycle.[1] Abnormal uterine bleeding was the leading indication for hysteroscopy. Tubal catheterization, although mentioned, was not practical. Tubal sterilization was suggested by von Mikulicz-Radecki and Freund and by Rubin.[14,15,25]

Although von Mikulicz-Radecki and Freund introduced instruments for biopsy of lesions found at hysteroscopy, operative hysteroscopy did not evolve until more refined and simple methods of uterine distention were introduced by Norment in the 1950s.[17] Hysteroscopic removal of endometrial polyps and biopsy of lesions suggestive of carcinoma became feasible with the type of cutting loop used by urologists.[18] In 1962 Silander used hysteroscopy for staging endometrial adenocarcinoma before therapy.[29] This new indication was adapted and extended by Joelsson and colleagues.[10]

MODERN HYSTEROSCOPY

The development of new media for uterine distention and the application of fiberoptics allowed high-intensity light to be delivered safely through endoscopes and broadened the indications for hysteroscopy.[5,12,24] Levine and Neuwirth used hysteroscopy to diagnose and treat intrauterine adhesions and established a method of management for this condition with concomitant laparoscopy.[11] In 1974 Porto enumerated the following indications for hysteroscopy: diagnosis of intrauterine lesions, biopsy of potentially malignant lesions, evaluation of the topography and extension of a cervical or uterine lesion, excision of adhesions and verification of the results of treatment, control and withdrawal of intrauterine devices (IUDs), and sterilization by tubal coagulation.[21] At the time, many clinical studies were underway to evaluate the feasibility and safety of sterilization by electrocoagulation of the uterotubal junction through hysteroscopy. All Porto's indications except hysteroscopic sterilization were practical and clinically applicable. Edström used hysteroscopic methods to divide uterine septae.[4]

As technologic refinements provided safety and simplicity and clinical experience grew,

Table 2-1
PRESENT INDICATIONS FOR HYSTEROSCOPY

Evaluation of unexplained abnormal uterine bleeding in premenopausal or postmenopausal patients

Diagnosis and transcervical hysteroscopic removal of suspected submucous leiomyoma or endometrial polyp

Location and retrieval of "lost" IUD or other foreign body

Evaluation of infertile patients with abnormal hysterogram

Diagnosis and surgical treatment of intrauterine adhesions

Exploration of endocervical canal, internal cervical os, and uterine cavity in patients with repeated miscarriages

Evaluation of patients with failed first-trimester elective abortions

Transcervical division of small uterine septae

hysteroscopy became more practical and new applications were developed. Present indications for hysteroscopy are numerous (Table 2-1). Dilatation and curettage may not be accurate for diagnosis of focal intrauterine lesions because they are either small or located in an area difficult to curet. Hysteroscopy can guide the curet and permit targeted biopsies of these lesions and their direct removal. The advantage of performing a biopsy under vision rather than by "blind" curettage has been amply demonstrated by Norment, Gribb, Burnett, Porto, and others.[2,6,8,17,22,30,33]

A common problem in gynecology is the management of patients with "lost" IUDs; that is, patients whose IUD filaments are not seen at the external cervical os. Hysteroscopy allows the physician to avoid haphazard transcervical manipulation and unnecessary radiation. The IUD can be located and then removed transcervically without unnecessarily damaging or injuring the surrounding endometrium.[34,36] Although hysterosalpingography is valuable in screening infertile patients, the technique, selection of contrast medium, and interpretation of findings may contribute to misinterpretation. Transient distortions of the uterine cavity may occur as a result of blood, mucus, debris, and air bubbles. Observation of the inside of the cavity allows direct evaluation of an abnormal shadow seen on the hysterogram and biopsy of abnormal lesions.[32,37] Dividing intrauterine adhesions by curettage is a "blind" approach; with hysteroscopy, diagnosis becomes more precise and therapy more effective. Adhesions can be divided under direct vision, ensuring completion of the procedure.[13,31]

Hysteroscopy is used to explore the endocervical canal of patients with repeated miscarriages. Anatomic defects of the endocervical canal can be seen, and many of these patients demonstrate a loss of the normal anatomic relations ·between the corpus and cervix, thus losing the sphincteric action of the internal os. Also, the uterine cavity can be searched for uterine anomalies or intrauterine adhesions. When a first-trimester elective abortion fails (histologic examination of the curettings does not reveal chorionic villi), tubal pregnancy should be suspected if the pregnancy test remains positive. If the laparoscopic examination reveals a normal pelvis, hysteroscopic findings might show an anomalous uterus with an early pregnancy in one of the horns and serve as a guide to suction curettage.[35]

Multiple applications of hysteroscopy are now being evaluated, particularly with the different types of hysteroscopes (Table 2-2).[9,20] The study of the early embryo by contact hysteroscopy might detect fetal anomalies or early embryonic life without the need for abortion. Anatomic and cytologic changes occurring in the endocervical canal and endometrium in normal and pathologic conditions are currently being studied by vital staining at ×150 magnification.[9]

CONCLUSION

Hysteroscopy is an adjunct to other techniques in the diagnosis and treatment of intrauterine lesions. The most common indications for its use are evaluation of abnormal, persistent, or recurrent uterine bleeding, abnormal hysterograms, diagnosis and management of intrauterine adhesions, and location and removal of misplaced IUDs. Experience in hysteroscopy will increase the operator's skill and confidence in interpretation, but observations must be accompanied by biopsy when abnormalities are seen. Therapeutic hysteroscopy requires additional experience and dexterity. It should be tailored to experience, particularly in the removal of submucous leiomyomas, the division of thick connective tissue adhesions or uterine septae, and tubal cannulation.

Table 2-2
INDICATIONS FOR HYSTEROSCOPY UNDER INVESTIGATION

Study of surface changes of endometrium during proliferative and secretory phase of menstrual cycle[37]

Evaluation and staging of endometrial adenocarcinoma as a step to appropriate therapy

Study of intratubal milieu, biochemistry of tubal secretions, and tubal motility with open-ended catheters directed through hysteroscopy[23]

Delivery at uterotubal junction of small endoscopes for intratubal observations[16]

Tubal occlusion by electrocoagulation, cryocoagulation, instillation of chemical substances, or placement of mechanical plugs[28]

REFERENCES

1. Ahumada JC, Gandolfo-Herrera R: Histeroscopia. Rev Med Latino Am 21:265, 1935
2. Burnett JE Jr: Hysteroscopy-controlled curettage for endometrial polyps. Obstet Gynecol 24:621, 1964
3. David C: Endoscopie de l'uterus aprés l'avortement et dans les suites de couches normales et pathologiques. Bull Soc Obstet 10:288, 1907
4. Edström KGB: Intrauterine surgical procedures during hysteroscopy. Endoscopy 6:175, 1974
5. Edström KGB, Fernström I: The diagnostic possibilities of a modified hysteroscopic technique. Acta Obstet Gynecol Scand 49:327, 1970
6. Englund SE, Ingelman-Sundberg A, Westin B: Hysteroscopy in diagnosis and treatment of uterine bleeding. Gynaecologia 143:217, 1957
7. Gauss CL: Hysteroskopie. Arch Gynakol 133:18, 1928
8. Gribb JJ: Hysteroscopy. An aid in gynecologic diagnosis. Obstet Gynecol 15:593, 1960
9. Hamou J: Microhysteroscopy. A new procedure and its original application in gynecology. J Reprod Med 26:375, 1981
10. Joelsson I, Levine RU, Moberger G: Hysteroscopy as an adjunct in determining the extent of carcinoma of the endometrium. Am J Obstet Gynecol 111:696, 1971
11. Levine RU, Neuwirth RS: Simultaneous laparoscopy and hysteroscopy for intrauterine adhesions. Obstet Gynecol 42:441, 1973
12. Lindemann HJ: Eine neue Untersuchungsmethode für die Hysteroskopie. Endoscopy 4:194, 1971
13. March CM, Israel R, March AD: Hysteroscopic management of intrauterine adhesions. Am J Obstet Gynecol 130:653, 1978
14. Mikulicz-Radecki F von: Experimentelle Untersuchungen über Tubensterilization durch Electrokoagulation. Z Geburtshilfe Gynaekol 94:318, 1928
15. Mikulicz-Radecki F von, Freund A: Ein neues Hysteroskop und seine praktische Anwendung in der Gynäkologie. Z Geburtshilfe Gynaekol 92:13, 1927
16. Mohri T, Mohri C, Yamadori F: Tubaloscope: Flexible glass fiber endoscope for intratubal observation. Endoscopy 2:226, 1970
17. Norment WB: The hysteroscope. Am J Obstet Gynecol 71:426, 1956
18. Norment WB, Sikes CH, Berry FX, et al: Hysteroscopy. Surg Clin North Am 37:1377, 1957
19. Pantaleoni D: On endoscopic examination of the cavity of the womb. Med Press Circ 8:26, 1869
20. Parent B, Toubas C, Doerler B: L'hystéroscopie de contact. J Gynecol Obstet Biol Reprod 3:511, 1974
21. Porto R: Pneumohysteroscopy: Instrumentation and

technique. In Sciarra JJ, Butler JC, Speidel JJ (eds): Hysteroscopic Sterilization, pp 51–58. New York, Intercontinental Medical Book Corporation, 1974

22. Porto R: Hystéroscopie. Travail de la Clinique Obstètricale et Gynécologique de la Faculté de Médicine de Marseille. Montrouge, France, Searle, 1975

23. Quiñones RG, Alvarado DA, Aznar RR: Tubal catheterization: Applications of a new technique. Am J Obstet Gynecol 114:674, 1972

24. Quiñones RG, Alvarado DA, Aznar RR: Histeroscopia. Una nueva téchnica Ginecol Obstet Mex 32:237, 1972

25. Rubin IC: Uterine endoscopy, endometroscopy with the aid of uterine insufflation. Am J Obstet Gynecol 10:313, 1925

26. Schack L: Unsere Erfahrungen mit der Hysteroskopie. Zentralbl Gynaekol 60:1810, 1936

27. Schroeder C: Über den Ausbau und die Leistungen zu der Hysteroskopie. Arch Gynäkol 156:407, 1934

28. Sciarra JJ, Droegemueller W, Speidel JJ (eds): Advances in Female Sterilization Techniques. Hagerstown, Harper & Row, 1976

29. Silander T: Hysteroscopy through a transparent rubber balloon in patients with carcinoma of the uterine endometrium. Acta Obstet Gynecol Scand 42:300, 1963

30. Stock RJ, Kanbour A: Prehysterectomy curettage. Obstet Gynecol 45:537, 1975

31. Sugimoto O: Diagnostic and therapeutic hysteroscopy for traumatic intrauterine adhesions. Am J Obstet Gynecol 131:539, 1978

32. Valle RF: Hysteroscopy in the evaluation of female infertility. Am J Obstet Gynecol 137:425, 1980

33. Valle RF: Hysteroscopic evaluation of patients with abnormal uterine bleeding. Surg Gynecol Obstet 153:521, 1981

34. Valle RF, Freeman DW: Hysteroscopy in the localization and removal of intrauterine devices with "missing" strings. Contraception 11:161, 1975

35. Valle RF, Sabbagha RE: Management of first trimester pregnancy termination failures. Obstet Gynecol 55:625, 1980

36. Valle RF, Sciarra JJ, Freeman DW: Hysteroscopic removal of intrauterine devices with missing filaments. Obstet Gynecol 49:55, 1977

37. Valle RF, Sciarra JJ: Current status of hysteroscopy in gynecologic practice. Fertil Steril 32:619, 1979

A Report of 560 Hysteroscopic Operations ■ 3

Hans Roll
Manuel Hilgarth

Using a cystoscope inserted through the cervical canal into the uterine cavity, Gauss and Schroeder thoroughly described physiologic changes of the endometrium during the menstrual cycle and many abnormalities in the uterine cavity.[1,4] They succeeded in probing and catheterizing the fallopian tube using hysteroscopy. Lindemann's idea of using carbon dioxide to distend the uterine cavity revitalized this diagnostic procedure. Together with modern optics and good light sources, the use of hysteroscopy has increased. This chapter will describe the results of hysteroscopy in 560 patients.

MATERIAL AND METHOD

Of 560 patients, 39% had primary infertility, 8% had secondary infertility, 36% had abnormal uterine bleeding, and 3% had a "lost" intrauterine device (IUD). The diagnosis of endometrial carcinoma had been made in 14%, and before starting therapy we tried to localize the site of the malignancy.

Most hysteroscopic procedures were done under general anesthesia. In the last 2 years we have used a prostaglandin E_2 derivative intramuscularly 6 hr before hysteroscopy. The widening and softening effect of prostaglandin E_2, even in postmenopausal women, is amazing, and cervical dilatation is unnecessary. We also used smaller diagnostic optics (4 mm).

RESULTS

Initially, technical problems in performing hysteroscopy caused inadequate observation in 27 patients, precluding a diagnosis. When we used an apparatus that insufflated carbon dioxide in a rather uncontrolled way, two women developed cardiovascular problems, the cause of which could not be ascertained definitively. With a carbon dioxide gas flow up to 100 ml/min, and with volumetric and manometric controls, cardiovascular problems have not recurred.

In 47% of 221 women with sterility, no abnormality was found, but 7% had arcuate uteri, 10% had fibroids, 7% had polyposis, 2% had severe intrauterine adhesions, and 2% had severe malformations of the müllerian ducts. Among 43 women with secondary infertility, no abnormality was detected in 40%, but 14% had arcuate uteri, 12% had fibroids, 12% had cervical abnormalities (*e.g.*, cervical incompetency), 9% had uterine synechiae, 7% had bicornuate uteri, and 7% had polyposis. Patients with primary infertility generally have ovarian dysfunction or tubal occlusion, and women with secondary infertility have more cervical and uterine abnormalities, although the high percentage of intrauterine adhesions reported from other countries could not be found in our patients.

In 34% of 204 patients with menometrorrhagia and perimenopausal and postmenopausal uterine bleeding, no abnormality was detected, but 21% had endometrial abnormalities (*e.g.,* endometritis). Endometrial atrophy was seen in 12%, myomas in 17%, and endometrial adenocarcinomas were localized in 11% of patients. In 8% we performed hysteroscopy after abortion to check the completeness of the previous curettage. To prove the hysteroscopic findings and for documentation in each patient with abnormal uterine bleeding, we performed curettage after hysteroscopy.

CONCLUSION

Carbon dioxide hysteroscopy is valuable in the office and hospital. When it is combined with other endoscopic procedures, mainly with laparoscopy, physicians can learn a good deal of important information about sterile patients. In locating and staging endometrial carcinomas and in differentiating between endometrial and endocervical adenocarcinoma, physicians should no longer omit hysteroscopy.

REFERENCES

1. Gauss CL: Hysteroskopie. Arch Gynaekol 133:18, 1928
2. Hepp H, Roll H: Die Hysteroskopie. Gynaekologie 7:166, 1974
3. Lindemann HJ: The use of CO_2 in the uterine cavity for hysteroscopy. Int J Fertil 17:221, 1972
4. Schroeder C: Über den Ausbau und die Leistungen der Hysteroskopie. Arch Gynaekol 156:407, 1934

Hysteroscopy in an Evaluation of 353 Patients ■

4

Chung Kun-chin

This chapter summarizes the hysteroscopic findings in 353 patients examined between May 1978 and October 1980. Abnormal uterine bleeding, infertility, and dislocated intrauterine devices (IUDs) were the main indications for the procedure.

MATERIALS AND METHODS

The hysteroscope was equipped with a glass fiber bundle and a liquid rinsing system to remove blood, mucus, and debris. Patients received meperidine for analgesia and a paracervical block as local anesthesia. I distended the uterine cavity with isotonic saline solution to obtain an adequate view of the endometrial surface. If it was difficult to distend the cavity with 50 cm of water pressure, a highly viscous dextran solution instilled under 50 mm Hg to 100 mm Hg pressure produced enough dilation for me to observe the entire endometrial surface (Figs. 4-1 and 4-2 on pgs. 30 and 31).

In every case of abnormal bleeding, I performed a hysteroscopic examination first and followed the visual diagnosis by biopsy of the abnormal tissue and dilatation and curettage. Most patients with trophoblastic disease and submucosal myomas received the necessary treatment immediately.

Hysteroscopic examination sometimes followed hysterograms that had shown intrauterine adhesions. I performed adhesiotomy with the outer sleeve of the hysteroscope or with Kelly forceps, inserting an Ota ring IUD postoperatively to prevent recurrence.

RESULTS

Of the 353 patients examined by hysteroscopy, 243 had abnormal bleeding of either anatomic or functional origin. Seventy-two percent of the 353 patients were women of reproductive age, while 28% were climacteric or postmenopausal; of the 243 patients, 88 (36%) had uterine bleeding of anatomic origin caused by retained secundines, silk, endometrial polyps, trophoblastic disease, submucosal myomas, endometritis, or uterine carcinoma (Fig. 4-1 and Table 4-1). Table 4-2 shows the causes of abnormal uterine bleeding in the menstruating and postmenopausal groups. The endometrial patterns of 155 women with dysfunctional uterine bleeding are shown in Table 4-3.

Sixty-five of the 353 patients were infertile and underwent hysteroscopic examination after preliminary hysterographic studies. Traumatic intrauterine adhesions (Asherman's syndrome) was the major problem (see Fig. 4-2). All patients with uterine synechiae were treated with both synechiolysis and supplementary therapy. After treatment, improved menstrual flow was found in 45% of patients and pregnancy occurred in 20% (Table 4-4).

Of the 353 patients, 40 underwent hyster-

Table 4-1

CAUSE OF UTERINE BLEEDING IN PREMENOPAUSAL AND POSTMENOPAUSAL WOMEN AS FOUND ON HYSTEROSCOPY

ABNORMAL UTERINE BLEEDING	PRE-MENOPAUSAL WOMEN		POST-MENOPAUSAL WOMEN		TOTAL	
	No.	%	No.	%	No.	%
Anatomic	61		27		88	(36)
Dysfunctional	113		42		155	(64)
Total	174	(72)	69	(28)	243	(100)

Table 4-2

ABNORMALITIES SEEN AT HYSTEROSCOPY IN PREMENOPAUSAL AND POSTMENOPAUSAL PATIENTS

ABNORMALITIES	PRE-MENOPAUSAL WOMEN		POST-MENOPAUSAL WOMEN		TOTAL	
	No.	%	No.	%	No.	%
Retained secudines or silk	34		0		34	(39)
Trophoblastic disease	9		0		9	(19)
Endometrial polyp	10		6		16	(18)
Endometritis	3		8		11	(12.5)
Submucosal myoma	3		5		8	(9)
Endocervical polyp	2		4		6	(7)
Endometrial carcinoma	0		4		4	(5)
Total	61	(69)	27	(31)	88	(100)

Table 4-3

ENDOMETRIAL PATTERNS IN DYSFUNCTIONAL UTERINE BLEEDING

ENDOMETRIAL PATTERN	PRE-MENOPAUSAL WOMEN		POST-MENOPAUSAL WOMEN		TOTAL	
	No.	%	No.	%	No.	%
Proliferative	80		24		104	(67)
Secretory	31		0		31	(20)
Hyperplastic	8		12		20	(13)
Total	119	(77)	36	(23)	155	(100)

Table 4-4

EFFECT OF SYNECHIOLYSIS ON MENSTRUATION AND FERTILITY

MENSES PREOPERATIVELY	NO.	AFTER THERAPY			
		Pregnancy	Eumenorrhea	Hypomenorrhea	Amenorrhea
Eumenorrhea	15	3	12	0	0
Hypomenorrhea	20	4	11	5	0
Amenorrhea	9	2	2	2	3
Total No. (and %)	44	9 (20)	25 (57)	7 (16)	3 (7)

Table 4-5

TYPES AND LOCATIONS OF "MISPLACED" IUDs

OCCULT IUD	OTA RING	LIPPES LOOP	CU-T	CU-7	METALLIC RING	TOTAL	
						No.	%
Thread missing, easily retrieved		15	5	14		34	(76)
Translocation into abdominal cavity	2	4				6	(13)
Intrauterine pregnancy		3	2			5	(11)
Total No. (and %)	2 (4)	22 (9)	7 (16)	14 (31)		45	(100)

oscopy because their IUD thread was missing (Fig. 4-3) and 5 did so to confirm an intrauterine pregnancy with an IUD in place. Table 4-5 describes the locations of the IUDs. Of the 40 patients with a missing thread, the IUD was located in 34 and removed easily. In the other six, the device had translocated into the abdominal cavity and laparoscopy was performed to remove it. In five patients who had an intrauterine pregnancy with an IUD *in situ*, the IUDs were removed smoothly under hysteroscopic guidance. No abortions occurred.

COMMENT

In patients with abnormal uterine bleeding, hysteroscopy provided the possibility for immediate diagnosis and prompt, effective treatment. It allowed me to ascertain the source of the bleeding and perform a directed biopsy of the suspected area, affording a more accurate diagnosis than dilatation and curettage.[5] For infertile patients, hysteroscopy provided significant advantages, especially in those with Asherman's syndrome. The hysteroscope could pinpoint the extent and location of the adhesions and thus afforded easier and effective synechiolysis.[2,6,7] In localizing and retrieving IUDs, hysteroscopy was more effective than radiography because in most cases it necessitated only one procedure. Radiography exposes the patient to radiation and is more costly than hysteroscopy, and a second procedure is required to remove the IUD. Observation of the location of the occult IUD endo-

scopically precludes unnecessary, possibly dangerous manipulation.[1,3,4,8,9]

ACKNOWLEDGMENTS

I am greatly indebted to Professor Osamu Sugimoto, MD, Department of Obstetrics and Gynecology, Osaka Medical College, Japan, for his encouragement and instruction. I also wish to thank the pathologist, Professor T.S. Huang, for his expert tissue diagnosis. Finally, I want to express my sincere thanks to the gynecologic and nursing staffs of Chung Shan Medical College Hospital, who have given me great support throughout this study.

REFERENCES

1. Devi PK, Gupta AN: Hysteroscopic removal of intrauterine contraceptive devices with missing threads. Indian J Med Res 65:5, 1977
2. Edström KGB: Intrauterine surgical procedures during hysteroscopy. Endoscopy 6:175, 1974
3. Neubuesser D, Vahrson H: Zur Diagnostik und Entfernung okkulter Intrauterinpessaren. Geburtshilfe Frauenheilkd 37:277, 1977
4. Siegler AM, Kemmann EK: Location and removal of misplaced or embedded intrauterine devices by hysteroscopy. J Reprod Med 16:139, 1976
5. Sugimoto O: Hysteroscopic diagnosis of endometrial carcinoma. Am J Obstet Gynecol 121:105, 1975
6. Sugimoto O: Diagnostic and Therapeutic Hysteroscopy. Tokyo, Igaku–Shoin, 1978
7. Sugimoto O: Diagnostic and therapeutic hysteroscopy for traumatic intrauterine adhesions. Am J Obstet Gynecol 131:539, 1978
8. Valle RF, Freeman DW: Hysteroscopy in the localization and removal of intrauterine devices with "missing strings." Contraception 11:161, 1975
9. Valle RF, Sciarra JJ, Freeman DW: Hysteroscopic removal of intrauterine devices with missing filaments. Obstet Gynecol 49:55, 1977

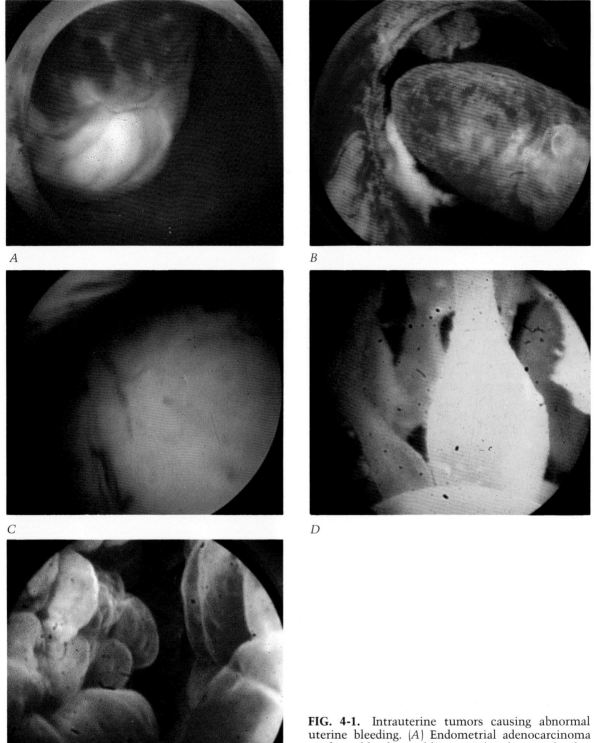

FIG. 4-1. Intrauterine tumors causing abnormal uterine bleeding. (*A*) Endometrial adenocarcinoma confirmed by directed biopsy. (*B*) Endometrial polyp occupies center of field. (*C*) Submucous myoma appears circumscribed and pink tan. (*D*) Hydatidiform mole has multiple vesicles. (*E*) Hyperplastic endometrium shows polypoid surface.

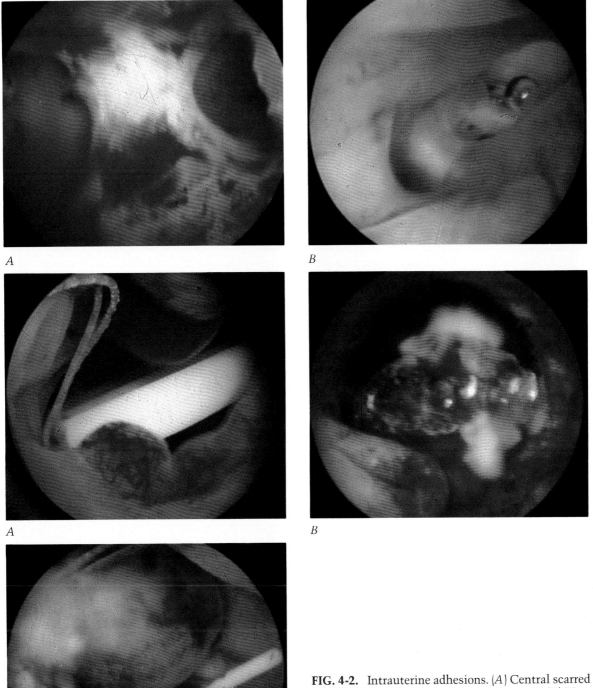

A

B

A

B

C

FIG. 4-2. Intrauterine adhesions. (*A*) Central scarred area divides cavity into two compartments. (*B*) Marginal and central adhesions are seen near the tubal ostium.

FIG. 4-3. IUDs with missing threads. (*A*) Lippes loop has thin overlying secretory endometrium. (*B*) Encrusted metallic ring is clearly visible. (*C*) Copper-T, with early intrauterine pregnancy beneath the device.

Selection of Patients for Hysteroscopy: Experience with 300 Operations ■

5

Roberto I. Tozzini
Rafael L. Pineda

The possibility of observing the uterine cavity *in vivo* is not new, but the development of fiberoptics and light transmission media has fostered the use of hysteroscopy.[10] Presently it constitutes a diagnostic and therapeutic procedure in operative gynecology. Reports on the technique and on its use and results have multiplied.[4,5,11–14,16,18,19] New models have facilitated observation of the uterine cavity and permitted the application of hysteroscopy to the ambulatory patient.[1–3,6–8]

Our first report on hysteroscopy was in 1975.[15] Knowledge of the uterine cavity and the endometrial surfaces obtained from hysteroscopic examinations has led us to use certain criteria in selecting patients for this operation.

MATERIALS AND METHODS

We performed 300 hysteroscopies between August 1974 and November 1981. Indications for the procedure are listed in Table 5-1. The hysteroscopes used were from American Cystoscope Maber Inc. and had a 7-mm oval stainless steel sheath, Hopkins optics, side stopcocks to instill the medium, an operating channel, and a Wolf's pneumohysteroscope.* Uterine distention was achieved with carbon dioxide instilled by a specially designed apparatus.† In the re-

maining patients, either a dextran 70 or a 5% dextrose solution was used to distend the uterine cavity.

Hysteroscopy was performed in the first half of the menstrual cycle in 87 patients (29%), in the second half in 133 (44.3%), in amenorrhea in 54 (18%), and during spotting in 26 (8.7%). The reason for the high incidence of studies during the second half of the cycle was the large group of sterile women who also underwent laparoscopy and endometrial biopsy. As a rule, the procedures were done under general anesthesia.

RESULTS

Observation of the uterine cavity and endometrium was good in 257 patients (85.7%), fair or incomplete in 40 (13.3%), and unsatisfactory in 3 (1%). In those three patients, partial or total perforation precluded any further attempt at observing the uterine cavity; the three patients had no other complications.

Among the most frequent indications for hysteroscopy was postcurettage amenorrhea or hypomenorrhea. Sixty-two patients constituted this group, 35 (56.5%) of whom had had hysterosalpingograms compatible with intrauterine adhesions or isthmic blockage. The view of the canal, isthmus, and uterine cavity disclosed adhesions in 43 patients (69.3%) as the only abnormality. Twenty five (58.1%) of

---

* Wolf lumina telescope, 25° vision, 4-mm diameter (8654.33).

† Metromat 2121. Hysteroscopy insufflator.

them were in the corpus, 11 (25.6%) were in the cervix and isthmus, and 7 (16.3%) were mixed. It was also possible to define the type of adhesion: endometrial, connective tissue and endometrium, and wall-to-wall severe synechiae. The features of these adhesions have been previously reported.[17] Nine patients (14.5%) had no adhesions, but their endometrium was atrophic; 5 patients (8.2%) showed adhesions and atrophic endometrium. Selective endometrial biopsy specimens confirmed the hysteroscopic finding. Placental remnants were found in 1 patient (1.6%). The uterine cavity was normal in 4 patients (6.4%), two of whom showed irregular endometrial surfaces.

The comparison between hysterographic and hysteroscopic findings in 35 patients with postcurettage amenorrhea or hypomenorrhea showed a high index (85.8%) of correlation (Table 5-2). Fifty-three women underwent hysteroscopy because of intrauterine filling defects. In 50, the defects had been found on hysterograms done during examination for sterility. The hysteroscopic findings are listed in Table 5-3. Hysterographic and hysteroscopic findings were similar in 66.7%. Abnormal uterine bleeding occurred in 58 patients, only 5 of whom had undergone previous hysterography and endometrial biopsy. Hysteroscopic findings are listed in Table 5-4. In 23 women

(39.7%), intracavitary abnormalities were not found, and the diagnosis was made by endometrial biopsy. Thirty-seven patients underwent hysteroscopy, laparoscopy with chromopertubation, and endometrial biopsy in a single surgical procedure (Table 5-5).[9]

Twenty-three women who had a clinical diagnosis of endocervical polyps underwent hysteroscopic examinations during polypectomy. Nine (39.1%) had endometrial polyps, and an endometrial biopsy specimen showed a polyp not seen at hysteroscopy in 1 instance

Table 5-1
INDICATIONS FOR HYSTEROSCOPY IN 300 PATIENTS

PREVIOUS DIAGNOSIS	NO. OF PATIENTS
Postcurettage amenorrhea	62
Abnormal uterine bleeding	58
Hysterographic filling defects	53
Sterility	37
Endocervical polyp	23
"Lost" IUD	22
Postmenopausal uterine bleeding	17
Uterine malformations	13
Abnormal menstrual cycle	7
Infertility (habitual abortion)	6
Endometrial pathologic condition suspected by cytologic study	2
Total	300

Table 5-2
CORRELATION OF HYSTEROGRAMS WITH HYSTEROSCOPIC FINDINGS IN 35 PATIENTS WITH POSTCURETTAGE AMENORRHEA*

HYSTEROSCOPY	HYSTEROGRAMS		TOTAL
	Filling Defect	Isthmic Obstruction	
Atrophic endometrium	4		4
Isthmic adhesions	2	5	7
Intrauterine adhesions	15		15
Intrauterine and isthmic adhesions	4	1	5
Intrauterine adhesions and atrophic endometrium	1	1	2
Uterine cavity with irregular endometrium surface	1		1
Normal uterine cavity	1	—	1
Total	28	7	35

* Agreement in 85.8%.

Table 5-3
HYSTEROSCOPIC FINDINGS IN 53 PATIENTS WITH HYSTEROGRAPHIC FILLING DEFECTS

HYSTEROSCOPY	PATIENTS	
	No.	%
Submucous leiomyoma*	11	(20.6)
Intrauterine adhesions†	9	(16.9)
Intramural leiomyoma††	8	(15.1)
Endometrial polyp	4	(7.5)
Large and irregular uterine cavity	2	(3.8)
Endocervical polyp	1	(1.8)
Submucous leiomyoma and endometrial polyp	1	(1.8)
Atrophic endometrium	1	(1.8)
Polypoid endometrium	1	(1.8)
Unilateral uterine horn (without abnormality)	1	(1.8)
Bicornuate uterus (without abnormality)	1	(1.8)
Normal uterine cavity	13	(24.5)
Total	53	(100)

* One case associated with intrauterine adhesions.
† One case associated with cervicoisthmic incompetence.
†† Two cases associated with uterine septum.

Table 5-4
HYSTEROSCOPIC FINDINGS IN 58 PATIENTS WITH ABNORMAL UTERINE BLEEDING

FINDINGS	PATIENTS	
	No.	%
Submucous leiomyomas	9	(15.5)
Intramural leiomyomas*	5	(8.6)
Endometrial polyp†	5	(8.6)
Thick and irregular endometrium††	3	(5.3)
Intrauterine adhesions	3	(5.3)
Uterine septum	3	(5.3)
Arcuate uterus	2	(3.4)
Adenomyosis	2	(3.4)
Endocervical polyp	1	(1.7)
Placental remnants	1	(1.7)
Isthmic adhesions	1	(1.7)
Normal uterine cavity	23	(39.5)
Total	58	(100)

* One case associated with adenomyosis, and another case associated with intrauterine adhesions.
† One case associated with uterine septum.
†† In one patient the histopathologic diagnosis was endometrial polyp.

Table 5-5
HYSTEROSCOPIC FINDINGS IN 37 PATIENTS WHO UNDERWENT HYSTEROSCOPY AND LAPAROSCOPY FOR STERILITY

FINDINGS	PATIENTS	
	No.	%
Intramural leiomyomas	4	(10.8)
Intrauterine adhesions	3	(8.1)
Incomplete uterine septum	2	(5.4)
Obstruction of the tubouterine ostium	2	(5.4)
Isthmic leiomyoma	1	(2.7)
Bicornuate uterus	1	(2.7)
Arcuate uterus	1	(2.7)
Normal uterine cavity	22	(59.5)
Procedure interrupted because of uterine perforation	1	(2.7)
Total	37	(100)

(Table 5-6). Twenty-two women complained of "lost" or broken intrauterine devices (IUDs). Two had ignored the presence of the IUD and presented with a chief complaint of sterility. In all cases the IUD was located at endoscopy and removed. There were nine Lippes loops, four rings, four Copper-Ts, two Saf-T-Coils, one Dalkon shield, one Majzlin-spring, and one homemade device. Seventeen patients were selected for hysteroscopy because of postmenopausal bleeding; only 1 patient showed a normal uterine cavity, and 1 localized endometrial carcinoma was found.

According to the results of hysterography, 13 patients with the diagnosis of uterine malformations were studied by endoscopy. Only one of four patients with arcuate uteri had a normal cavity (Table 5-7). In the remaining patients, hysteroscopy confirmed the hysterographic diagnosis, and it was useful to measure the diameters of the cavities and the length and thickness of the septum in anomalous uteri. Finally, a miscellaneous group of 13 patients who presented with infertility, menstrual abnormalities, and abnormal cytologic findings suggestive of endometrial origin were subjected to endoscopy. Two patients had com-

Table 5-6
HYSTEROSCOPIC AND HISTOLOGIC FINDINGS IN 23 PATIENTS WITH ENDOCERVICAL POLYPS

HISTOLOGIC FINDINGS	HYSTEROSCOPY		
	Normal Uterine Cavity	Endometrial Polyps	Total
Endocervical polyps and proliferative or secretory endometrium	9	2	11
Endocervical polyps and hyperplastic endometrium	2		2
Endocervical polyps and inactive endometrium	1		1
Isthmic polyps	1	3	4
Endocervical and endometrial polyps	1	4	5
Total	14	9	23

municating adenomyosis among the six infertile women, and one endometrial polyp was located in the patient with abnormal cytologic findings.

COMMENT

Hysteroscopy is a valuable, simple, low-risk operation that allows an adequate exploration of the uterine cavity under visual control. One of its chief indications is postcurettage amenorrhea, since the presence, extension, and nature of synechiae can be seen and the possibility of their lysis under visual control can be assessed with great accuracy.

Endometrial atrophy is a diagnosis made by hysteroscopy and not by hysterography. Endometrial biopsy specimens in women with endometrial atrophy do not always yield a positive diagnosis, and there is always a risk of worsening the condition. Filling defects detected by hysterography and infertility constitute other indications for hysteroscopy. In metrorrhagia, endoscopy frequently shows endometrial polyps or small leiomyomas that would otherwise go undetected. During endocervical polypectomy, hysteroscopy might disclose endometrial abnormalities. Finally, in patients with postmenopausal uterine bleeding, the technique of hysteroscopy involves a risk

Table 5-7
HYSTEROSCOPIC FINDINGS IN 13 PATIENTS WITH UTERINE MALFORMATIONS ON HYSTEROGRAPHY

HYSTEROSCOPIC FINDINGS	PATIENTS	
	No.	%
Complete uterine septum and bicornuate uterus	4	(30.7)
Incomplete uterine septum	3	(23.1)
Arcuate uterus	3	(23.1)
Unilateral uterine horn	1	(7.7)
Fundal leiomyoma	1	(7.7)
Normal uterine cavity	1	(7.7)
Total	13	(100)

of dissemination of malignant cells, and because of this endoscopy is not used routinely to study these patients.

ACKNOWLEDGMENT

We wish to thank Dr. Guillermo Reeves for help in translating this chapter.

REFERENCES

1. Baggish MS: Contact hysteroscopy: A new technique to explore the uterine cavity. Obstet Gynecol 54:350, 1979

2. Barbot J, Parent B, Dubuisson JB: Contact hysteroscopy: Another method of endoscopic examination of the uterine cavity. Am J Obstet Gynecol 136:721, 1980

3. Brueschke EE, Wilbanks GD: A steerable fiberoptic hysteroscope. Obstet Gynecol 44:273, 1974

4. Lindemann HJ, Mohr J: CO_2 hysteroscopy: Diagnosis and treatment. Am J Obstet Gynecol 124:129, 1976

5. Neuwirth RS, Amin HK: Excision of submucous fibroids with hysteroscopic control. Am J Obstet Gynecol 126:95, 1976

6. Newell JW: Comparative study of various hysteroscopes. In Sciarra JJ, Butler JC Jr, Speidel JJ (eds): Hysteroscopic Sterilization, p 27. New York, Intercontinental Medical Book Corporation, 1974

7. Parent B, Doerler B, Barbot J, et al: Metrorragies postmenopausiques: Diagnostic par l'hystéroscope de contact. Acta Endoscopy 8:13, 1978

8. Parent B, Toubas C, Doerler B: L'hystéroscopie de contact. J Gynecol Obstet Biol Reprod 3:511, 1974

9. Pineda RL, Tozzini RI: Histeroscopía en esterilidad e infertilida. Obstet Ginecol Latin Am 38:139, 1980

10. Pineda RL, Tozzini RI: Estado actual de la histeroscopía en esterilidad. Obstet Ginecol Latin Am 39:169, 1981

11. Pous—Ivern LC: La histeroscopía con CO_2. Técnica, indicaciones y contraindicaciones. Reproduccion 3:275, 1976.

12. Siegler AM, Kemmann EK, Gentile GP: Hysteroscopic procedures in 257 patients. Fertil Steril 27:1267, 1976

13. Sugimoto O: Diagnostic and therapeutic hysteroscopy for traumatic intrauterine adhesions. Am J Obstet Gynecol 131:539, 1978

14. Taylor PJ, Cumming DC: Hysteroscopy in 100 patients. Fertil Steril 31:301, 1979

15. Tozzini RI, Pineda RL: La histeroscopía como método diagnóstico en ginecologia. Presented at the Actas de la XX@ Reunión Anual Nacional de FASGO, Resistencia, Argentina, September 1975

16. Tozzini RI, Pineda RL: Histeroscopía en esterilidad. Presented at the Actas del IX Congreso Latinoamericano de Obstetricia y Ginecologia, Lima, Peru, October 1978

17. Tozzini RI, Pineda RL: El sindrome de amenorrea postraspado uterino estudio y tratamiento de 50 casos. Obstet Ginecol Latin Am 36:114, 1978

18. Valle RF: Hysteroscopy in the evaluation of female infertility. Am J Obstet Gynecol 137:425, 1980

19. Valle RF, Sciarra JJ: Current status of hysteroscopy in gynecologic practice. Fertil Steril 32:619, 1979

Methods of Uterine Distention 6

Jacques E. Rioux

Although hysteroscopy is the oldest gynecologic endoscopic procedure, it has not been frequently used.[7] For a long time inadequate instruments, poor illumination, and inefficient optical systems existed. The inability to obtain and sustain adequate distention of the uterine cavity precluded its adequate observation. Fear of introducing infection into the peritoneal cavity through the tubes and of initiating uncontrollable bleeding were other objections to hysteroscopy.[8] With the development of versatile instruments enabling consistent reproducible results and with media to distend the cavity, hysteroscopy may become a routine gynecologic endoscopic procedure.[4]

Although choice of medium seems arbitrary, whatever agent is used requires sufficient intrauterine pressure to obtain the necessary distention and to prevent or stop endometrial bleeding. With the contact hysteroscope, the instrument is inserted without a medium and exploration is possible despite bleeding, since only the few millimeters of endometrium in contact with the end of the hysteroscope can be evaluated. The types of hysteroscopic techniques depend on the medium and the instruments.

PANORAMIC HYSTEROSCOPY

To obtain a panoramic view of the uterine cavity, the potential cavity with the anterior and posterior walls in apposition must be enlarged. Performing a hysteroscopy without adequate distention would be like performing a laparoscopy without pneumoperitoneum. The three most commonly used media are carbon dioxide, dextran 70 (Hyskon), and low-viscosity fluids.

Carbon dioxide requires a special insufflator that limits the flow of gas to 100 ml/min. A reducing valve ensures the rate. The volume of gas required for a procedure is not significant. The maximal intrauterine pressure never exceeds 200 mm Hg.[6] The insufflator used for laparoscopy should never be used for hysteroscopy.

To proceed, insert the sheath around the hysteroscope into a suction cup that is fixed on the cervix by vacuum to prevent escape of gas through the cervix. With the suction cup fixed on the cervix, insert the hysteroscope into the sheath. Under direct vision, using carbon dioxide as the cervical dilator, slowly ad-

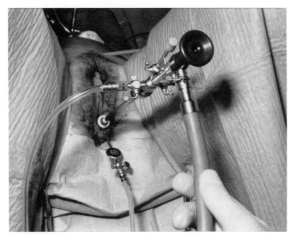

FIG. 6-1. The hysteroscope is inserted into the suction cup that is fixed to the cervix by vacuum. The continuous flow of carbon dioxide is provided by a special insufflator (not shown) through the tubing.

vance the instrument into the cervical canal. The continuous flow of carbon dioxide compensates for loss through the tubes and absorption. Complete exploration of the cervical canal and uterine cavity is possible after distention is obtained. Close the stopcocks on the sheath and secure the hysteroscope in its sheath to prevent gas loss during the procedure (Fig. 6-1).

The advantages of using carbon dioxide to distend the uterine cavity are its perfect transmission of the image, its availability, its long history of safety in tubal patency tests, and its rapid absorption. Some of the disadvantages of using carbon dioxide include the need for the complicated, expensive insufflating apparatus, a perfect cervical occlusion with the instrument, a flow rate that does not exceed 100 ml/min, extreme care to avoid provoking bleeding or bubbles, and maintaining uterine distention even with easy escape of carbon dioxide through patent tubes. Although carbon dioxide hysteroscopy gives excellent images, it is not always successful because of bleeding or the presence of thick, viscous secretions. In such patients, other media can be useful.[5]

Dextran 70(Hyskon) is a colorless liquid of 70,000 molecular weight with high viscosity and excellent optical qualities.[1] To proceed,

use a 50-ml plastic syringe and a 25-cm piece of tubing with Luer-Lok connections (Fig. 6-2). To avoid bubble formation, slowly pour the medium into a sterile container and then aspirate it with the 50-ml plastic syringe. Connect the tubing from the syringe to the sheath and load the sheath with the solution; introduce the hysteroscope through the previously dilated endocervical canal. Maintain manual pressure on the syringe to ensure a continuous flow, thus preventing accumulation of blood and mucus. Less than 100 ml generally suffices for a procedure. Some of the solution accumulates in the cul-de-sac with no untoward effects. Thoroughly clean instruments immediately after use to prevent crystallization of this viscous material, sticking of the various valves, and occlusion of the channels.

The advantages of dextran 70 are that the transmission of light is very good, only a simple apparatus is required (50-ml syringe and tubing), blood in the cavity forms droplets in the medium and flows slowly out of the tubal orifices, allowing for sustained uterine distention and a good operative field. Its main dis-

FIG. 6-2. A 50-ml plastic syringe filled with dextran 70 (Hyskon) and a 12-in piece of tubing with Luer-lock connections are the only pieces of equipment needed to do dextran 70 hysteroscopy.

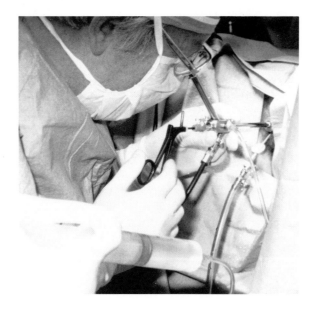

advantages are that it is very viscous, so that instruments require immediate washing in warm water and flushing to prevent permanent bonding, the rate of its reabsorption and reactivity in the abdominal cavity is unknown, and occasional allergic manifestations have been reported. Hysteroscopy with dextran 70 is probably the easiest technique to master, gives the most reproducible results, can always be performed, and may often be the procedure of choice.

Dextrose 5% and 10%, dextran 4% and 6%, and *normal saline* also provide adequate distention. To proceed, put one of these fluids in a plastic bag and place a pressure cuff around the bag; inflate the cuff to obtain and maintain adequate pressure, thus enabling fluid to flow through the tubing and into the uterine cavity (Fig. 6-3). The view initially is clear, but the field clouds rapidly, necessitating frequent rinsing. Quiñones has devised a small electric pump to regulate the flow automatically to achieve sufficient intrauterine pressure, thus preventing intrauterine bleeding and maintaining clarity of the medium (see Chap. 7). When using electrosurgical instruments, do not use saline.

The low-viscosity fluids are advantageous in that they are readily available and inexpensive, the insufflating apparatus is simple (a bag, a pressure cuff, and tubing), their reabsorption from the peritoneal cavity is rapid and physiologic, and they are used to lavage the uterine cavity and bleeding is not a contraindication. Some disadvantages are the need for frequent rinsing to maintain a clear image and the use of large amounts of fluid because these media pass easily through the tubes. I frequently use 5% dextrose and water to rinse the uterine cavity during a carbon dioxide hysteroscopy when bleeding is a problem, but I have little experience with it as the principal medium for hysteroscopy.

CONTACT HYSTEROSCOPY

The contact hysteroscopic system is called *Hysteroser.** The instrument and technique

* Advanced Biomedical Instruments.

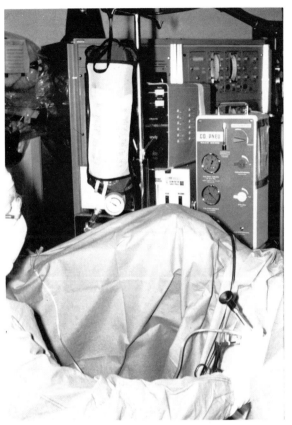

FIG. 6-3. A pressure cuff placed around a bag of low-viscosity fluid provides adequate pressure to obtain and maintain uterine distention.

are simple compared to panoramic hysteroscopy because no distention of the uterine cavity is necessary and no light source or cable is required. The Hysteroser collects, traps, and transmits room or directed light through the previously dilated cervical canal.[2] No panoramic view is possible because only surfaces in contact with the tip of the hysteroscope are visible. Vision is not obstructed by blood or other fluids. Attachments for directed biopsies have become available. I have had no experience with the Hysteroser, but the simplicity of the instrument and facility of the technique make it a worthwhile addition to gynecologic endoscopic procedures.

The *contact microcolpohysteroscope†* developed by Hamou can be used as a panoramic hysteroscope with a distending medium and as a contact hysteroscope.[4] As a contact hysteroscope without its sheath it is only 4 mm in diameter. A speculum and a light source and fiberoptic cable are required. Contact observation of the surfaces of the endocervical canal and the endometrial cavity can be meticulously performed using $\times 60$ or $\times 150$ magnification after staining the tissues appropriately (see Chap. 13). Adding a sheath with a valve enables the insufflation of carbon dioxide and an excellent panoramic view at unit and $\times 20$ magnification.

CONCLUSION

Thanks to the array of very good instruments and a broad choice of distending media, hysteroscopy is on its way to becoming a routine gynecologic endoscopic procedure.[3]

REFERENCES

1. Neuwirth, RS: Hysteroscopy. In Friedman EA (ed): Major Problems in Obstetrics and Gynecology, Vol 8. Philadelphia, W B Saunders, 1975
2. Parent B, Toubas C, Doerler B: L'hystéroscopie de contact. J Gynecol Obstet Biol Reprod 3:511, 1974
3. Phillips JM: Endoscopy in Gynecology. Downey, California, American Association of Gynecologic Laparoscopists, 1977
4. Rioux JE, Yuzpe AA: Gynecologic endoscopic equipment. In Levinthal JM (ed): Current Problems in Obstetrics and Gynecology. Chicago, Year Book Medical Publishers, 1981
5. Sciarra JJ, Butler JC, Speidel JJ: Hysteroscopic Sterilization. New York, Intercontinental Medical Book Corporation, 1974
6. Semm K: Atlas of Gynecologic Laparoscopy and Hysteroscopy. Philadelphia, W B Saunders, 1977
7. Siegler AM, Kemmann EK: Hysteroscopy. Obstet Gynecol Surv 30:567, 1975
8. Sugimoto O: Diagnostic and Therapeutic Hysteroscopy. Tokyo, Igaku–Shoin, 1978

† Storz Instruments, Tuttlingen, West Germany.

Hysteroscopy with a New Fluid Technique ■ 7

Rodolfo G. Quiñones

Currently the four media used for distending the uterine cavity to have a clear image in hysteroscopy are dextran, carbon dioxide, saline, and glucose solutions.[1–4,6] All require a proper pressure to obtain optimal results and overcome two of the major problems in making hysteroscopy a practical technique for intrauterine diagnosis and surgical procedures, namely, uterine distention and bleeding.

MATERIALS AND METHODS

Quiñones and colleagues started hysteroscopy with the Silander technique and later tried saline, glucose 5% and 10%, and dextran 4% and 6% solutions, injecting the solutions into the uterine cavity at a proper pressure by squeezing a rubber bulb attached to the receptacle of the solutions to increase the pressure inside the bottle (Fig. 7-1). The uterine cavity was dilated by increasing the flow of the solution.

Intrauterine pressures were recorded during hysteroscopy.[5] Although images of the uterine cavity are possible with a pressure of 40 mm Hg, the pressure must be increased to 100 mm Hg or 110 mm Hg to identify the tubal orifices. Occasionally during hysteroscopy small blood clots or mucus were aspirated by inserting a polyethylene catheter through the surgical channel of the hysteroscope sheath and aspirating through the catheter with a syringe. This

maneuver required the withdrawal of biopsy forceps, scissors, or electrodes during surgery so that the catheter could be introduced. Hysteroscopy is sometimes prolonged, and bleeding is annoying because intrauterine pressure diminishes.

Physicians have had difficulties in obtaining adequate uterine dilatation in hysteroscopy with the glucose technique because only with experience can proper pressure be applied to the bulb. To obviate this problem a metallic bridge with two surgical channels was constructed by Storz, one channel to aspirate blood or mucus and the other for biopsy forceps, scissors, or electrodes (Fig. 7-2). In addition, a device consisting of a small air compressor with a regulator system modifies the amount of air introduced into the receptacle of the glucose solution and an anaeroid manometer continuously measures the pressure of the air chamber in the fluid container. With this device, enough 5% glucose solution is constantly available to dilate the uterine cavity, permitting a clear endoscopic view and diminishing uterine bleeding considerably.

The regulator, added to the small compressor, maintains the pressure needed (Fig. 7-3), even though almost 20% of the total amount of glucose solution injected into the uterus passes to the pelvic cavity through the tubes when they are patent. A small amount is lost through the cervical conduit unless a cervical cup fixed

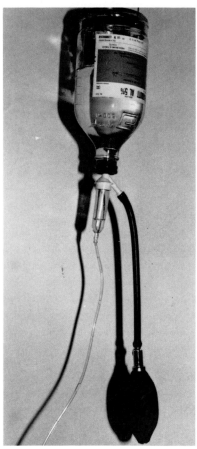

FIG. 7-1. Original setup for instillation of liquid media.

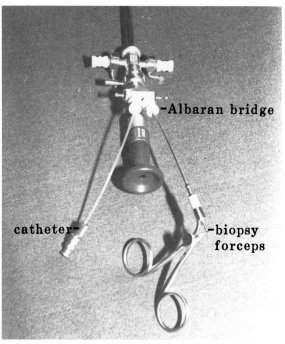

FIG. 7-2

FIG. 7-3

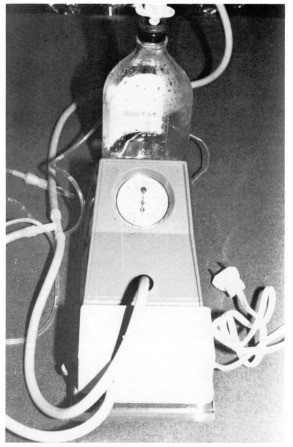

FIG. 7-2. Storz metallic bridge with two surgical channels. One channel contains a biopsy forceps, and the other has a catheter.

FIG. 7-3. Air compressor with an anaeroid manometer to measure pressure.

with negative pressure is used, as in the carbon dioxide technique. The intrauterine pressure remains between 100 mm Hg and 180 mm Hg.

COMMENT

When a paracervical block is used, patients complain only of minimal discomfort in the lower abdomen as the uterus is distended. The pain is not greater than that occurring when dextran or carbon dioxide is used. Hysteroscopy must be simple to be practical. Adding two surgical channels to the hysteroscope and the uterine insufflator system have simplified the procedure. Five percent glucose solution is used as a distending medium because of its availability, low cost, and effectiveness in enabling good endoscopic views.

Improvement of hysteroscopic instruments and safety and effectiveness of uterine-distending media are the main reasons for physicians' acceptance of hysteroscopy as a practical diagnostic and therapeutic endoscopic procedure. The potential indications for hysteroscopy are increasing, and the therapeutic methods are becoming standardized.

ACKNOWLEDGMENTS

I wish to thank Karl Storz, K.G. Gmbh & Co., who manufactured the metallic bridge with two surgical channels, and Jose Antonio Velazquez, who manufactured the uterine insufflator system.

REFERENCES

1. Edström K, Fernström I: The diagnostic possibilities of a modified hysteroscopic technique. Acta Obstet Gynecol Scand 49:327, 1970
2. Lindemann HJ: Pneumometra für die Hysteroskopie. Geburtshilfe Frauenheilkd 33:18, 1973
3. Porto R: Pneumohysteroscopy: Instrumentation and technique. In Sciarra JJ, Butler JC Jr, Speidel JJ (eds): Hysteroscopic Sterilization. New York, Intercontinental Medical Book Corporation, 1974
4. Quiñones RG, Alvarado DA, Esperanza AR: Histeroscopia (reporte preliminar). Ginecol Obstet Mex 27:683, 1970
5. Quiñones RG, Alvarado DA, Aznar RR: Tubal catheterization: Applications of a new technique. Am J Obstet Gynecol 114:674, 1972
6. Sugimoto O: Diagnostic and therapeutic hysteroscopy for traumatic intrauterine adhesions. Am J Obstet Gynecol 131:539, 1978

Carbon Dioxide Hysteroscopy: Principles and Physiology ■   8

Adolf Gallinat

To look into the uterine cavity with a hysteroscope it is necessary to distend the narrow slit between the front and rear walls. Two different media, liquids and carbon dioxide, are used.[1,2,6,8] After more than 10,000 hysteroscopies, I find the carbon dioxide method preferable because it allows for better visibility and a clean, fast operation in a dry medium. No allergic manifestations have occurred.

MATERIALS AND METHODS

Carbon dioxide gas in gynecology was first used for tubal perflation by Rubin in 1920.[7] In 1971 Lindemann introduced the use of controlled carbon dioxide gas insufflation in hysteroscopy.[2] Special equipment, such as the Hysteroflator or the Metromat, is required (Fig. 8-1). With a constant insufflation pressure of 200 mm Hg (150*), carbon dioxide flows into the uterus. The flow is increased until the uterus is completely distended, and then it decreases to a constant level as the gas escapes through the tubes.[3] This steady state is reached within 20 to 40 sec. The flow is a function of time (Fig. 8-2). The maximal flow rate is limited to 100 ml/min. During the initial dynamic phase (O-B) the flow increases up to maximum (O-A) and then decreases because of pressure

built up in the cavity. A steady state is reached, and the cavity is distended and remains open even though gas flows out of the tubes. The inside pressure remains constant. The hatched area shows the gas required for complete distention (see Fig. 8-2). With an insufflation pressure between 150 mm Hg and 200 mm Hg and a preselected maximal gas flow of 70 ml/min with normal tubal patency, stability is reached at approximately 30 ml/min to 40 ml/min at an intrauterine pressure of 40 mm Hg to 80 mm Hg. Hysteroscopic procedures lasting about 5 min cause 200 ml of carbon dioxide to flow through the tubes into the peritoneal cavity. Figure 8-3 shows the development of intrauterine pressure. The flow is limited to 100 ml/min, but it can be adjusted on the Hysteroflator by the gas-flow regulator as needed. The Metromat has no adjusting valve, and the flow rate is fixed.[4] When tubes are blocked, the intrauterine pressure increases to the insufflation pressure of 200 mm Hg (150 mm Hg*), while flow decreases to zero.[3]

RESULTS

Early uses of carbon dioxide for hysteroscopy resulted in some serious complications. Gas insufflation apparatus and machines for lapa-

---

* Refers to the Metromat.

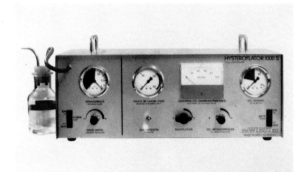

A

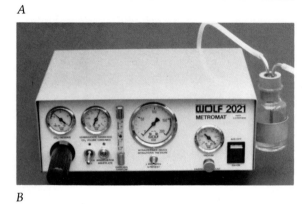

B

FIG. 8-1. Carbon dioxide apparatus is used for insufflating and distending the uterine cavity. (*A*) Hysteroflator. (*B*) Metromat.

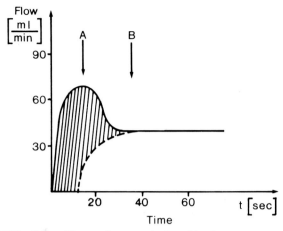

FIG. 8-2. Chart shows relationship between rate and duration of carbon dioxide flow.

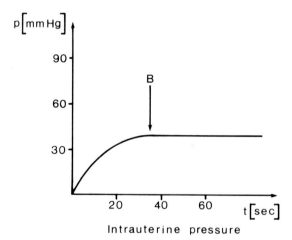

Intrauterine pressure

FIG. 8-3. A steady state is reached in 40 sec (*point B*).

roscopy were used without special installations for limiting pressure and flow rates. Such equipment could deliver a gas flow from 300 ml/min to 1000 ml/min. Cardiac arrhythmias and arrests were reported. Excess gas cannot be eliminated by the normal body buffer systems and regulatory mechanisms.

German shepherds were used with or without general anesthesia to check the effect of carbon dioxide in the body.[5] Direct insufflation of 200 ml/min into the femoral vein for 5 min caused a slight increase of pulse rate and a deepening of breathing. The initial increase in breathing soon returned to normal. There was no change of pH or pco_2 within 15 min of gas insufflation. At insufflation of 400 ml/min, toxic signs appeared. The lethal dosage was established at 1000 ml/min after 60 sec (Fig. 8-4).

Buffer systems and regulatory mechanisms collapsed, but there was no sign of gas embolism. Even after insufflation of 90 ml/min for 10 min into the carotid artery, no embolism occurred. pH, pco_2, po_2, and bicarbonate were checked in patients undergoing hysteroscopy under general and local anesthesia. No significant changes of these levels were found, even in women who had some uterine bleeding.

Carbon dioxide is cleared by breathing at its first passage through the lungs, and it is not detectable in the arterial system (Fig. 8-5). I have

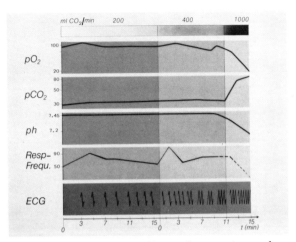

FIG. 8-4. Chart shows effects of increasing carbon dioxide flow rate in German shepherds. ECG = electrocardiogram.

not seen any complications from carbon dioxide in 10,000 hysteroscopic examinations with either the Hysteroflator or the Metromat. Rubin reported results from 80,000 carbon dioxide tubal perflations by 380 different authors without any untoward sequelae.[8]

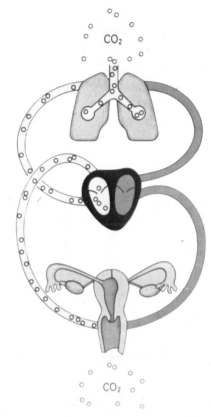

FIG. 8-5. Mechanism for clearing insufflating carbon dioxide from the body.

REFERENCES

1. Edström K, Fernström I: The diagnostic possibilities of a modified hysteroscopic technique. Acta Obstet Gynecol Scand 49:327, 1970
2. Lindemann HJ: Eine neue Untersuchungsmethode für die Hysteroskopie. Endoscopy 4:194, 1971
3. Lindemann HJ, Gallinat A: Physikalische und physiologische Grundlagen der CO$_2$-Hysteroskopie. Geburtshilfe Frauenheilkd 36:729, 1976
4. Lindemann HJ, Gallinat A, Lueken, RP: Metromat. A new instrument for producing pneumometra. J Reprod Med 23:73, 1979

5. Lindemann HJ, Mohr J, Gallinat A, et al: Der Einfluss von CO$_2$-Gas während der Hysteroskopie. Geburtshilfe Frauenheilkd 36:153, 1976
6. Quiñones RG, Alvarado DA, Aznar RR: Histeroscopia. Una nueva téchnica. Ginecol Obstet Mex 32:237, 1972
7. Rubin IC: The nonoperative determination of patency of fallopian tubes. JAMA 74:1017, 1920
8. Rubin IC: Uterotubal Insufflation. St. Louis, C V Mosby, 1947

Carbon Dioxide Hysteroscopy Without Anesthesia in 478 Patients ■

Rene Marty

Hysteroscopy is indicated in women who have abnormal shadows on hysterography to ascertain the cause of the defect. The findings can help determine whether subsequent gynecologic surgery is necessary. In addition, hysteroscopy can monitor the results of previous surgical procedures, including the quality of a cesarean section scar and the effect of a metroplasty, myomectomy, or tubal cornual implantation. It should certainly be used routinely before an intrauterine device (IUD) is inserted because 10% to 15% of women choosing this method of birth control have uterine abnormalities that preclude normal acceptance of an IUD.

This chapter will report on 478 hysteroscopic operations with carbon dioxide performed without anesthesia in patients from the Hôpitaux de Paris Université XIII University Hospital, and private practice.

MATERIALS AND METHODS

The instruments for hysteroscopy include sheaths* (3 mm and 5 mm), fiberoptic, foroblique telescopes (2.7 mm and 4 mm), a source of light, and a Hysteroflator.† A special plastic probe is graduated in centimeters; a 35-mm miniature camera, full frame, also has an electric motor drive. Instruments are disinfected between patients with 2% benzalkonium dimethyl ammonium (Stericline) for 30 minutes in cold water.

Before beginning hysteroscopic examination without anesthesia, a physician should learn the technique from an experienced gynecologist. Initially, the physician should perform hysteroscopy with the patient anesthetized and using a teaching attachment.

The optimal time in the menstrual cycle for examination is the proliferative phase. To proceed, sound the uterus in the cycle before hysteroscopy. Prescribe vaginal suppositories for 7 days before the procedure and disinfect the vulva and vagina before the hysteroscopic examination. Counsel patients, show them the instruments, and let them watch the operation through the teaching attachment. Document each operation with photographs and fill out a report on a special form. Allow the patient to rest for 30 min postoperatively.

I performed hysteroscopic examination in 478 patients: in 231 (48.3%) for gynecologic indications, in 202 asymptomatic women who were scheduled for insertion of IUDs, and in 45 because of lost or troublesome IUDs. Not more than 5 or 10 min was needed to perform the examination. As the intrauterine pressure rose to between 80 mm Hg and 100 mm Hg, the gas

* Storz, Tuttlingen, West Germany.
† F. Wiest, West Berlin, West Germany.

flowed in at 35 ml/min. Carbon dioxide did not reduce the optical quality of the view. If the patient has significant uterine bleeding, use liquid for uterine distention.

RESULTS

Polyps (Fig. 9-1) appeared in 51 patients, and submucous myomas appeared (Fig. 9-2) in 57. I examined 24 postoperative patients, including 13 who had had cesarean section, 4 who had undergone metroplasty, four who had undergone tubal implantation (Fig. 9-3), 2 after a myomectomy, and 1 after a uterine perforation. Abnormal uterine bleeding was the main complaint in 18 women; 23 others were infertile, and 10 patients had hysteroscopy to stage endometrial adenocarcinoma.

In 203 instances, I performed a hysteroscopic examination in asymptomatic patients before inserting an IUD, and I found intracavitary abnormalities in 13 women (6%). These included polyps (six), myomas (five), synechiae (two), and endometrial hyperplasia (two). Forty-five women with IUDs complained of abnormal bleeding (23), retraction of the string (11), pelvic pain (9), or possible expulsion of the device (2). Most of the IUDs were the Cu-7 type, and a few were multiload; most were first insertions. Two IUDs were seen in one patient (Fig. 9-4). None had had an intrauterine investigation before placement of the IUD. I removed the IUD uneventfully in each instance. Six women had some uterine abnormality.

I found no significant changes in the endometrial mucosa of 80 women who had worn their IUDs for 2½ years. Any local change the IUD causes is transient and does not affect the basal endometrial layer. Complications included mild postoperative bleeding in three patients and shoulder and pelvic pain in three others. Incomplete studies or failed examinations occurred in seven instances.

COMMENT

An IUD is generally inserted without a prior investigation into the shape of the uterine cavity. However, the medical press and many authors note that some complications are induced by the presence of an IUD in the uterine cavity. Since hysterography is time consuming and irradiates the ovaries, I decided to perform a routine hysteroscopy just before inserting an IUD. Of 202 patients, 13 had abnormalities. These patients were asymptomatic. Because of these results, in some cases I delayed IUD insertion to treat the abnormality; in other instances, alternative methods of contraception were chosen. At least 6% of the IUD complications were predictable as a consequence of preexisting uterine disease.

The uterine cavity, after 2½ years of exposure to an IUD, showed no significant changes in the endometrium in 80 women. These hysteroscopic examinations were performed after a 1-month delay. If some local modification caused by the IUD presence occurred early, it did not last more than one cycle and did not involve the basal endometrium. The abnormal uterine findings on routine hysteroscopy in asymptomatic women before IUD insertion and those found during the removal of troublesome IUDs seem to justify routine hysteroscopy before IUD insertion.

Hysteroscopy is no longer an experimental technique, and the extended indications for its use suggest that it will be performed more often. Carbon dioxide hysteroscopy is a safe outpatient procedure and certainly is feasible without anesthesia. Its greater use will lower the need for hysterography and curettage.

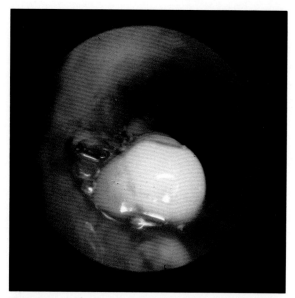

FIG. 9-1. Polyp is present in lower uterine segment.

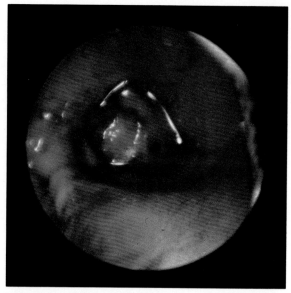

FIG. 9-3. Tubal implantation in cornual region. Original ostium is to the right.

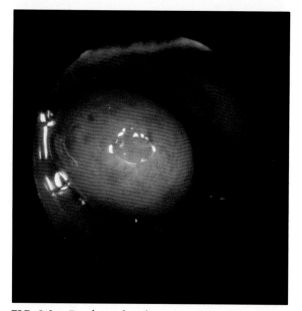

FIG. 9-2. Pendunculated myoma along lateral wall.

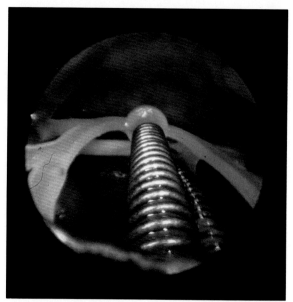

FIG. 9-4. Two IUDs are present in this uterine cavity.

Instruments ■ 10

Harry Van der Pas

Instruments for hysteroscopy must fulfill three principles. To transform the slit-shaped uterine cavity into a hollow cavity, a distending medium and apparatus are needed. To illuminate this cavity, a source of light must be available. To permit a view into this illuminated cavity, an endoscope is essential.

DISTENTION MEDIUM AND APPARATUS

Either gas or liquid is used to distend the uterine cavity. Although gas is usually used in Europe, liquid is the usual medium in other parts of the world. In principle, any gas could distend the cavity if the danger of a gas embolism did not exist. In this context Buchwald distinguishes between primary and secondary factors predisposing to embolism.[1] The primary factor is the solubility and diffusion constant of a gas. The secondary factor depends on the pressure used to apply the gas, the quantity per minute, and the patient's condition and position.

Carbon dioxide is the only gas currently used in hysteroscopy. It is colorless, nonpoisonous, and nonconducting. It is not flammable and does not support combustion. It has good solubility in water. At 37C, 54.1 ml of carbon dioxide is soluble in 100 ml of blood, and thus the carbon dioxide is an almost negligible primary factor. A good insufflation apparatus is necessary. Most accidents have been caused by unadjusted insufflation apparatus used without concern for the danger of carbon dioxide insufflation in the bloodstream or the possibility of embolism. Two alternatives are possible to obtain safe carbon dioxide insufflation: an apparatus that functions at a constant volume, 100 ml/min of carbon dioxide under variable pressure regulated between 0 mm Hg and 100 mm Hg, or one that functions under a constant pressure of 100 mm Hg at a variable volume between 0 ml/min to 100 ml/min of carbon dioxide. The Metromat limits the pressure to 150 mm Hg and the volume to 70 ml/min. As a result, the supply of gas needs no regulation because the apparatus automatically adds carbon dioxide in case of loss. If this apparatus is used, the dangers of hypercarbia or embolism are nonexistent. Using an unadjusted insufflation apparatus can lead to catastrophic complications. Lindemann and colleagues insufflated carbon dioxide gas intravenously (IV) into a dog that had not been anesthetized. Introduction of 200 ml/min over 15 min caused minor changes of pO_2, pCO_2, and pH values. At 400 ml/min for 9 min, tachypnea occurred; pO_2, pCO_2, and pH remained normal. The electrocardiogram (ECG) showed arrythmias. At 1000 ml/min for 60 sec pCO_2 increased, pO_2 diminished, and pH fell. The breathing frequency fell, and the arrythmia increased. The animal died without any indication of embolism. These tests distinctly prove that the fatal accidents in hysteroscopy were not caused by the carbon dioxide itself but by improper use of the gas and incorrect instruments.

LIGHT SOURCE

Most sources of cold light are fitted with halogen or xenon lamps. The power varies between 100 and 300 watts. The light is transmitted to the endoscope by a fiberglass, loses its heat component entirely, and keeps its intensity of light. The difference of quality of the light-conducting cords lies in the content of fiber rods and in the index of refraction. A loss of light occurs when the conduction cord is connected to the endoscope, especially if intermediate parts for adaptation are used. For that reason an integral bundle hysteroscope has recently been constructed; the fiberglass transporting light is continuous from the source of light to the distal end of the hysteroscope. This connection ensures a greater intensity of light. More light is needed for photographic documentation. Modern sources of light are fitted with a flash generator, supplying 500 watts/sec. Film and video require light of 1000 watts with a lighting temperature of 6000 K. Persons desiring both kinds of documentation, photos and videotapes, need two sources of light, a flash generator and a source of cold light of 1000 watts. This problem can be avoided with an Olympus photocamera OM-2. The camera is set at automatic and loaded with a film of 400 ASA. Sufficient light is given to get good colored slides. Video shots can be obtained with the aforementioned source of light but only with the integral hysteroscope.

ENDOSCOPE

The hysteroscope is an endoscopic instrument consisting of an optical and a mechanical part to inspect the uterine cavity. The optics of an endoscope built for a source of cold light consist of two parts, the system of lenses transmitting the image and the fiberglass conducting the cold light. More trials are underway to build thinner optics. Since it is not possible to discuss all available hysteroscopes, only general characteristics will be described here. The optical system can be flexible or rigid. The flexible endoscope consists of conducting fibers for light and others for the image put together into one shaft. The quality of the image is rather granular for its weaker resolution. At the moment, the use of flexible endoscopes in hysteroscopy is controversial. The price and fragility of the instrument are deterrents to wider acceptance. A positive point is the possibility of penetrating into the tubal ostium with greater facility. Mohri and associates have built a tubaloscope in the style of Machida. In Europe no flexible hysteroscopes were commercialized.

The rigid hysteroscope consists of a shaft of fiberglass bundle that conducts light along a system of lenses. In Europe three optical systems are used to manufacture endoscopes: the Hopkins optics, the Lumina optics, and the Olympus optics. The extremely strong resolution of the image enables a pronounced contrast. The image remains definite even if the distance between the optics and the organ diminishes. The image at 2 mm of the optics comes to $\times 0.25$ magnification. At a greater distance, the magnification and intensity of light diminish. At a distance of 20 mm or 30 mm the image keeps its full size, and a very good view of the intrauterine cavity is obtained. The brightness and accurate reproduction of colors have been improved a good deal compared to the results obtained with the former optics. The most important advantage is that the diameter of the optics has been decreased. The thinnest hysteroscope at the moment, the so-called needle hysteroscope, has a diameter of 2 mm.

Each optical system has its own direction of view and its own eyefield. The direction of view varies between 0 (180) degrees and 30 (150) degrees. Most hysteroscopes have a direction of 30 degrees. The largest field, 90 degrees, is obtained with the Hopkins optics. There is a great advantage for inspecting the uterine cavity with wide-angle optics, but this field has not yet been built up. The diameter of the hysteroscope ranges between 2 mm and 8 mm. The operating hysteroscope built for Porto has a diameter of 8 mm. The shaft is a circular stainless steel tube through which the optic is pushed. Through this shaft the distending medium, gas or liquid, is injected through a stopcock at the proximal end of the shaft. The hole must be airtight if carbon dioxide is used. The operating shaft has a supplementary channel, also airtight with a stopcock and usually with an extra rubber cap, through which the ancillary instruments are introduced (Fig. 10-1). The shaft is 30 cm long, and the diameter varies between 11 and 20 on the Charrière scale depending on the thickness of the optics and the purpose or the introduction of the hysteroscope. Some shafts are fitted out with an Albaran bridge in their distal end (Fig. 10-2).

COMMENT

The outline of these three principles of hysteroscopy leads to the question of how to introduce the hysteroscope into the uterine cavity, since the cervical channel is closed by the external and internal os. There are various methods of penetrating the uterine cavity, depending on the purpose of the hysteroscopic intervention. If hysteroscopy is for diagnosis only, the physician can insert a thin hysteroscope into the uterine cavity without any analgesia, anesthesia, or cervical dilatation. A hysteroscope 5-mm thick is appropriate for all multiparas and for most nulliparas. To take a biopsy or to retrieve a "lost" intrauterine device (IUD), a work shaft and dilatation of the cervical channel are necessary. Hegar dilators that increase by half sizes are best with carbon dioxide; a cervical adapter is important to prevent loss of carbon dioxide during operative hysteroscopy.

Auxiliary instruments can be rigid or flexible (Fig. 10-3). For major intrauterine interventions such as cutting septae or excising submu-

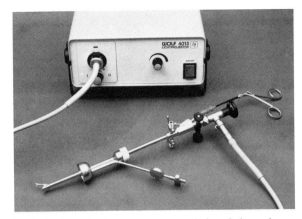

FIG. 10-1. The hysteroscope and sheath have been inserted into a metal suction cup. A biopsy forceps has been introduced through the accessory channel on the sheath. The light source is in the rear.

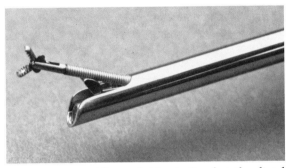

FIG. 10-2. An Albaran bridge is fitted at the distal end to manipulate the operating instrument.

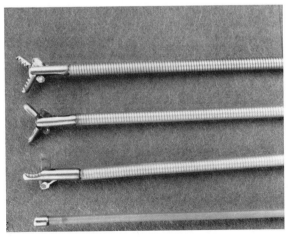

FIG. 10-3. Some ancillary instruments, shown from top to bottom, are a grasping forceps, a biopsy forceps, a scissors, and a coagulating probe.

cous myomas, the rigid instruments are preferable. The latter can only be used through the channel of the Porto operating hysteroscope. It has the advantage of introducing auxiliary instruments into the center of the field instead of alongside. Flexible instruments can be used through the smaller operating shaft even under local anesthesia. Grasping an IUD with the classic forceps is often very difficult. An adapted "chased" instrument with clamping nicks would be desirable because it is more reliable. To remove extraneous objects or excise small myomas from the cavity, the urologic stone dislodger is useful.

Practical training in hysteroscopy is urgently needed in the development of young physicians, since even the best instruments can cause serious complications if handled by untrained persons.

REFERENCES

1. Buchwald W: Die Verwendung schnell resorbierbarer Gase bei diagnostischen Gasinsufflationen. Fortschr Röntgen 103:187, 1965
2. Lindemann HJ, Mohr J, Gallinat A, et al: Der Einfluss von CO_2-gas während des Hysteroskopie. Geburtshilfe Frauenheilkd 36:153, 1976
3. Mohri T, Mohri C, Yamadori F: Tubuloscope: Flexible glass fiber endoscope for intratubal observation. Endoscopy 2:226, 1970

A Teaching Aid ■

11

Richard K. Kleppinger

As subspecialization within the medical specialties develops, required skills become more demanding and physicians' perception must become more critical. Neither my basic medical training nor my training in gynecology adequately prepared me for the nuances of hysteroscopy. During a 1974 research project under Lindemann's direction, I saw for the first time intrauterine anatomy heretofore seen only in the bisected extirpated specimen. Orientation to a new perspective of uterine anatomy, interpretation of observed structures, and consideration for visual limitation of the optical system were areas Lindemann stressed. Siegler has described hysteroscopy as "a new kind of anatomic exploration and that's the first thing to realize. The gynecologist sees structures in a setting, in situ, that have hitherto not been accessible endoscopically. The pelvis and internal genitalia are quickly identified at laparoscopy. But looking at the uterine cavity through the hysteroscope is quite new. The landmarks are unfamiliar and the manipulative techniques are different."[1]

MATERIALS AND METHODS

I recognized the need to become familiar with the "landscape" and the technique. An extirpated uterus would allow practice and provide experience. Colleagues and the pathology department at Reading Hospital cooperated in making extirpated specimens accessible. I performed initial examinations by placing the extirpated uterus on a stack of towels. Because the addition of an elastic bandage over the fundus proved no substitute for ligamentous attachments, a 3-in belt of nylon webbing was constructed to support varying sized uteri suspended within the cutout portion of an examination table. Greater stability was required, so a more secure support was designed of plywood. A tiltable stage and some support for the cervical adapter were required. When this prototype fulfilled its mechanical purpose, a nonpermeable material of 0.14-cm stainless steel was chosen for construction of several permanent models, since there were obvious additional uses for this tool within the teaching program.

Although this teaching aid was patented as an educational exercise for the college-aged inventor, it has not been manufactured and there is no intention to do so. The patent describes the teaching aid as "an anatomical display device for use in learning and teaching . . . hysteroscopy under nonoperating room conditions and utilizing an extirpated specimen."

The patent lists as ancillary uses the instruction and demonstration of the proper technique for insertion of various intrauterine devices (IUDs), menstrual extraction and aspi-

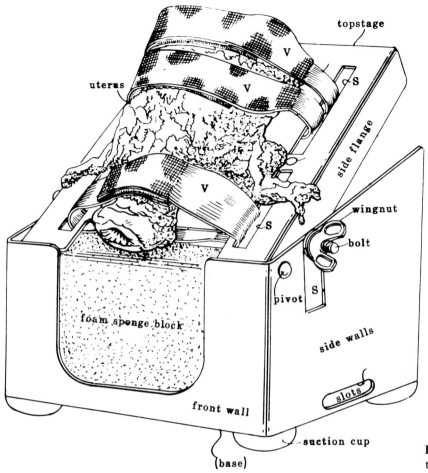

Fig. 11-1.   Hysteroscopy teaching aid with an extirpated uterus anchored to the stage by elastic Velcro straps. S = slots; V = velcro.

S - slots
V - velcro

ration, endometrial biopsy, cervical dilatation and curettage, uterine suction aspiration of early intrauterine pregnancy, thermal or cryosurgical cervical cauterization, cervical biopsy, cervical conization, colposcopy and colpomicrobiopsy, and the carbon dioxide laser vaporization technique.

Described in United States Patent Number 4,001,952, filed Oct. 24, 1975, the teaching aid (Fig. 11-1) consists of a boxlike base with downward-facing suction cups for engaging the top surface of a suitable table. Alternately, the base may be fastened to a table by passing a fastening strap around the tabletop and through horizontal slots provided centrally on the lower portions of the side walls. The stage or top portion of the boxlike base is pivotally connected to the upper corner portions of the side walls by adjustable bolts. These pivotal connections are located so that the stage may be rotated through a 75-degree arc. The rotation enables simulation of uterine anteflexion through retroversion.

The stage, at each of its opposite side portions, contains a pair of elongated rectangular slots, allowing the passage of elastic straps for anchoring the extirpated uterus. The straps are provided at their overlapping surfaces with Velcro pads for appropriate adjustment to accommodate the size of the specimen. The front wall of the base and the stage contain a U-shaped cutout, into which is inserted a large, rectangular, foam sponge block. This foam sponge serves as a resilient support for the cervix of the extirpated uterus. The cutout portions are large enough to accommodate a suction adapter applied to the cervix when carbon dioxide is the medium for uterine distention.

COMMENT

In vitro practice in hysteroscopy can be valuable as an early learning experience. It gives the physician the opportunity to gain confidence and a measure of competence in the unfamiliar aspects of this procedure before operating on patients. Such a teaching aid can be used for review before operative hysteroscopy. The prime purpose of this teaching aid is to provide a display device primarily designed for the practice of hysteroscopy under nonoperating room conditions using an extirpated uterus and either a liquid or gas medium for uterine distention. It allows self-learning, teaching, and demonstration of the various techniques of diagnostic and operative procedures, especially the technique of transuterine catheterization of the tubal ostia for sterilization procedures.

REFERENCE

1. Siegler AM: A symposium on advances in fiberoptic hysteroscopy. Contemp Obstet Gynecol 3:115, 1974

Contact Hysteroscopy with the Universal 4-mm Hysteroscope ■

12

Valentin Marleschki

Contact hysteroscopy was introduced by Marleschki in 1956, at a time when most physicians performed endoscopic examinations of the uterine cavity by dilating the cervical canal, expanding the uterine cavity with carbon dioxide or a liquid, and using some form of anesthesia.[1,3]

MATERIALS AND METHODS

Marleschki's Universal Hysteroscope, which has an outer diameter of 4 mm, obviates the necessity for cervical dilatation and anesthesia, even in nulliparas.[4] Inasmuch as it is a contact hysteroscope, uterine distention is unnecessary. Among its many applications are the identification of intracervical and intrauterine anomalies, neoplasia, premalignant and malignant changes, polyps, synechiae, intrauterine causes of infertility, sources of bleeding, and misplaced intrauterine devices (IUDs).[2] In pregnant women, contact hysteroscopy is useful in amnioscopy in selected high-risk patients and in identifying ruptured membranes, finding the source of bleeding, and locating residual chorionic tissue (benign, molar, or malignant).

Apart from its clinical applications, the contact hysteroscope is a diagnostic method for the clarification of many abnormalities associated with gynecologic and obstetric problems.[6] It is also used to study changes in endometrial vessels (Fig. 12-1).[5] Contact hysteroscopy is indicated in searching for the causes of dysmenorrhea, menorrhagia, and metrorrhagia and in examining the cavity in a missed or incomplete abortion, after a spontaneous abortion, in suspected uterine perforation after manipulation for a misplaced IUD (Fig. 12-2) or abnormal hysterogram, and in patients who may have Asherman's syndrome. The technical and optical construction of the Universal Hysteroscope makes it usable during uterine bleeding.

It is possible to find a submucous myoma (Fig. 12-3) or endometrial polyps (Fig. 12-4) or to locate intrauterine adhesions with this hysteroscope. In a patient who has had an incomplete or missed abortion (Fig. 12-5) or in one with a suspected hydatidiform mole, hysteroscopy is recommended. Contact hysteroscopy is useful after such intrauterine procedures as sounding, curettage, dilatation, or the insertion of an IUD and suspected uterine perforation. Localization of inadvertent perforation by hysteroscopy and its evaluation by laparoscopy can determine management.

In 1964, Marleschki used the contact hysteroscope for amnioscopy.[5] In cases of suspected intrauterine fetal asphyxia, the color of the amniotic fluid can be significant. In postpartum hemorrhage, the physician can search for retained placental tissue. For research purposes, contact hysteroscopy can be performed as embryoscopy (Fig. 12-6) and used to study uterine perfusion during both normal delivery and delivery with abdominal decompression.[7]

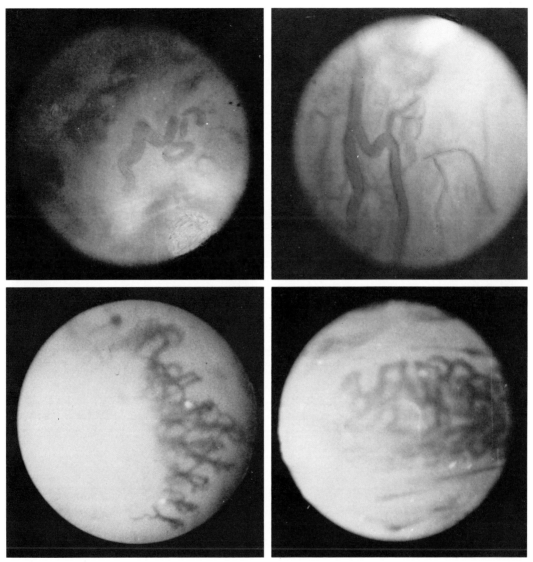

FIG. 12-1. Vascular patterns seen in the endometrium with contact hysteroscopy. (*A*) Normal vessels of the proliferative phase. (*B*) Decidua vessels are typical. (*C*) Endometrial hemangioma. (*D*) Atypical vessels caused by vascular occlusion.

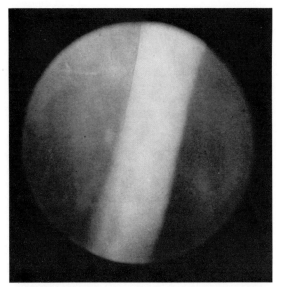

FIG. 12-2. Part of an IUD seen with endometritis and bleeding.

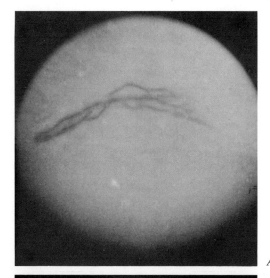

A

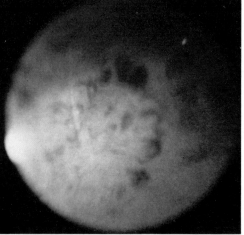

B

C

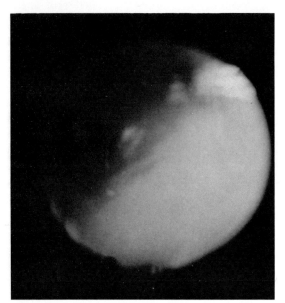

FIG. 12-3. Myoma and bleeding.

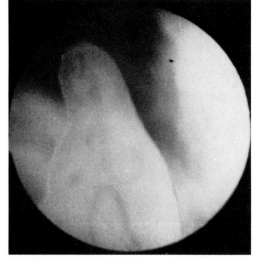

FIG. 12-4. Endometrial polyp. (*A*) Central vessel is present with scanty stroma and draining vessels. (*B*) Top of an endometrial polyp is noted, with atypical vessels, bleeding, and endometritis. (*C*) Top of a polyp in the cervical canal with a central vessel.

FIG. 12-5. Intrauterine adhesion is seen with contact hysteroscope.

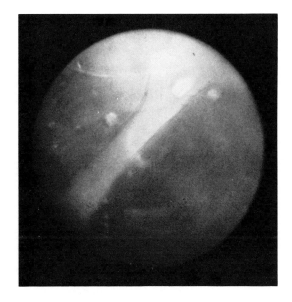

FIG. 12-6. Intrauterine pregnancy. (*A*) Imminent abortion with bleeding. (*B*) Missed abortion with calcification. (*C*) Normal pregnancy, 8th week, with normal vascular pattern. (*D*) Normal pregnancy, 12th week, with large vessels.

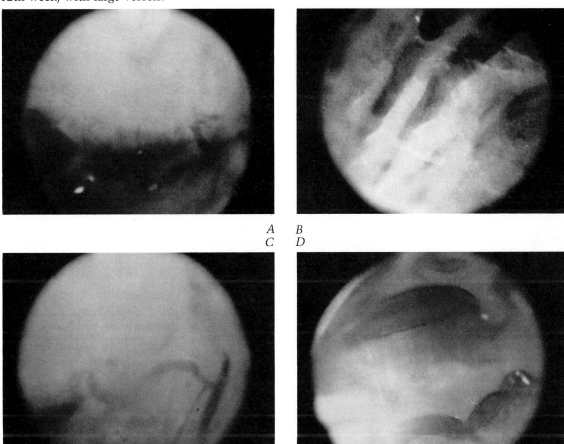

A   B
C   D

CONCLUSION

Based on personal experience with contact hysteroscopy for more than 20 years and in more than 6400 examinations, I recommend this method for examination of selected gynecologic and obstetric outpatients and for scientific research purposes.

REFERENCES

1. Marleschki V: Die moderne Zervikoscopie und Hysteroskopie. Zentralbl Gynaekol 88:637, 1966
2. Marleschki V: Eine weiterer Schritt in der Frühdiagnose des Intracervikal und Korpuskarzinomas: Der Krebsarzt 3:159, 1966
3. Marleschki V: Moderne Cervikoscopie und Hysteroskopie. Abhandlungen der deutschen Akademie der Wissenschaften zu Berlin. Akademic Verlag Berlin 3:421, 1966
4. Marleschki V: Das Universal Hysteroskop nach Marleschki. Urania 6:34, 1971
5. Marleschki V: Geburtserleichterung unter Kontrolle. Urania 11:34, 1971
6. Marleschki V: Hysteroscopy in Gynecological and Obstetrics Emergencies: Urgent Endoscopy of Digestive and Abdominal Diseases, p 248. Basel, S Karger, 1972
7. Marleschki V: Hysteroscopic study of uterine circulation in normal labor and in labor involving the use of abdominal decompression. 1973 World Congress of Obstetrics and Gynecology. Abstracts of Papers. Int Cong Series 279:50, 1973
8. Marleschki V: The hysteroscopic method of Marleschki. 1973 World Congress of Obstetrics and Gynecology. Abstracts of Papers. Int Cong Series 279:263, 1973
9. Marleschki V: Hysteroskopische Feststellung der spontanen Perfusionsschwankungen am menschlichen Endometrium. Zentralbl Gynaekol 90:1094, 1980

Advanced Hysteroscopy and Microhysteroscopy in 1000 Patients ■   13

Jacques E. Hamou
Jacques Salat-Baroux

Conventional hysteroscopy as recently reported by other investigators throughout the world employs a 7-mm sheathed endoscope.[7,12,14] This diameter and, even more important, the crossing of the cervical canal and internal os require prior dilatation and general anesthesia or paracervical nerve block. Dilatation causes minimal bleeding; to prevent impaired vision and bubbles, higher carbon dioxide flow rates or, preferably, liquid media are needed. Microhysteroscopy is a painless procedure, and no anesthesia is required. The absence of induced bleeding helps keep the gas flow rate to a minimum.

MATERIALS AND METHODS

Between January 1980 and June 1980 we performed 680 hysteroscopic and 320 microcolpohysteroscopic examinations on patients aged 15 to 71 years. The indications are listed in Table 13-1. Whenever possible, for each indication we compared hysteroscopic results to the results of other diagnostic studies.

The instrument used was the Harnou microcolpohysteroscope,* conceived in 1979 and built in 1980.[6] It has a 4-mm diameter and is 25-cm long (Fig. 13-1) with a 90-degree field angle and a 30-degree foroblique lens. It offers

* Storz Endoscopy America, Culver City, CA.

panoramic and contact vision with four magnifications, which are obtained by adjusting the ocular. They are as follows:

Unit magnification (position 1) gives a conventional panoramic endoscopic view.
Magnification $\times 20$ (position 2) permits a detailed panoramic view of the mucosa equivalent to colposcopy.
Magnification $\times 60$ (position 3) gives contact, microscopic views with a depth of field of about 80 μm and shows superficial layers.
Magnification $\times 150$ (position 4) is a contact microscopic view that shows the nucleus and cytoplasm.

An important quality in an optical instrument is its resolution, or smallest visible detail, which is 1.5 μm for microhysteroscopy, comparable to a conventional microscope. Eye resolution is 75 μm and the colposcope has a resolution of 15 μm. The Japanese miniature endoscope and the French contact hysteroscope cannot be used for panoramic viewing. Light is supplied by a 150-watt lamp through a fiberoptic cable. Carbon dioxide is insufflated from a Hysteroflator, with a control of maximal gas flow rate of 100 ml/min and a pressure between 90 mm Hg and 100 mm Hg, through a sheath whose external diameter is 5.2 mm. This technique is used in position 1 for panoramic vision.

Table 13-1

INDICATIONS FOR HYSTEROSCOPY AND MICROHYSTEROSCOPY

PRESUMPTIVE DIAGNOSIS	HAMOU AND SALAT-BAROUX (1000 PATIENTS)		VALLE[17] (350 PATIENTS)		SCIARRA AND VALLE[11] (320 PATIENTS)	
	No.	%	No.	%	No.	%
Hysteroscopy (680 patients)						
Abnormal uterine bleeding						
Premenopausal	164	16.4	109	31.1	104	32.5
Postmenopausal	51	5.1	36	10.3	36	11.2
After pregnancy	40	4	4	1.1	4	1.2
Infertility						
Synechiae	27	2.7	55	28.6	47	14.7
Abnormal hystero-salpingogram	39	3.9				
Unknown cause	62	6.2				
Intrauterine abnormalities						
Polyps and myomas	64	6.4	18	5.1	18	5.6
Abnormal hysterogram	98	9.8	21	6	16	4.9
Adenocarcinoma						
Patent	4	0.1				
Screening	52	5.2	0			
Other						
IUD	27	2.7	102	29.1	95	29.7
Pelvic pain	18	1.8				
Amenorrhea	6					
Malformations	5					
Molar pregnancies	3					
After surgery	9		5	1.5		
Salpingoscopy	7					
Embryoscopy	4					
Microcolpohysteroscopy (320 patients)						
Abnormal smears	27	2.7				
Screening	293	29.3				

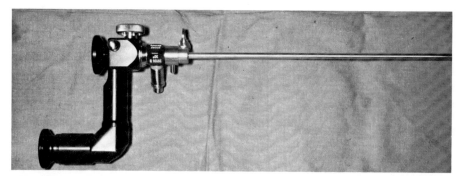

FIG. 13-1.   Hamou microcolpohysteroscope.

The procedure is as follows. No premedication is required. The pelvic examination indicates the uterine position. Use either a Colin or a disposable speculum to expose the cervix, which is cleansed with cotton balls soaked with saline. A tenaculum holds the cervix near the external os and helps to hold and straighten the uterus. The major step of the procedure is crossing the cervical canal to perform an atraumatic, simple, well-accepted hysteroscopy. The instrument offers very close and magnified vision for a cervical crossing under strict visual control. Create a small carbon dioxide cavity in front of the endoscope to avoid trauma to the endocervical mucosa as the scope is advanced (Fig. 13-2). Locate the direction of the internal os by withdrawing the scope a few millimeters, then directing the distal sharp edge into the opening under contact $\times 60$ magnification. The lens will slide smoothly on the endometrium. Enter the uterine cavity and reestablish a panoramic view (Fig. 13-3).

At unit magnification, assess the morphology and size of the cavity. At $\times 20$ magnification, study disposition and density of endometrial gland openings, capillary vascularization, and any abnormalities. Also at this magnification, evaluate tubal ostia and the first millimeters of the intramural segment (Fig. 13-4). High magnification ($\times 60$ and $\times 150$) requires prior staining. Methylene blue solution, 0.1 ml to 0.2 ml of 1%, is instilled through a 1-mm catheter (Fig. 13-5). The gas flow is lowered to 10 ml/min to avoid uterine contractions when the procedure is long or is associated with bleeding or an incompetent os.

Cervicoscopy (Fig. 13-6), a new application, allows a better evaluation of cervicoisthmic filling defects on hysterosalpingography. It will also detect normal, atrophic (Fig. 13-7), or fibrous aspects of glandular structures of the endocervix and the quality of mucus.

Contraindications to hysteroscopy are pregnancy, pelvic infection, or profuse bleeding. Microhysteroscopy can be performed when bleeding is moderate. The distal end of the endoscope creates a retrograde distention by entering the fundal region to avoid causing bubbles. This creates a carbon dioxide cavity and aids in locating the origin of the bleeding.

An average procedure does not exceed 10 min. The average amount of carbon dioxide used and recorded does not exceed 400 ml, which is 10% to 20% of the amount used for tubal insufflation. Arterial measurements of pH, Pa_{O_2}, and Pa_{CO_2} before and after the procedure have shown no significant variations (see Chap. 22). Tubal passage of carbon dioxide and risks of infection are insignificant. Twenty-one patients complained of shoulder pain, and 5 had mild pelvic infections. We had 16 failures (2.3%) because of severe cervical atresia in 680 patients in whom we attempted hysteroscopic examination. The procedure was completely painless in 410 women, similar to menstrual discomfort for 215, and more painful than menses in 39 patients.[1]

RESULTS

Abnormal uterine bleeding constituted the largest indication for hysteroscopy (Table 13-2). In 164 patients who complained of premenopausal bleeding, hysteroscopy primarily revealed endometrial dystrophy, polyps, and submucous myomas. Polyps (Fig. 13-8) and myomas (Fig. 13-9) were evaluated for shape, vascularization, consistency, and location. High magnification permitted a precise evaluation of endometrial glandular structures, vascular patterns, and endometrial thickness by simply touching the endoscope on the structure. Hyperplasia was found in 39 women; atrophy was found in 24 others. In five instances the atrophy was so severe that myometrium could be seen. Endometrial adenocarcinoma was found in one patient, but neither Siegler nor Sciarra reported any in their two series.[11,12]

Postmenopausal bleeding (51 patients) revealed that endometrial hyperplasia was less common than atrophy (55%). Endometrial adenocarcinoma was seen in 8%; polyps, myomas, and vascular abnormalities were found in 37% of patients.

Abnormal uterine bleeding is frequently encountered in gynecologic practice, with the underlying possibility of cancer, particularly in the postmenopausal patient. Often these patients require a hysterography and fractional

(Text continues on p. 68)

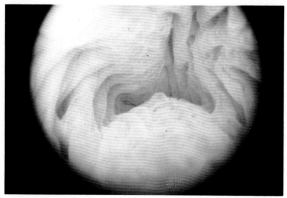

FIG. 13-2. Endocervical canal is entered under visual control.

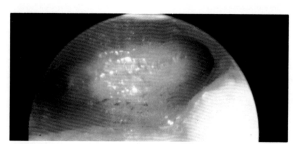

FIG. 13-3. Normal uterine cavity.

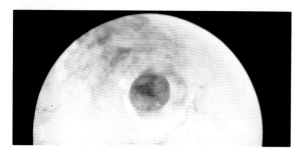

FIG. 13-4. Intramural segment.

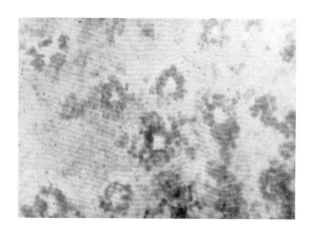

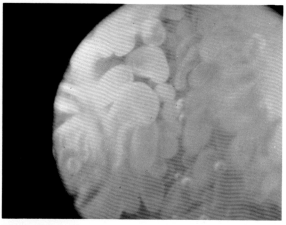

FIG. 13-6. Cervical canal shows glandular and papillary structures. (Original magnification ×20)

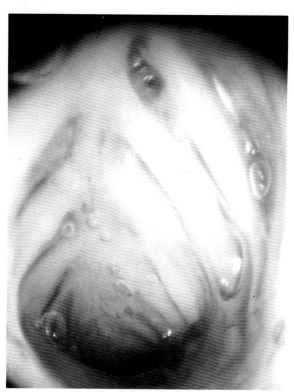

FIG. 13-7. Cervical canal reveals atrophic glandular structure. (Original magnification ×20)

FIG. 13-5. Endometrium reveals glandular openings surrounded by cells stained in methylene blue 1%. (Original magnification ×150)

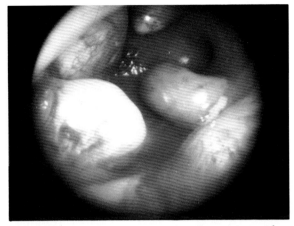

FIG. 13-8.   Polyps are present in the cavity with a submucous myoma.

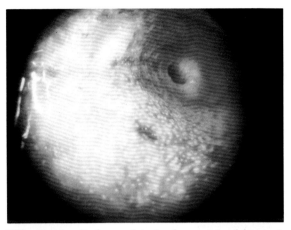

FIG. 13-11.   Endometritis is characterized by periglandular congestion.

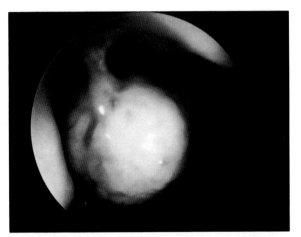

FIG. 13-9.   Pedunculated submucous myoma.

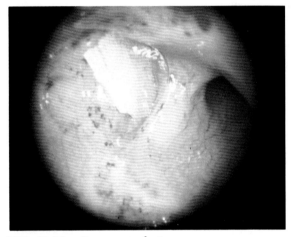

FIG. 13-12.   Bone metaplasia.

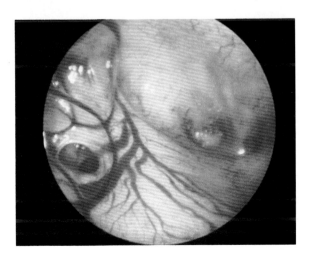

FIG. 13-10.   Abnormal and superficial endometrial vascularization.

Table 13-2

HYSTEROSCOPIC FINDINGS IN PATIENTS WITH PREMENOPAUSAL ABNORMAL UTERINE BLEEDING

FINDING	HAMOU AND SALAT-BAROUX (164 PATIENTS)	SIEGLER AND COLLEAGUES[12] (36 PATIENTS)	SCIARRA AND VALLE[11] (104 PATIENTS)
Normal cavity	9	15	30
Polyps	15	10	42
Submucous myomas	49	6	18
Hyperplasia	39		4
Atrophy	24		
Vascular dystrophy	12		
Adenomyosis	3		
Synechiae	0	1	2
Adenocarcinoma	1	0	0
Uterine septum	0	1	4
Cesarean section scar	2		4
Endometritis	10		

curettage. Office hysteroscopy can negate the need for hospitalization in many instances, and it offers the possibility of directed biopsy. During bleeding, hysterography is contraindicated and endometrial smears are not reliable. Microhysteroscopy can explain the bleeding by locating its source and thus enable the physician to make a diagnosis.

Sixty-two women with unexplained infertility underwent microhysteroscopy. In six instances severe vascular abnormalities made the endometrium unfit for nidation (Fig. 13-10). Acute endometritis (Fig. 13-11) with severe periglandular congestion and suspicious secretions was found in three patients. Nonspecific chronic infection with formations near the horns was seen in two women; bone metaplasia and cartilage (Fig. 13-12) was found in one patient. The findings of microhysteroscopy explained the reasons for infertility in 20% of patients with previously unknown causes. Further experience and more observation with high magnification may disclose additional significant factors. Thirty-nine infertile patients were referred to us because of an abnormal hysterogram. The diagnosis of polyps and submucous myomas was made in 22 instances; treatment depended on intrauterine location.

The high percentage of discrepancies between hysterographic and histologic findings has been described by Sweeney in a study of 218 patients.[15] Histologic examination did not confirm hysterographic results in 55% of patients. Other investigators comparing hysterosalpingography to hysteroscopy found similar rates of discrepancy.[3,8,10]

Hysteroscopy is preferred for detection of intrauterine abnormalities because of some of the shortcomings of hysterosalpingography, such as the need for an iodinated, liquid medium that may "wash" the cavity and can cause infections, dissemination of neoplastic cells, and allergic reactions. Roentgenograms have adverse effects, and repeated examinations are of limited value. Direct observation and magnification $\times 20$ can provide valuable data and locate glandular structures, infectious processes, vascular patterns, and dysplastic or precancerous endometrial lesions. It offers to the gynecologist an area heretofore not accessible by other investigation. Since most intrauterine abnormalities are poorly echogenic, microhysteroscopy can be very helpful in locating retained products of conception.

Comparison between hysterosalpingograms and hysteroscopy in 144 patients showed that hysterosalpingograms were often misinterpreted (Table 13-3). The correlation with regard to polyps or submucous myomas was good, showing agreement in 75%. It was less reliable for synechiae in that the x-ray shadow usually led the physician to overestimate the lesion. Hysterography could not detect either endometrial hyperplasia or atrophy.

In eight patients in whom proximal obstruction was reported, hysteroscopy with or without the help of intramural catheterization (3 on the Charrière scale) revealed spasm. Postoperatively, hysteroscopy was performed in removal of catheters (Fig. 13-13), for tubal implantation by microsurgery in eight patients and after a Bret–Palmer procedure (septal re-

Table 13-3

CORRELATION OF HYSTEROSCOPIC AND HYSTEROSALPINGOGRAPHIC FINDINGS

ABNORMALITY	POLYPS, SUBMUCOUS MYOMAS Chapter authors	ATROPHY, HYPERPLASIA Chapter authors	SYNECHIAE Chapter authors	Porto[10]	Edstrôm and Fernstrôm[3]	March et al[8]
No. of patients	64	53	27	134	30	39
Confirmation of hysterography (%)	75	52	62	70	53	63
Rectification (%)	11	16	27	30	47	27
Complete discordance (%)	14	32	11			10

moval) in one patient. Hysteroscopy was used to view the uterus two months postoperatively in four women who had had complicated cesarean sections.

Salpingoscopy (Fig. 13-14) is also an application for the new endoscope, and we have performed it seven times during laparotomy before tubal microsurgery for infertility. The gas flow is set at 10 ml/min and between 40 mm Hg and 50 mm Hg. The hysteroscope is carefully inserted into the distal tubal opening and slowly advanced under vision without touching the mucosa. The tube is explored from the ampulla to the ampulloisthmic junction. In four patients who had distal tubal obstruction, the endosalpinx and folds were altered, patches of fibrosis were observed, and some intratubal adhesions were freed under contact vision. These procedures were done after the salpingostomy was completed. In the three other patients, normal primary and secondary folds structures with normal vascularity were seen.

Microhysteroscopy will allow reevaluation of the pathogenesis, diagnosis, management, and follow-up study of intrauterine synechiae. Our results on the extension and age of synechiae are shown in Table 13-4. The generally recognized hypothesis of their cause, documented by Musset and Netter, has been observed and confirmed in our previous study (see Chap. 51).[9] It implicates myometrial adhesions subsequent to trauma by postpregnancy curettage. Sequential hysteroscopy in some patients shows residual formations, which will be vascularized and then organized into bridgelike synechiae (Fig. 13-15). Hysteroscopy will confirm their topography and extension, but high magnification may reveal the histologic nature (endometrial, fibrous, or myometrial) of the adhesion. Treatment immediately follows the diagnosis. The use of $\times 20$ and $\times 60$ magnifica-

(Text continues on p. 72)

Table 13-4

RESULTS OF HYSTEROSCOPY IN 27 PATIENTS WITH PRESUMPTIVE DIAGNOSIS OF SYNECHIAE

SYNECHIAE	NO. OF PATIENTS	ADHESIOLYSIS Complete	Under General Anesthesia and Laparoscopy	Normal Menstruation	FERTILITY Pregnancies Desired	Pregnancies Obtained	Delivered at Term
Isthmic	6	5	1	5	4	4	2
Marginal	7	6	1	7	5	3	2
Central	10	10	0	9	6	4	4
Severe or total	4	1	3	2	3	1	1
Total	27	22	5	23	18	12	9
Percentage				85			50

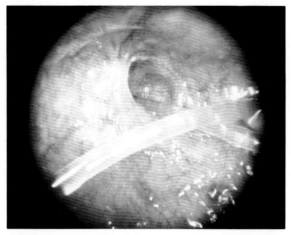

FIG. 13-13. Tubal splint coming from tubal ostium before removal 8 days after tubal microsurgery.

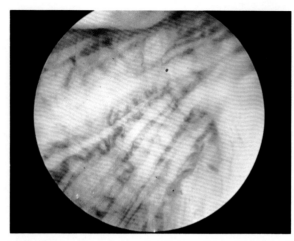

FIG. 13-14. Normal endosalpinx shows folds and vascularization on salpingocopy.

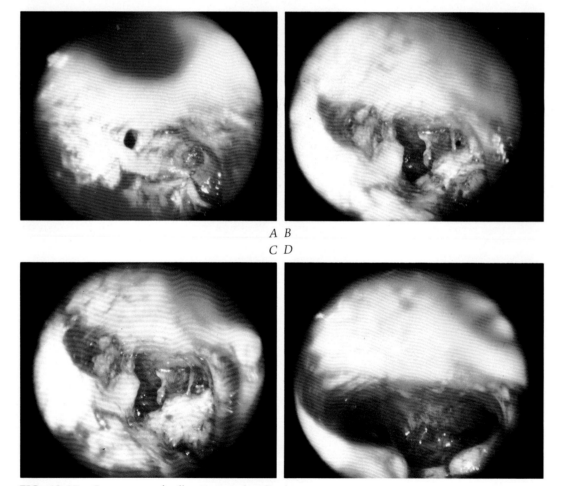

A B
C D

FIG. 13-15. Sequences of adhesiotomy by dissection with the distal sharp end of the microhysteroscope.

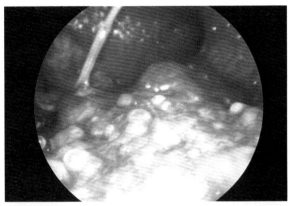

FIG. 13-16. Follow-up examination on the 15th postevacuation day of a molar pregnancy shows residual vesicles.

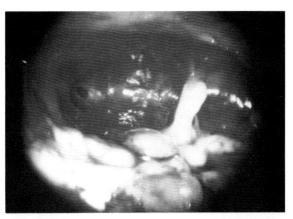

FIG. 13-19. Uterine cavity seen at 15 days after curettage of an uncomplicated first-trimester elective abortion.

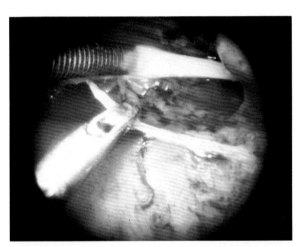

FIG. 13-17. Removal of a lost IUD is possible.

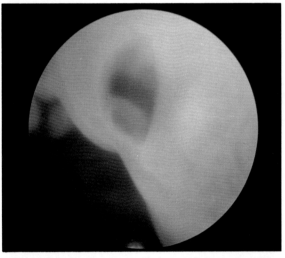

FIG. 13-20. Embryoscopy of an embryo at 6 weeks shows the eye in detail. (Original magnification ×20)

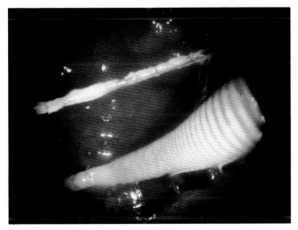

FIG. 13-18. Altered IUD with calcium carbonate deposit.

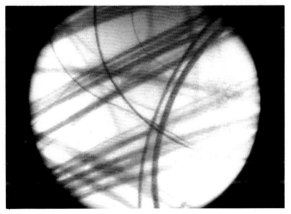

FIG. 13-21. Amnioscopy shows hair of fetus.

Table 13-5
HYSTEROSCOPIC FINDINGS AFTER PREGNANCY IN 40 PATIENTS

HYSTEROSCOPIC FINDINGS	TYPE OF PREGNANCY			
	Elective Abortion	Spontaneous Abortion	Postmolar Pregnancy	Postpartum
Normal		3	1	2
Moderate residual formation	9	6	1	
Important residual formation	8	2		
Endometritis	2			
Atrophy	4	1		1
Total	23	12	2	3

tion helps locate the least vascular zone of connective tissue. With the sharp distal edge of the hysteroscope, microsurgical resection is done under contact microscopy at ×60 magnification until a satisfactory cavity is obtained (Fig. 13-15). This procedure causes minimal bleeding or discomfort, since it deals with poorly vascularized and innervated tissue, and a control hysterogram is not needed.

In five patients with extensive, fibrous, old, or marginal synechiae, adhesiolysis was performed under general anesthesia and with laparoscopy. The aim in synechiectomy is to restore normal menses; this was achieved in 23 patients (85%). The results are comparable to those reported by Sugimoto and by March and colleagues.[8,14] Eighteen women wished to conceive; 12 did, and 9 had term deliveries (50%). This result remains disappointing, but it constitutes progress when compared to the results with conventional hysteroscopy (Sugimoto, 41%; March, 26%).[8,14] Microhysteroscopy does not traumatize the adjacent endometrium and allows more careful dissection. Patients received a sequential cyclic treatment for 2 months of 100 μg of ethinyl estradiol and 100 μg of mestranol. When adhesions were extensive or located in the isthmus, an intrauterine device (IUD) (Lippes loop) was inserted (10 patients). A previous study showed that IUDs were unnecessary in milder cases. Monthly hysteroscopies were done until the cavity appeared normal.

Hysteroscopy was performed in 18 patients who complained of pelvic pain, but no intrauterine cause was found. Hysteroscopy was done on six women with amenorrhea, of whom three were postabortal; isthmic synechiae without any intracavitary adhesions were detected. In one instance, 2 mo after an elective abortion, hematometra was found. In two patients, atrophic endometrium suggested premature menopause. In one patient, no cause was found. Uterine malformations were discovered in five patients, and the findings on hysteroscopy influenced the surgical treatment. Three patients who had had curettage for hydatidiform mole had a monthly hysteroscopy and human chorionic gonadotropin (hCG) assays. In two instances, the cavities returned to normal within 2 mo; one patient showed vesicles (Fig. 13-16) and was scheduled for chemotherapy.

Misplaced IUDs were located and retrieved in 20 patients by hysteroscopy; 7 women decided to retain them. When the occult filament is visible, it can be caught by a 1-mm forceps passed through an operative sheath (Fig. 13-17). Copper alterations, calcification (Fig. 13-18), and adjacent endometrial changes can be followed.

In afebrile patients complaining of postabortal moderate bleeding (40 patients), hysteroscopy can show a normal cavity, negating the need for curettage and avoiding the potential for subsequent synechiae (Table 13-5). Postabortal curettage can be dangerous when atrophy or endometritis is present, and most decidual elements will be spontaneously resorbed or shed within 1 cycle, as has been reported in a previous study concerning 151 patients who underwent postabortal hysteroscopies (see Chap. 51) (Fig. 13-19). Echography is reliable only if the vacuity line is clearly identified. Embryoscopy was done in three instances before elective abortion (Fig. 13-20). Magnification ×20 locates a small portion of clear amnion, which is used as a window to focus on the embryo. The technique is easy, and the risk to the amnion is minimal. Since it is not possible to avoid light on the retina, the procedure has limited indications. However, this technique is recommended for near-term pregnant women as an alternative to amnioscopy (Fig. 13-21).

Microcolpohysteroscopy can be performed alone or as the last step in hysteroscopy. To proceed, clean the cervix with saline to remove cellular debris, mucus, and secretions. Apply cotton balls soaked with Lugol's iodine solution, 2%. Perform a colposcopic examination at ×20 magnification. Use Waterman blue at pH 5 to stain the nuclei and cytoplasm of the squamous epithelium. This dye will not stain columnar epithelium because of the mucus in the cells. Start observing promptly. After a prior scanning with ×60 magnification and evaluation of glandular and epithelial structures, localize the squamocolumnar junction and the transformation zone. Perform the second step at ×150 magnification to detail nucleocytoplasmic structures. The major step is the screening of the transformation zone by a simple, complete rotation of the instrument. This zone is vital, since any cervical neoplasia begins here. After each procedure, record results on a special form to facilitate the collection of data with this new technique.

Microhysteroscopy introduces an important, intermediate step in cytology, colposcopy, and histology. The squamocolumnar junction will always be located, living cells can be seen in their anatomic context, biopsy will be directed precisely on the "epicenter," and effective, conservative management can be performed and diagnostic conization and unnecessary hysterectomy thus abandoned. This technique will be largely applied only if the cervical cellular aspects are accessible to the clinician who is not a cytologist or pathologist. Experience with several thousands of microhysteroscopies indicates this possibility. The cellular aspects on the cervix are limited and concern only superficial layers. There is no spatial reconstitution of cellular disposition.

Microcolpohysteroscopy is the most recent and probably the most important application of this instrument. It will enable the clinician to perform, during the same simple, quick, atraumatic procedure, a colposcopic (×20 magnification), cytologic (×60 magnification), and histologic (×150 magnification) study. After a macroscopic examination of cervical mucosa and localization of a suspicious area, the clinician can proceed to a microscopic, cellular observation *in vivo*. Until now, effective magnification above ×10 (colposcopy) was not possible.[5]

NORMAL ASPECTS

After vital staining with Lugol's iodine solution, 2%, and Waterman blue at pH 5, the squamous epithelium shows a very regular arrangement of the pyknotic cells (Fig. 13-22) when there is good endogenous estrogen. As in cytologic examination, intermediary or younger cells are found in accordance with hormonal status or infection. The transformation zone (Fig. 13-23) shows a regular transition of superficial, intermediary, and parabasal cells. The squamocolumnar junction appears clearly as a blue tract. A complete scanning of this area is done by full rotation of the instrument; all dysplasias begin in this zone. The columnar epithelium (Fig. 13-24) covers the endocervix and the ectopia. It appears with its characteristic glandular and papillary structure; its cellular layer and the mucus load of the apical pole can also be seen. This unicellular layer is transparent, making it possible to see the terminal capillary vascularization and the circulating red blood cells (RBCs) (Fig. 13-25).

PATHOLOGIC ASPECTS

After reviewing more than 200 patients with abnormal cytologic findings, we consider the following criteria pathologic for microhysteroscopy (Fig. 13-26):

Irregular arrangement of superficial cells
Anisonucleosis
Dyskaryosis with asynchronic nucleocytoplasmic maturation

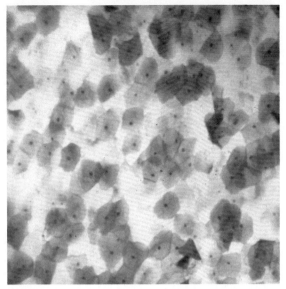

FIG. 13-22. Normal squamous cells are stained and examined *in vivo*.

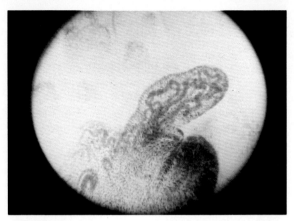

FIG. 13-24. Columnar epithelium overlies a papillary projection.

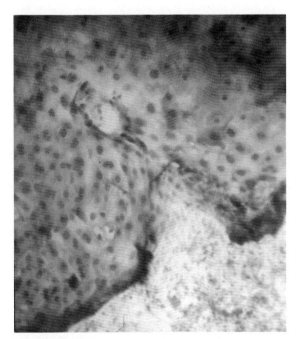

FIG. 13-23. The transitional zone is clearly demarcated after proper staining.

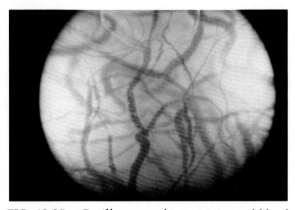

FIG. 13-25. Capillary vessels containing red blood cells (RBCs).

Mitotic activity
Dyschromia
Koilocytosis (ballooned cells; (Fig. 13-27)
Severe nuclear abnormalities (shape, size)

In our study, four grades were defined:

Grade 0 (G0) if no abormality is detected

Grade 1 (G1) if leukoplakia, punctation, or one abnormality is noted with exclusion of the two last ones
Grade 1⁺ (G1⁺) if koilocytes are present whether or not associated to last one
Grade 2 (G2) when the last criterion is noted or the others are not present

The first 27 patients were referred to us with smears of class III or worse. During this comparative study it became clear that the features revealed by microhysteroscopy would complement those offered by colposcopy, cytology, and histology (Table 13-6). Microhysteroscopy will naturally show the exact topography of the lesion. It can distinguish within the same lesion a gradation of aspects ranging from dystrophy to dysplasia. The most advanced lesion is considered the "epicenter." A directed biopsy on the epicenter becomes feasi-

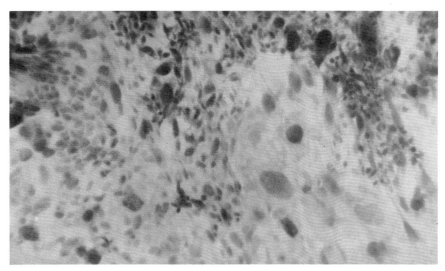

FIG. 13-26. Atypical cells are characteristic of carcinoma *in situ in vivo.*

FIG. 13-27. Balloon cells are typical of condyloma seen *in vivo.*

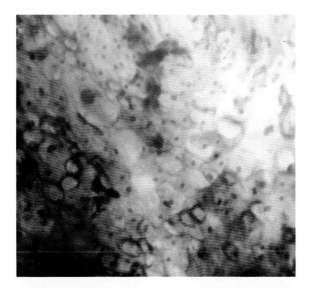

ble. Microhysteroscopy can locate the squamo-columnar junction or upper border of the neoplasm even if it ascends into the endocervix, as it did in 12 patients. A group of 293 patients had a screening microhysteroscopy before a Papanicolaou (Pap) smear, and the results appear in Table 13-7.

No patients with grades G0 or G1 had neoplasia, but two patients had condylomas. Grade 1 patients must be carefully followed in a prospective study. All patients with grade G1+ showed cytologic evidence of condylomas (see Fig. 13-27), and one patient showed moderate dysplasia. Four patients were graded G2. This small series reveals the same difficulties with cytology, namely, in distinguishing clearly severe dysplasia, condyloma, and carcinoma *in situ.* The more significant feature is that the only patient in this series with carcinoma *in situ* was grade G2.

Fig. 13-28 on the following page.

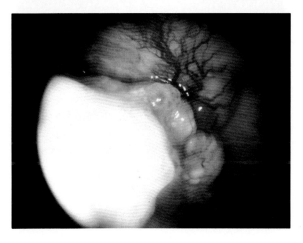

FIG. 13-29. Endometrial adenocarcinoma at an early stage.

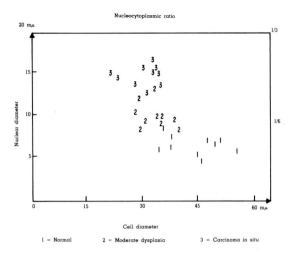

Nucleocytoplasmic ratio

FIG. 13-28. Nuclear–cytoplasmic ratio on colpomicrohysteroscopy.

1 = Normal   2 = Moderate dysplasia   3 = Carcinoma *in situ*

Because of the limited normal and pathologic aspects and criteria offered by microhysteroscopy, a tentative study was designed to measure by a simple planimetric technique the mean size of the ten most representative cells in each microhysterophotograph in ten patients with a normal cervix, ten with moderate dysplasia, and ten with carcinoma *in situ*. Three main areas were located in relation to normality, moderate dysplasia, and carcinoma *in situ*. Mean cellular size could not constitute a reliable criterion, since the three zones sometimes overlap (Fig. 13-28). The nucleocytoplasmic ratios are more reliable, but they still can show slight overlap and cause misinterpretation. The mean nuclear size of the superficial layer shows very distinct areas between normal and pathologic and therefore constitutes a significant criterion for microhysteroscopy. When mean nuclear diameter is over 15 μm, the lesion is G2. The clinician must refer to histologic studies for the definite diagnosis. Only a prospective, randomized, multicentric, ongoing study can assess the value of microhysteroscopy for screening cervical intraepithelial neoplasia.

Microhysteroscopic histology is more significant than microhysteroscopy and cytology or cytology and histology. We obtained no false-negative results with microhysteroscopy thus far. Four patients had carcinoma *in situ* and a junction out of colposcopic range. Normally they might have been scheduled for diagnostic blind conization or hysterectomy, but 3 of them were under 32 years of age and wished to maintain their child-bearing capacity. Directed, therapeutic, limited conization was possible. An appropriate therapeutic conization is more likely, and the new transformation zone can be followed by microhysteroscopy. Approximately half the cases of carcinoma *in situ* involve the endocervix. Townsend and colleagues specified 65.7%; other estimates range from 40.8% to 62.9% and are out of range of colposcopy.[16] "Blind" diagnostic conization should no longer be performed and should be replaced by controlled, limited conization, made possible with microhysteroscopy. The results for these 27 patients are tabulated in Table 13-6.

Symptomatic endometrial adenocarcinoma (four patients) is of limited interest for physicians using microhysteroscopy. Hysteroscopy can give the topography and assess any extention into the endocervix. On the contrary, microhysteroscopic screening for precancerous lesions or preclinical adenocarcinoma is a promising approach, as in cervical neoplasia. Retrospective and prospective studies have assessed the permanence of dystrophic or dysplastic aspects of the endometrium before adenocarcinoma, and these aspects may constitute precancerous or border lesions.[2,4] This atraumatic technique should initially be performed only on high-risk patients (*e.g.*, obese, hypertensive, diabetic, or receiving estrogen therapy). Of 52 such patients who had a screening microhysteroscopy, 2 preclinical adenocarcinomas (Fig. 13-29) were isolated and confirmed by directed biopsy.

Table 13-6

RESULTS OF HYSTEROSCOPY IN 27 PATIENTS WITH ABNORMAL PAP SMEARS; CORRELATION OF FIVE MAIN PARAMETERS (CYTOLOGY, COLPOSCOPY, HISTOLOGY, MICROHYSTEROSCOPY, AND THERAPEUTIC)

HISTOLOGIC EXAMINATION	NO. OF PATIENTS	MICROHYSTEROSCOPY			
		Grade 0	Grade 1	Grade 1+	Grade 2
Normal	5	2F	2F 1F		
Moderate dysplasia	6		1ER 2F	2F 1C	
Severe dysplasia and carcinoma *in situ*	16			2C 1L	3C 4L 4C 2H
Invasive	0				0

* F, follow-up study; ER, electroresection; C, conization; H, hysteroscopy; L, laser; ☐, junction not seen colposcopically.

Table 13-7

RESULTS OF SCREENING MICROHYSTEROSCOPY IN 293 PATIENTS

CYTOLOGIC PLUS HISTOLOGIC EXAMINATION	MICROCOLPOHYSTEROSCOPY			
	Grade 0	Grade 1	Grade 1+	Grade 2
Normal	267	16		1
Condylomas	1	1	3	2
Moderate dysplasia			1	
Carcinoma *in situ*				1

REFERENCES

1. Beutler HK, Decherty MA, Ranall, LM: Precancerous lesions of the endometrium. Am J Obstet Gynecol 86:433, 1963
2. De Brux J: Histopathologie Gynécologique. Paris, Masson, 1971
3. Edström K, Fernström I: The diagnostic possibilities of a modified hysteroscopic technique. Acta Obstet Gynecol Scand 49:327, 1970
4. Gusberg SB: Endometrial cancer. Int Surg Dig 76:497, 1976
5. Hamou J: Microhysteroscopy. A new procedure and its original application in gynecology. J Reprod Med 26:375, 1981
6. Hamou J: Hysteroscopy and microhysteroscopy with a new instrument: The microhysteroscope. Acta Eur Fertil 12:29, 1981
7. Lindemann HJ: The use of CO_2 in the uterine cavity for hysteroscopy. Int J Fertil 17:221, 1972
8. March CM, Israel R, March AD: Hysteroscopic management of intrauterine adhesions. Am J Obstet Gynecol 130:653, 1978
9. Musset R, Netter A: Traitement des synéchies utérines. Encycl Méd-Chirurgie 140:A10, 1972
10. Porto R: Correlation hystérographiques et hystéroscopiques. Faculté de Médecine Broussais, Paris, June 15, 1974
11. Sciarra JJ, Valle RF: Hysteroscopy: A clinical experience with 320 patients. Am J Obstet Gynecol 127:340, 1977
12. Siegler AM, Kemman EK, Gentile GP: Hysteroscopic procedures in 257 patients. Fertil Steril 27:1267, 1976
13. Siegler AM: Hysterography and hysteroscopy in the infertile patient. J Reprod Med 18:143, 1977
14. Sugimoto O: Diagnostic and therapeutic hysteroscopy for traumatic intrauterine adhesions. Am J Obstet Gynecol 135:539, 1978
15. Sweeney WJ: Accuracy of preoperative hysterosalpingograms. Obstet Gynecol 11:640, 1958
16. Townsend DE, Ostergard DR, Mischell D Jr, et al: Abnormal Papanicolaou smears. Am J Obstet Gynecol 108:429, 1970
17. Valle RF: Hysteroscopy: Diagnostic and therapeutic applications. J Reprod Med 20:115, 1978

Uses of the Hamou Microcolpohysteroscope in Clinical Practice ■ 14

Philip G. Brooks
Stephen L. Corson
Duane E. Townsend

Interest in hysteroscopy has intensified because of reports of unsuspected uterine abnormalities, some missed by curettage.[2,4] In addition, new evidence shows that dilatation and curettage causes more cervical damage than previously believed.[3] Finally, the Hamou microcolpohysteroscope has features that increase the use of and indications for hysteroscopy.[1] This chapter will discuss the uses of the Hamou microcolpohysteroscope in clinical practice.

MATERIALS AND METHODS

The characteristics of the microcolpohysteroscope have been described in Chapter 13. A cold light* is transmitted through a fiberoptic bundle. The xenon light is used for photography. We perform most hysteroscopic examinations in the office without anesthesia or a cervical cap, and cervical dilatation is rarely required. A Kidde carbon dioxide cartridge tubal insufflator is used to instill the carbon dioxide (Fig. 14-1A). The cost of the apparatus is far less than a Hysteroflator, and the small cartridges (Fig. 14-1B) of carbon dioxide cost about $0.55 each; 6 to 10 procedures can be performed with each cartridge. The rate of flow is between 30 ml/min and 90 ml/min and is adjustable. The insufflator delivers carbon dioxide at a maximal pressure of 200 mm Hg, controlled by the weight of a piston (Fig. 14-1C). At flow rates of 30 ml/min to 50 ml/min the intrauterine pressure is sufficient to distend the cavity but inadequate, in most cases, to open the tubal ostia. This results in minimal passage of carbon dioxide through the tubes. Only slight intraoperative discomfort results, with almost no postoperative shoulder pain, even in patients with patent tubes.

From March 1981 to December 1981 we used the microcolpohysteroscope in 88 patients. Initially we performed hysteroscopy in the operating room under general anesthesia. At present, it is almost exclusively an office procedure without anesthesia. Table 14-1 lists the indications for the procedure. Abnormal uterine bleeding was present in 44 patients (50%) and infertility or repeated abortions existed in 30 others. The 14 other operations were done to evaluate complications of intrauterine devices (IUDs), secondary amenorrhea, cervical neoplasia, and pelvic pain. Cervical and endocervical epithelia were stained, and cellular morphologic changes were observed at high magnification ($\times 150$).

* Storz Miniature Cold Light Fountain.

Table 14-1
RESULTS IN 88 PATIENTS WHO UNDERWENT HYSTEROSCOPY

Primary Indications	
Abnormal bleeding (premenopausal)	37
Menopausal bleeding	7
Infertility	16
Pregnancy wastage	14
IUD complications	
Lost or embedded IUD	3
Bleeding with IUD	1
Pregnant with IUD	1
Secondary amenorrhea	2
Pelvic pain	1
Anomaly associated with DES	2
Cervical neoplasia	3
Metastatic cancer, search for primary site	1

Table 14-2
FINDINGS OF ABNORMAL BLEEDING IN 37 PATIENTS*

Normal hysteroscopy	6
Endometrial polyps	17
Endometrial hyperplasia	4
Submucous myoma	4
Pedunculated myoma	3
Endocervicitis	2
Uterine anomaly	
DES	1
Rudimentary horn	1

* One patient had multiple causes of bleeding.

RESULTS

Hysteroscopy in 37 premenopausal women who had abnormal uterine bleeding revealed only 6 normal uterine cavities (Table 14-2). Endometrial polyps were found in 17 women, myomas in 7, endometrial hyperplasia in 4, endocervicitis in 2, and rudimentary horn and anomalies associated with diethylstilbestrol (DES) in 2. In the seven women who complained of perimenopausal bleeding, two patients had atrophic endometria and two had endometrial polyps; endometrial hyperplasia and endocervical carcinoma were discovered in

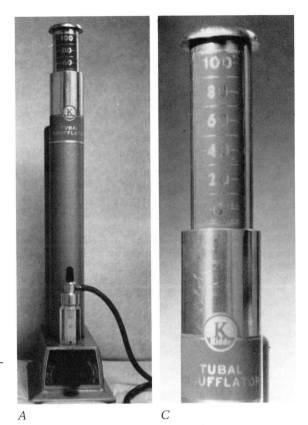

A   *C*

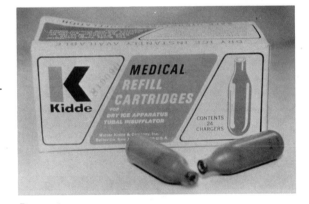

B

FIG. 14-1. (*A*) Kidde carbon dioxide cartridge tubal insufflator. (*B*) Carbon dioxide cartridges. (*C*) Weighted piston.

Table 14-3
FINDINGS OF MENOPAUSAL BLEEDING IN SEVEN PATIENTS

Normal hysteroscopy (atrophic)	2
Endometrial polyps	2
Endometrial hyperplasia	1
Endocervical carcinoma	1
Stenotic vagina (found cervix)	1

Table 14-4
FINDINGS OF INFERTILITY IN 16 PATIENTS*

Normal hysteroscopy	3
Endometrial polyps	7
Cornual obstruction	3
Endometrial hyperplasia	1
Synechiae	4
Submucous myoma	4
Uterine anomaly	3

* Eight patients had multiple causes of infertility.

Table 14-5
FINDINGS OF PREGNANCY WASTAGE IN 14 PATIENTS

Normal hysteroscopy	2
Uterine synechiae	4
Chronic endometritis	1
Endometrial polyps	1
Uterine deformity	
Septum	4
DES related	1
Myomas	1

two other women. In another patient, the hysteroscope helped to locate the cervical canal, which was obscured because of a severely stenotic upper vagina (Table 14-3).

Of the 16 infertile women, a normal cavity was identified only in 3 instances (Table 14-4). Endometrial polyps, synechiae, submucous myomas, and uterine anomalies were the most common abnormalities. Cornual obstructions were identified in three women. Eight of these patients had more than one defect. Fourteen patients underwent hysteroscopic examination

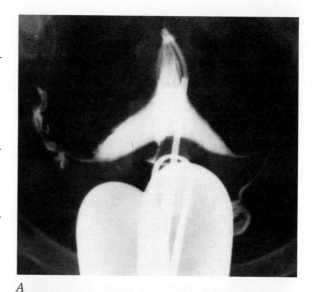

A

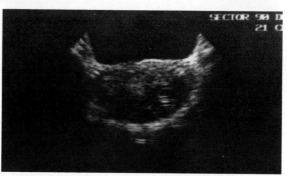

B

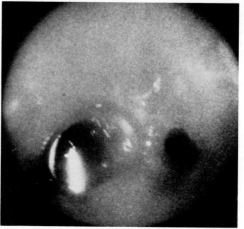

C

FIG. 14-2. Patient examined for synechiae. (*A*) Hysterogram shows a normal cavity. (*B*) Pelvic sonogram is suspicious for uterine defect. (*C*) Two uterine cavities and a wide septum are shown at hysteroscopy.

because of repeated abortions, and only two had normal cavities; synechiae and fundal septae were present in four others. Chronic endometritis, endometrial polyps, myoma, and a deformed cavity caused by exposure to DES *in utero* were found in four other women (Table 14-5).

Of the nine women who had synechiae discovered at hysteroscopy, only one had associated amenorrhea. Four had a history of postabortal curettage, three were asymptomatic, and four had infertility as their only symptom. One of the patients had a normal hysterogram (Fig. 14-2*A*) and a sonogram suggestive of an intrauterine defect (Fig. 14-2*B*). At hysteroscopy an unsuspected midline septum with two narrow horns was discovered (Fig. 14-2*C*).

There were no complications in these 88 procedures. When bleeding obscured the view, a soft 3-mm nasotracheal suction catheter was attached to a wall section or a syringe to remove blood and debris.

CONCLUSION

The microcolpohysteroscope has a double optical system and can function as a panoramic hysteroscope and a microcolposcope. It can be used in the office and in the operating room to evaluate the epithelial surfaces of the endocervix and endometrium. The high incidence of unsuspected abnormalities detected with this instrument suggests that hysteroscopy should be integrated into gynecologic examination.

REFERENCES

1. Hamou J: Microhysteroscopy. A new procedure and its original applications in gynecology. J Reprod Med 26:375, 1981
2. Taylor PJ, Cumming DC: Hysteroscopy in 100 patients. Fertil Steril 31:301, 1979
3. Taylor PJ, Graham G: Is diagnostic curettage harmful to women with unexplained infertility? Br J Obstet Gynecol 89:296, 1982
4. Valle RF: Hysteroscopy in the evaluation of female infertility. Am J Obstet Gynecol 137:425, 1980

Echoscopy and Microhysteroscopy for the Evaluation of Physiopathologic Endometrial Changes ■

15

Gianfranco Scarselli

Luca Mencaglia

Roberto Nannini

Francesco Branconi

Carlo Tantini

Luciano Savino

Elisabetta Chelo

Hamou's microcolpohysteroscope permits direct observation of histologic changes during the menstrual cycle and identifies intracavitary abnormalities (Fig. 15-1).[1,2] Diagnostic ultrasound is useful in evaluating the endometrium, which appears on the sonogram as a white phantom of the uterine cavity, clearly in contrast to the myometrial image in pictures taken at low gains. The endometrium is not identifiable by sonography in prepubertal girls, and, if seen, is always a sign of abnormal hormonal stimulation. During the reproductive age endometrial hyperplasia can be detected by the abnormally thick "phantom" relative to the uterine volume (Figs. 15-2 and 15-3). In postmenopausal women the endometrium is not normally seen on sonograms. Inasmuch as such women are at risk for endometrial carcinoma, the finding of either a homogeneous or an irregular endometrium calls for further investigation.

Hysteroscopy and microhysteroscopy provide definitive diagnoses by direct observation and by study of biopsy specimens taken under vision; abnormal areas of endometrium might be missed by curettage (Figs. 15-4 and 15-5). Moreover, some lesions can be treated during hysteroscopy, and needless curettage can thus be avoided. Hysteroscopy can also detect abnormalities not seen on sonograms.

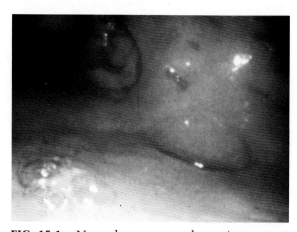

FIG. 15-1. Normal secretory endometrium.

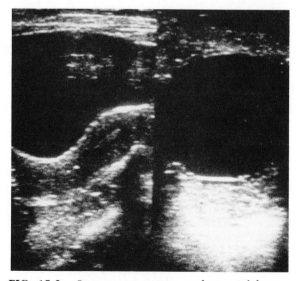

FIG. 15-2. Sonogram suggests endometrial hyperplasia associated with an ovarian cyst.

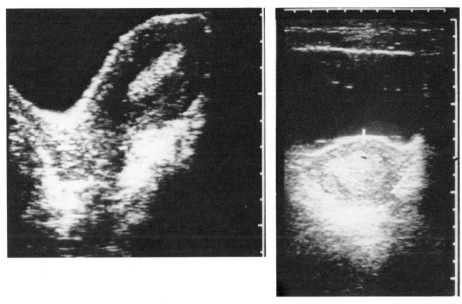

FIG. 15-3. Sonogram shows endometrial hyperplasia. (A) Longitudinal scan. (B) Transverse scan.

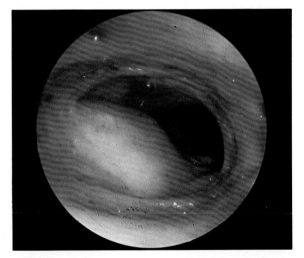

FIG. 15-4. Submucous myoma located in the lower uterine segment.

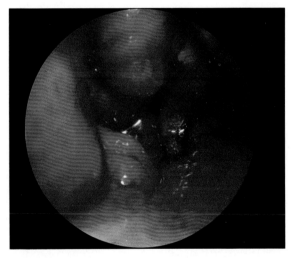

FIG. 15-5. Endometrial polypoid hyperplasia.

REFERENCES

1. Hamou J: Hystéroscopie et microhystéroscopie avec un instrument nouveau, le microhystéroscope. In Albano V, Cittadini F, Quartararo P (eds): Endoscopia Ginecologica, p 131. CoFeSe Palermo, Sicily, 1980
2. Scarselli G, Mencaglia L, Hamou J: Atlante de Microcolpoisteroscopia. CoFeSe Palermo, Sicily, 1981

Hysteromicroscopy ■

16

Kimiyasu Ohkawa
Ryoki Ohkawa

Attempts have been made with a special endomicroscope using high magnification to study cells *in vivo* without biopsy.[1,2,4–6] Ohkawa and Ohkawa reported that endomicroscopy makes it easy to discover cancer early and to delineate its extent in the uterine cavity with supravital staining of nuclei with cresyl violet acetate and thionin.[7,8] In 1981 Hamou reported clinical applications of a contact microhysteroscope.[3]

MATERIALS AND METHODS

Panendomicroscopes permit forward and lateral observation; the endomicroscope for forward observation has a lens provided at the tip, and the other has a lens provided at the lateral side of the top. Both scopes have an 8-mm diameter and are 360 mm long (Fig. 16-1). The contact microhysteroscope has a 4-mm diameter (Fig. 16-2). For photomicrography with a panendomicroscope, an Olympus OM2, an extension ring (83 mm), and adapter were used. Images on the film are magnified ×190; images on the paper, ×671. Consequently, atypical cells are easily distinguished from normal

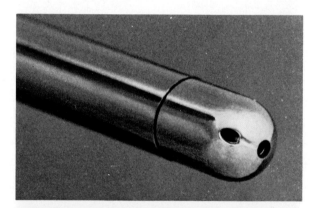
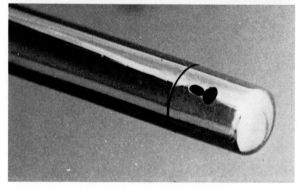

FIG. 16-1. Miniature panendomicroscope has forward (*A*) and lateral (*B*) observation tips.

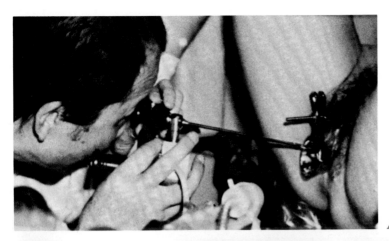

FIG. 16-2. The contact microhysteroscope has a 4-mm diameter and can magnify. (A) Observations being made through the microhysteroscope. (B) Original magnification ×20. (C) Original magnification ×50. (D) Original magnification ×150.

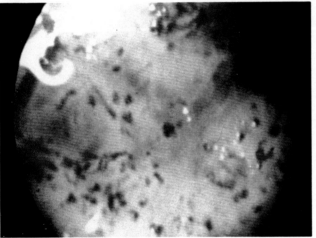

B

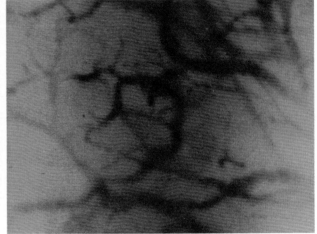

C

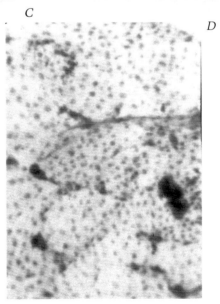

D

ones. For photomicrography of contact microhysteroscope, one converter (×2), an adapter (zoom 170), and an Olympus OM2 are used. Images on the film are magnified ×74 and ×212 on the paper. When an Olympus OM2 and adapter (zoom 170) are used (Fig. 16-3), images on the film become magnified ×30 and atypical vessels are clearly seen.

In supravital staining, the nuclei of living cells are stained. The staining of deoxyribonucleic acid (DNA) is essential to the technique of endomicroscopy. Dyes having an affinity for DNA should be used. For this purpose, cresyl violet acetate and thionin should be used.

The staining solution is made by combining 8 ml of a saturated solution of cresyl violet acetate in 50% ethanol with 2 ml of a saturated

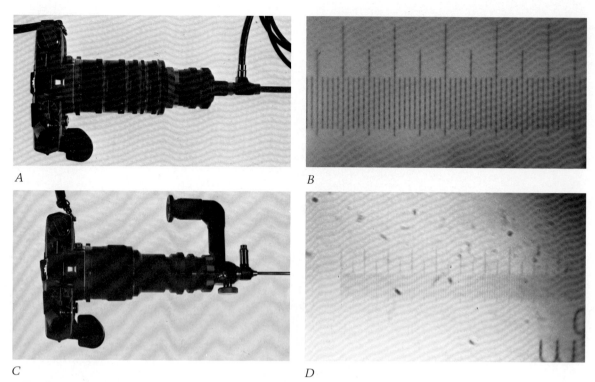

A   *B*

C   *D*

FIG. 16-3.   Photomicrography by panendomicroscopy Olympus OM2 adapter exten-sion ring (82 mm). (*A*) Original magnification ×190 on film. (*B*) Original magnification ×671 on paper (interval 10 μm). (*C*) Photography by contact microhysteroscopy Olympus OM2 adapter lens (zoom 170); original magnification ×30. (*D*) Photography by contact microhysteroscopy Olympus OM2 converter and adapter lenses (zoom 170); original magnification ×74 on film and ×212 on paper.

solution of thionin in 50% ethanol and 90 ml of distilled water. The solution is passed through a millipore filter for sterilization. The toxicity of this solution is very low: lethal dose ×50 of this solution in a mouse is 83 ml/kg. For hysteromicroscopy, the cervical canal is di-lated using Laminaria and the dye solution is infused into the uterine cavity through a poly-ethylene tube.

RESULTS

NORMAL

The nuclei in both the proliferative and secre-tory phases are uniformly small, and the ar-rangement of cells is regular (Fig. 16-4). No di-lated vessels are observed.

Table 16-1
ENDOMICROSCOPIC AND HISTOLOGIC FINDINGS IN ENDOCERVIX COMPARED IN 244 PATIENTS

MICROENDOSCOPY	HISTOLOGY			
	Normal	Metaplasia	Dysplasia	Cancer
Normal	125	52	0	0
Atypical epithelium I	0	24	10	0
Atypical epithelium II	0	0	22	11

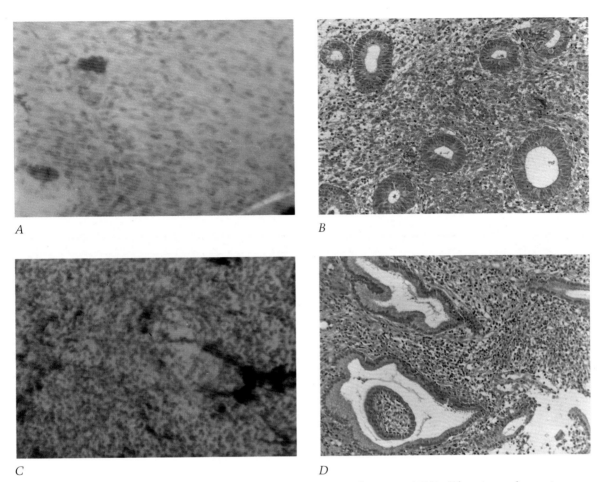

FIG. 16-4. Proliferative and secretory endometria. (A) Proliferative endometrium seen at hysteroscopy. (B) Proliferative phase. (C) Secretory endometrium seen at hysteroscopy. (D) Secretory phase.

ENDOMETRIAL HYPERPLASIA

Using hysteroscopy, we observed polypoid proliferation of the endometrium in patients with endometrial hyperplasia. Using the endomicroscope (×190 on the film), we observed dilated blood vessels (Figs. 16-5 and 16-6). Nuclei of endometrial cells show enlargement but no atypia. A more severe form of endometrial hyperplasia shows enlarged nuclei and papillary changes in the glands (Fig. 16-7).

ENDOMETRIAL CANCER

Endometrial cancer was found in the right side of the uterine cavity. With the endomicroscope at the position of the cancer, nuclei were large and irregular (Fig. 16-8). The contact microhysteroscope shows an atypical vascular pattern in endometrial carcinoma (Fig. 16-9). On endomicroscopy, atypical nuclei are irregular in size and shape (Fig. 16-10).

Of 113 women who had endometrial evaluation, 23 had histologic evidence of adenocarcinoma. Microendoscopy suggested the disease in 21 of these instances because of atypical type II cells, but in one case, only hyperplasia was suspected, and in another, only type I cells were seen. In one instance, an adenocarcinoma was suggested by abnormal findings on microendoscopy, but a biopsy specimen revealed only hyperplasia. The remaining patients showed a good correlation between histologic and microendoscopic findings (Table 16-1).

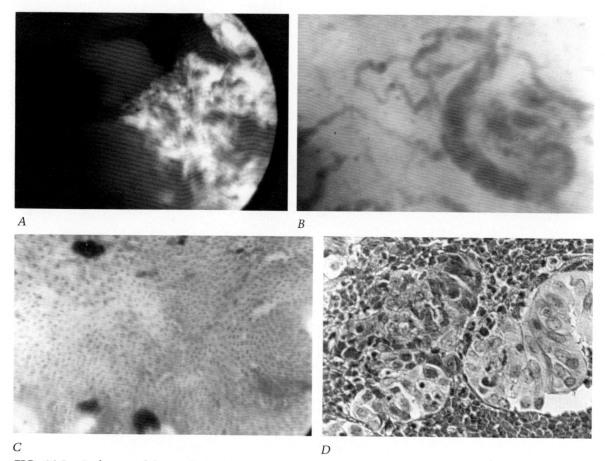

A

B

C

D

FIG. 16-5. Endometrial hyperplasia. (*A*) Gross appearance during hysteroscopy. (*B*) Atypical vessels. (Original magnification ×190) (*C*) Hysteromicroscopy. (Original magnification ×190) (*D*) Endometrial hyperplasia present histologically.

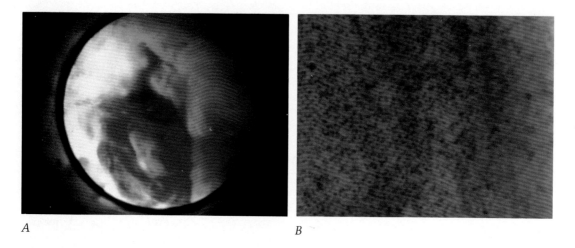

A

B

FIG. 16-6. (*continued facing page*)

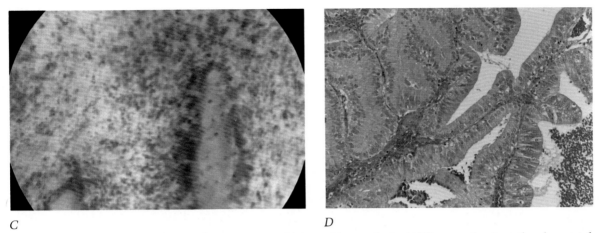

C

D

FIG. 16-6. Adenomatous endometrial hyperplasia. (*A*) Panoramic view of endometrial hyperplasia. (*B*) Contact microhysteroscope shows same area. (Original magnification ×74) (*C*) Endomicroscopy shows nonmalignant appearance. (*D*) Histology reveals endometrial hyperplasia.

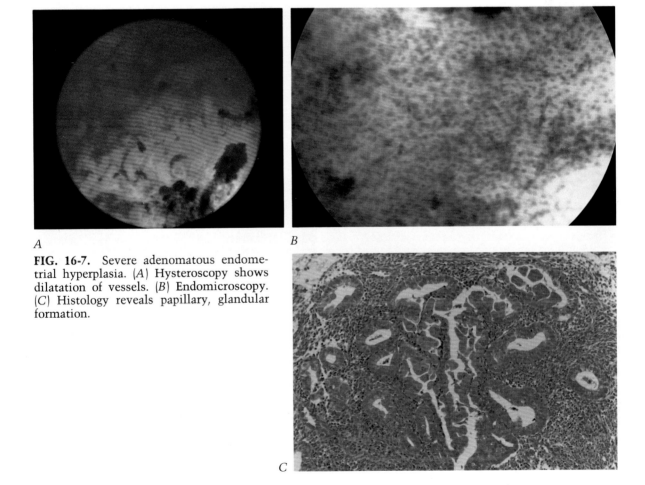

A

B

FIG. 16-7. Severe adenomatous endometrial hyperplasia. (*A*) Hysteroscopy shows dilatation of vessels. (*B*) Endomicroscopy. (*C*) Histology reveals papillary, glandular formation.

C

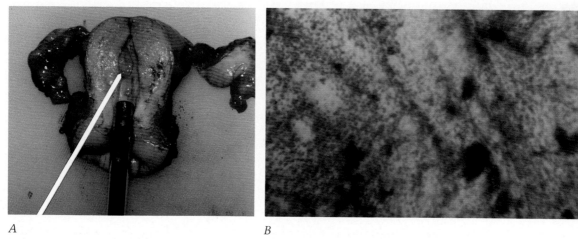

FIG. 16-8. Endometrial adenocarcinoma. (*A*) Tumor appears at right side of uterine cavity. (*B*) Endomicroscopy of endocervix is within normal limits.

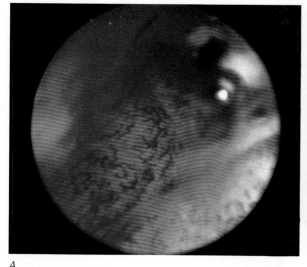

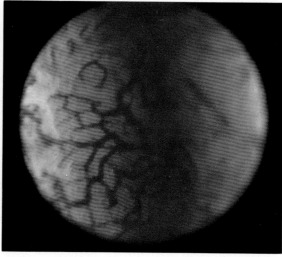

FIG. 16-9. Atypical vessels are relatively specific for malignant change. Area with atypical vessels must be examined by endomicroscopy. (*A*) Original magnification ×12. (*B*) Original magnification ×30.

CHORIOCARCINOMA

In patients with choriocarcinoma, hysteroscopic examination revealed polypoid protuberance and white, necrotic, hemorrhagic areas, but no atypical vessels. Cresyl violet acetate staining shows large and irregular nuclei (Fig. 16-11).

CHORIOADENOMA DESTRUENS

The findings in patients with chorioadenoma destruens are almost similar to those in choriocarcinoma (Fig. 16-12).

ENDOCERVICAL DYSPLASIA

In patients with endocervical dysplasia, atypical capillaries were observed along the endocervical canal 2 cm up from the external os

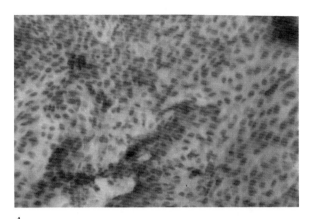

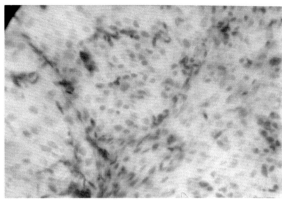

A   *B*

FIG. 16-10. Endometrial adenocarcinoma. (*A*) Endomicroscopy. (*B*) Atypical nuclei are seen. (*C*) Adenocarcinoma was confirmed on histology.

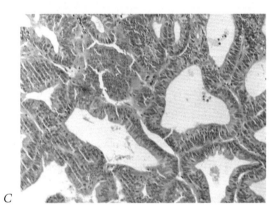

C

Table 16-2
ENDOMICROSCOPIC AND HISTOLOGIC FINDINGS IN ENDOMETRIUM COMPARED IN 113 PATIENTS

MICROENDOSCOPY	HISTOLOGY		
	Normal	Hyperplasia	Adenocarcinoma
Normal	50	15	0
Hyperplasia	0	12	1
Atypical I	0	12	1
cells II	0	1	21

(Fig. 16-13). The endomicroscope (lateral-observation type) revealed the extent of dysplasia after the nuclei were stained (Fig. 16-14).

Eleven patients who had histologic evidence of squamous cell carcinoma of the cervix were also identified by microendoscopy. On histology, 177 women had either normal or metaplastic squamous epithelium, and none of these was considered as significantly atypical as on microendoscopy (Table 16-2). In general, the results of the two diagnostic tests were quite similar.

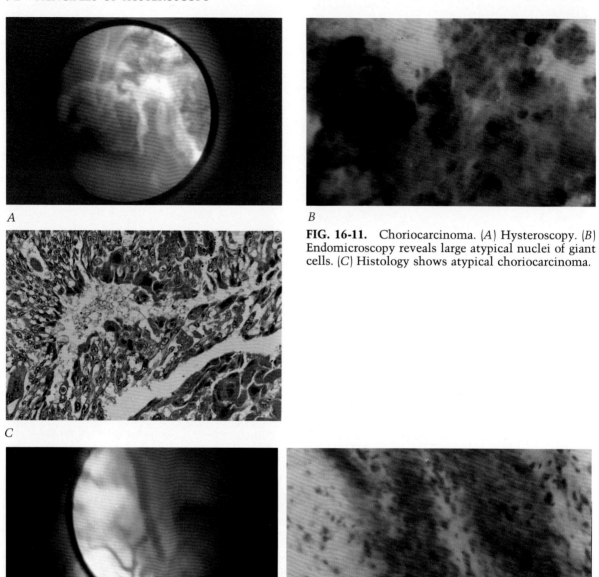

FIG. 16-11.   Choriocarcinoma. (*A*) Hysteroscopy. (*B*) Endomicroscopy reveals large atypical nuclei of giant cells. (*C*) Histology shows atypical choriocarcinoma.

FIG. 16-12.   Chorioadenoma destruens. (*A*) Hysteroscopy. (*B*) Endomicroscopy reveals atypical nuclei. (*C*) Histology shows multinucleated giant cells.

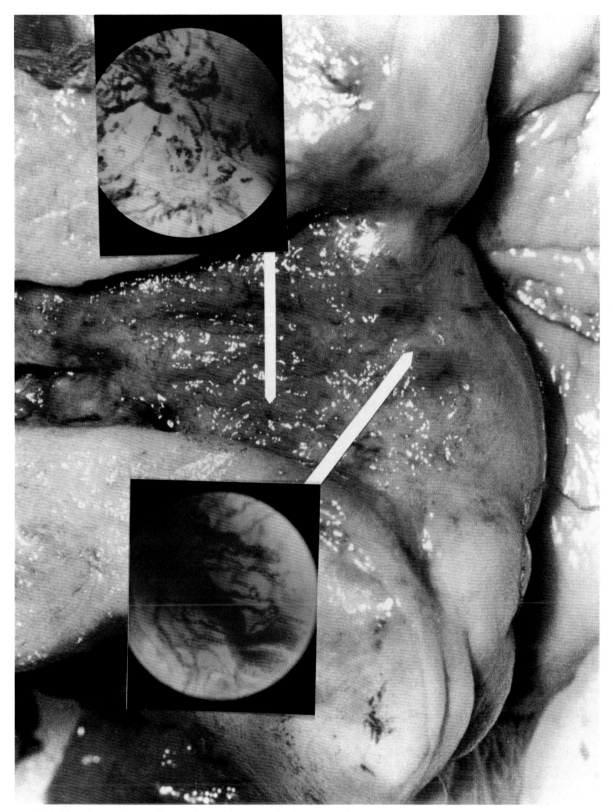

FIG. 16-13. Atypical capillaries (*inset*) seen with the panendoscope.

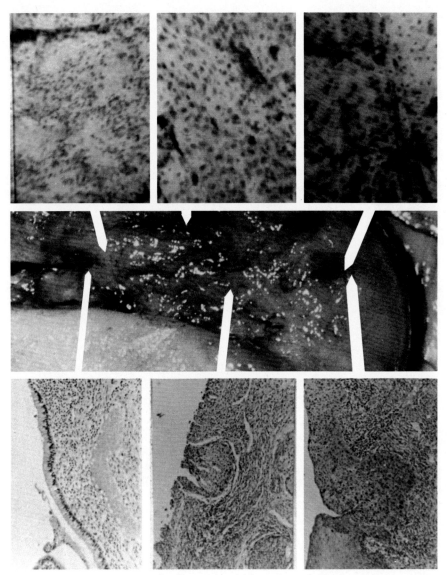

FIG. 16-14.   Comparison of endoscopic and histologic findings in early squamous cell carcinoma of the cervix.

DISCUSSION

Endomicroscopic diagnoses can be made at cellular levels, since the panendomicroscope has a $\times 100$ magnifying lens. Images $\times 190$ magnification appear on the film; they are $\times 671$ on paper. Abnormal cells can be differentiated from normal ones by specifically staining nuclei with a dye having affinity for DNA, such as a mixture of cresyl violet acetate and thionin. The panendomicroscope discloses the stained nuclei on the photomicrograph. The contact microhysteroscope has two different magnifications, low and high. Panoramic observations are possible using this scope. Using ×30 magnification to examine the endometrium, atypical vessels are visible in endometrial adenocarcinoma. Intrauterine abnormalities should be diagnosed at the cellular level; the endomicroscope enables the physician to make an immediate diagnosis.

CONCLUSION

An endomicroscopic method that facilitates the early detection of cancer has been developed and improved. With high magnification, microscopic study at cellular levels is possible. Living cells, especially during cell division, are spray stained *in situ* with cresyl violet acetate and thionin solution. The stain distinguishes normal from abnormal cells. The endomicroscopic method allows the physician to identify and localize lesions precisely. In addition, precancerous atypical changes missed by standard cytologic study can be found.

REFERENCES

1. Antoine T: Der heutige Stand der Auflichtmicroskopie in der Gynäkologie. Arch Gynaekol 180:62, 1951
2. Fujimori H: Fujimori colpomicroscope in the early diagnosis of the cancer of the uterine cervix. J Jpn Obstet Gynecol Soc 7:207, 1960
3. Hamou J: Microhysteroscopy. A new procedure and its original application in gynecology. J Reprod Med 26:375, 1981
4. Masubuchi K, Tenzin M: Colpomicroscope. Clin Obstet Gynecol 13:1705, 1959
5. Noda S: Studies on colpomicroscopy, especially on the visible depth of stained epithelia of the vaginal portion of the uterus. J Osaka City Med Center 11:179, 1962
6. Ohkawa K, Ohkawa R: Early detection and prevention of cancer development from dysplasia of uterine cervix. In Nieburgs HE (ed): International Symposium on Prevention and Detection of Cancer. New York, Marcel Dekker, Inc 1978
7. Ohkawa K, Ohkawa R: Panendomicroscope and its clinical use. Colposcopist, Spring 1–3, 1980
8. Ohkawa K, Ohkawa R: Pan-endomicroscope and its clinical use. Scientific Exhibition Monograph, Ninth World Congress of Gynecology and Obstetrics, 34:86, 1980

Hysterosonography: A New Approach for Extending Endoscopic Observations ■

17

Lothar W. Popp
Rolf Peter Lueken

The purpose of this chapter is to describe the use of a hysteroscope combined with a rotating ultrasound transducer. In 1976 Kratochwil proposed similar instruments for vaginal and rectal examinations.[2] A rotating ultrasound probe replaces the hysteroscope. The ultrasound beam cuts through the environs like a rotating lighthouse reflector. On the screen, the semi-real-time imaging of the sectional echographic plane is performed in true scale. By moving the probe back and forth, all 360-degree sectional scans in a right angle to the long axis of the uterus appear on the monitor (Fig. 17-1).

The ultrasound transducer rotates in a 8-mm stainless steel tube and has a convenient length of 24 cm. The transducer projects about 25 mm in front of the tube. A Luer-lock valve allows the uterine cavity to fill with liquid. The number of revolutions of the ultrasound transducer can be between 6 rps and 10 rps. We used a 5.5 MHz transducer focused at 3 cm to 4 cm. The ultrasound penetration depth is 3 cm to 4 cm from the first tissue barrier. On the screen, distance measurements can be done. The ultrasound unit* is seen with monitors, operative elements, and a camera (Fig. 17-2).[4] Video recordings are possible. Figure 17-3 shows the scanning probe, consisting of the motor unit, the shaft with the filling facilities, and the rotating ultrasound transducer. In Figure 17-4 the transducer is demonstrated in detail. The equipment was originally designed for use in urology.[1,5] The procedure is easy to perform and is without any additional risk. After dilatation of the cervix to Hegar 8, the probe is inserted and scanning can begin.

Figure 17-5 is a typical hysterosonogram of the cervix. The big white spot in the middle of the picture corresponds to the rotating ultrasound transducer. The thin cervical mucosal layer is outlined in a stockade pattern. A sharp outside border is surrounded by vaginal tissue. Figure 17-6 shows a hysterosonogram through the fundus of a retroflexed uterus of normal size. The endometrium is thicker than the endocervical epithelium, and its stockade pattern is less distinct. The demarcation between the dense endometrium and the less compact myometrium can be seen. Figure 17-7 shows a less distinct barrier between the endometrium and the coarse and broad myometrium. The histologic finding was adenomyosis. Figure 17-8 presents an enlarged uterus with multiple fibroids. The solid, sound-absorbing fibroids show the sonographic sign of shadowing. In Figure 17-9, an encapsulated ovarian mass is seen close to the uterus with internal echos. The laparoscopic finding was a follicular cyst. Figure 17-10 shows the "igloo," and Figure 17-11 presents the corresponding hysteroscopic view in a woman 7 wk pregnant.[3] Figure 17-12 shows the inside of the "igloo." A longitudinal scan through the embryo in the amniotic fluid is clearly seen. The uterine cavity was filled with liquid for hysterosonography before abortion in the seventh week of pregnancy. Decidua has a much higher density than normal endometrium.

* Manufactured by Brüel & Kjaer, Naerum, Denmark.

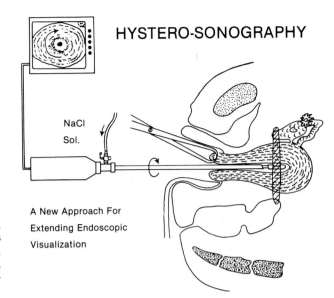

HYSTERO-SONOGRAPHY

NaCl
Sol.

A New Approach For
Extending Endoscopic
Visualization

FIG. 17-1. Hysterosonography. The rotating ultrasound transducer protrudes in front of the 8-mm stainless steel tube of the probe. The transducer is rotated by a motor in the handle. During rotation, echo information is collected from the sectional plane and displayed on the monitor. The uterine cavity can be filled with liquid.

FIG. 17-2. The ultrasound unit has monitors, operative elements, and a camera.

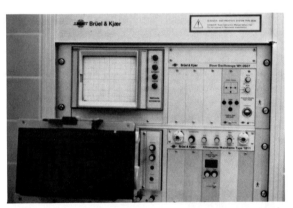

FIG. 17-3. The scanning probe consists of the motor unit, the shaft with the filling facilities, and the rotating ultrasound transducer.

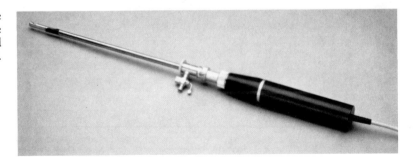

FIG. 17-4. Rotating ultrasound transducer.

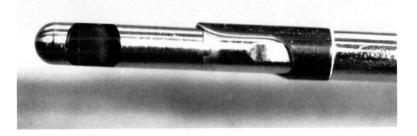

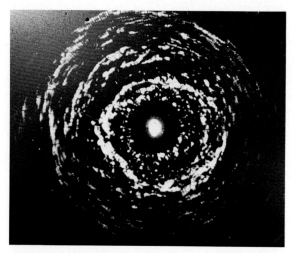

FIG. 17-5. The thin cervical mucosal layer is outlined in a stockade pattern.

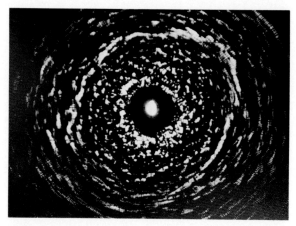

FIG. 17-7. There is a less distinct barrier beween the endometrium and the coarse and broad myometrium in adenomyosis.

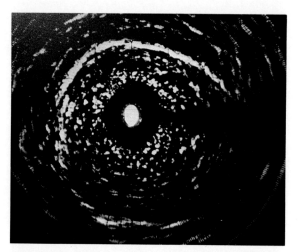

FIG. 17-6. There is a clear demarcation between the endometrium and the myometrium in the hysterosonogram through the fundus.

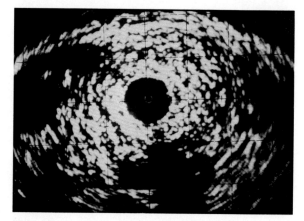

FIG. 17-8. Uterus with multiple fibroids.

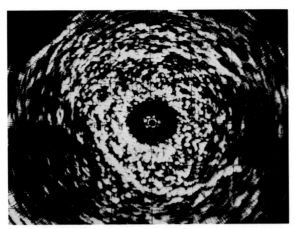

FIG. 17-9. An encapsuled ovarian mass appears close to the uterus.

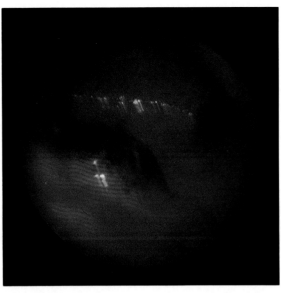

FIG. 17-11. Hysteroscopic view shows the "igloo" in early pregnancy.

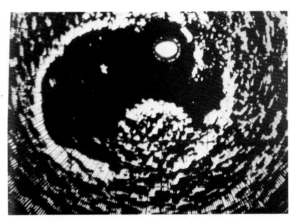

FIG. 17-10. The uterine cavity was filled with liquid. The "igloo" is clearly demonstrated at 7 weeks' gestation.

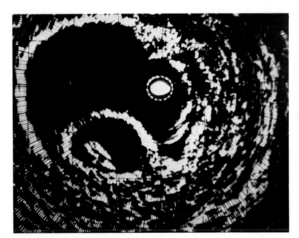

FIG. 17-12. Longitudinal scan through the embryo in the amniotic fluid.

REFERENCES

1. Gammelgaard J, Holm HH: Transurethral and transrectal ultrasonic scanning in urology. J Urol 124:863, 1980
2. Kratochwil A: Ultraschalldiagnostik in der Gynäkologie. Gynakologe 9:166, 1976
3. Lindemann HJ, Gallinat A, Lueken RP, et al: Atlas der Hysteroskopie. Untersuchungstechnik, Diagnostik, Therapie der Gebärmutterhöhle. Stuttgart, Gustav Fischer, 1980
4. Popp LW, Lueken RP, Lindemann HJ: Hysterosonographie. Diagn Intens Therap 4:69, 1982
5. Schüller V, Walther G, Staehler G, et al: Beurteilung von Blasenwandveränderungen mit der intravesikalen Ultraschalltomographie. Urology 20:204, 1981

Choice of Anesthesia ■

18

Milan Buros
Gerlinde Partecke

General anesthesia with endotracheal intubation has become the most widely accepted method of anesthesia for laparoscopy. Local anesthesia alone or in combination with systemic analgesia is sufficient for most hysteroscopic examinations. The combined operations of hysteroscopy and laparoscopy require general anesthesia for adequate observation. From our experiences with 8350 general and 1750 local anesthesias for gynecologic endoscopy (Fig. 18-1), we are convinced that the risk from the endoscopy is low. The result depends on a properly administered and monitored anesthesia in combination with a carefully performed endoscopic procedure.

Many types of anesthesia for hysteroscopy are possible, but some surgeons perform the operation without any anesthesia.[4] Many authors find value in using analgesia and sedation only. The introduction of local anesthesia followed that of general anesthesia by almost 40 yr. The techiques of administration are simple, the costs are reasonable, and the equipment required is minimal. The need for postoperative care of the patient is lessened. Most of the undesirable effects of general anesthesia are avoided. The method is ideal for the ambulatory patient.[1,3,13]

Careful discussion with the patient preoperatively will alert her to the procedure of hysteroscopy and a paracervical nerve block. It is a most practical method for this endoscopic operation because the area can be easily anesthetized with relatively small amounts of the agent and the effects are almost immediate. The operative procedure is short and easily completed before the effect of the drug wears off. Local anesthesia is preferable for hysteroscopy.[1,4] It should be administered by the endoscopist. Equipment and drugs for the treatment of complications must be prepared and available. Skill and gentle handling prevent some untoward reactions.

The patient scheduled for a paracervical nerve block should not eat for 4 hr preoperatively. A sedative dose of a short-acting barbiturate or diazepam can be prescribed to alleviate apprehension. Patients should be questioned for untoward reactions to local anesthesia, and their general physical condition should be known.

To proceed, use the minimal effective dose and concentration. Wait long enough for the anesthetic to take effect. Interrupt the injection with frequent aspiration for blood. Continuous conversation serves to reassure the patient and allows detection of toxic manifestations. After completing the procedure, observe the patient for some time to detect delayed complications. Finally, keep a record of the procedure as protection for both physician and patient.

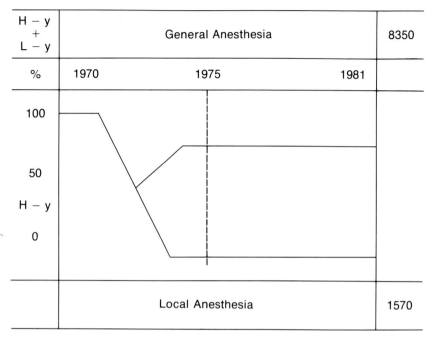

| H − y + L − y | General Anesthesia | 8350 |

FIG. 18-1. Types of general anesthesia and drugs used. Premedication: atropine, 0.5 mg; promethazine, 50 mg to 75 mg. Intraoperative medication: Diazepam, 5 mg to 10 mg; Alloferin, 3 mg; Brevimytal, 100 mg; Pantolax, 50 mg to 60 mg; Intubation. Manual hyperventilation: 1.5 1.O$_2$: 3.5 1 N$_2$O luothane; repeat Pantolax, 25 mg, or Alloferin, 7 mg

Adverse, systemic reactions principally affect the central nervous system (CNS). Patients may be lightheaded, drowsy, or euphoric or have blurred vision, tremors, and even convulsions. Unconsciousness, respiratory depression, and even cardiac arrest have been reported. With severe reactions, obviously no further injections are given, and resuscitative measures are initiated. An ultra-short-acting barbiturate is needed. Adverse reactions result from high plasma levels because of rapid absorption, inadvertent intravascular injection, or excessive doses. Other causes of reactions include hypersensitivity, idiosyncrasy, or decreased tolerance. Reactions caused by overdose are usually systemic, primarily involving the CNS and the cardiovascular system. Allergic reactions are characterized by cutaneous erythema of delayed onset and general manifestations of allergy. Treatment of patients with toxic manifestations consists of maintaining an airway and supporting ventilation using oxygen and assisted or controlled respiration as required. Supportive treatment of the cardiovascular system consists of using vasopressors (*e.g.*, ephedrine) and intravenous (IV) fluids.

With a paracervical block, 5 ml to 10 ml of 1% to 2% solution of local anesthetic is injected.[3,5,11] At the Elisabeth Hospital in Hamburg, West Germany, the injections are made behind the cervix, 2.5 ml into each uterosacral ligament. Intracervical infiltration is also used by injecting 6 doses each of 1.5 ml of 1% carticaine (Ultracain) or, in pregnant women, 6 doses each of 3 ml of 1% mepivacaine (Scandicain, Carbocaine) with epinephrine (Fig. 18-2).

Regional anesthesia is not required for hysteroscopy. Neither with local anesthesia (Table 18-1) nor with general anesthesia (Tables 18-2 and 18-3) has a clinically significant change in acid−base balance been found by Lindemann in a series of patients, some with bleeding uteri, who underwent hysteroscopy if reasonable volumes of carbon dioxide were used and enough time taken. If hysteroscopy and laparoscopy are performed together, then regional anesthesia certainly has value; some authors do use it.[2] However, the long preparation, the delayed onset of analgesia, and the need for high levels and a skillful anesthesiologist are limiting factors. A comprehensive description of the method has been published by Moore and by others.[5,10] Regional anesthesia is indi-

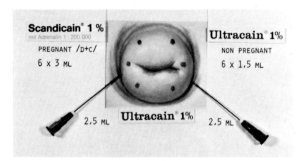

FIG. 18-2. Sites for injection of local anesthetic agent.

Table 18-1
EFFECTS OF HYSTEROSCOPY ON BLOOD GASES UNDER LOCAL ANESTHESIA IN PATIENTS WITH INTACT AND BLEEDING UTERI

DURATION	pH	pCO_2	pO_2	BICARBONATE
0 min	7.37	37	76	22
5 min	7.38	39	81	24
10 min	7.40	34	87	21

Table 18-2
EFFECTS OF GENERAL ANESTHESIA ON BLOOD GASES DURING HYSTEROSCOPY IN PATIENTS WITH INTACT UTERI

DURATION	pH	pCO_2	pO_2	BICARBONATE
0 min	7.35	43	129	23
5 min	7.31	45	122	23.7
10 min	7.33	46	129	24

Table 18-3
EFFECTS OF GENERAL ANESTHESIA ON BLOOD GASES DURING HYSTEROSCOPY IN PATIENTS WITH BLEEDING UTERI

DURATION	pH	pCO_2	pO_2	BICARBONATE
0 min	7.38	43.2	107	22.6
5 min	7.35	47	96	23
10 min	7.35	47.7	101	22.5

cated for the patient with chronic pulmonary disease. Its disadvantages for therapeutic hysteroscopy and laparoscopy are that a mild to moderate discomfort could result if the patient has some pelvic inflammation or restrictive adhesions. For laparoscopy, intra-abdominal adhesions are a definite contraindication to local anesthesia, according to Fishburne and Keith.[6]

When Lindemann and Gallinat started using hysteroscopy with carbon dioxide in 1976, they used general anesthesia. Operations lasted almost 1 hr, and the amount of insufflated carbon dioxide was appreciable. Controlled respiration was maintained by mask and rarely by endotracheal tube. Under exceptional circumstances, general anesthesia is now administered for combined hysteroscopy and laparoscopy without endotracheal intubation. The incidence of cardiac arrhythmias during gynecologic endoscopies that use carbon dioxide has been reported by several authors.[6] Hypercarbia, especially in connection with some degree of hypoxia, provokes a release of catecholamines with their sequelae, namely, vasoconstriction, increased central venous pressure (CVP), positive inotropy and chronotropy of the myocardium, pulsus bigeminus, and multiple extrasystoles.

In 1972, during a combined hysteroscopy–laparoscopy in a healthy young woman, tachyarrhythmia appeared. Hyperventilation and oxygen were increased, and 2 ml of propranolol was injected slowly.[12] Nevertheless, cardiac arrest followed in a few seconds. After 0.4 mg of atropine and two firm blows on the precordial area, regular cardiac action returned. No reason for this accident was ascertained. Another cardiac arrest in 1977 occurred in a healthy woman, 34 years of age, who was undergoing hysteroscopy and laparoscopy. Suddenly bradycardia was detected, followed a few seconds later by cardiac arrest. A balloonlike abdomen was discovered. After reversal of the Trendelenburg position, release of the intra-abdominal gas and a dose of atropine, the operation continued uneventfully.

Lindemann and colleagues, in experimental work with dogs, showed that 400 ml/min of

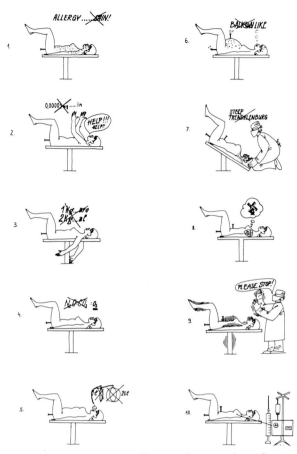

FIG. 18-3. Recommendations for anesthesiologist giving anesthesia for gynecologic endoscopy.

carbon dioxide insufflated IV caused recognizable toxicity.[9] Höffken used carbon dioxide for pneumoradiography without signs of a gas embolism. For the anesthesiologist giving anesthesia for gynecologic endoscopy, we recommend (Fig. 18-3) the following:

Avoid nonindicated drugs (*i.e.*, check for allergy)

Avoid shallow anesthesia to prevent cardiac irregularities

Avoid excessive or deep anesthesia to prevent cardiovascular depression and unnecessarily prolonged recovery

Avoid a steep Trendelenburg position

To ensure proper oxygenation, we recommend the following:

Hyperventilate patients adequately

Be aware of the dangers caused by extremely high intra-abdominal pressure

Be alert for the possibility of gas embolism

If some cardiorespiratory difficulties appear and do not disappear shortly, stop the operation, reverse the Trendelenburg position, and release the gas from the abdomen.

REFERENCES

1. Andersen PK, Stokke DB, Hole P, et al: Carbon dioxide tension in manually ventilated, prone patients. Anaesthetist 12:610, 1981

2. Aribarg A: Epidural analgesia for laparoscopy. J Obstet Gynaecol Br Commonw 80:567, 1973

3. Auberger HQ: Praktische Lokalanästhesie, p 116. Stuttgart, Georg Thieme, Verlag, 1974

4. Barbot J, Parent B, Dubuisson JB: Contact hysteroscopy: Another method of endoscopic examination. Am J Obstet Gynecol 136:721, 1980

5. Bonica JJ: Principles and Practice of Obstetric Analgesia and Anesthesia, p 567. Santa Cruz, Davis, 1967

6. Fishburne JI Jr, Keith L: Laparoscopy, pp 69–85. Baltimore, Williams & Wilkins, 1977

7. Höffken W, Junghans R, Zylka W: Die Grundlagen der Pneumoradiographie des rechten Herzens mit Kohlendioxyd. ROFO 86:292, 1957

8. Lindemann HJ, Gallinat A: Physikalische und physiologische Grundlagen der CO_2 Hysteroskopie. Geburtshilfe Frauenheilkd 36:729, 1976

9. Lindemann HJ, Mohr J, Gallinat A, et al: Der Einfluss von CO_2-Gas während der Hysteroskopie. Geburtshilfe Frauenheilkd 36:153, 1976

10. Moore DC: Regional Block. Springfield, IL, Charles C Thomas, 1957

11. Nolte H: Indikationen und Methoden der Regionalanästhesie in der Geburtshilfe. Klin Anästhesiol 4:189, 1974

12. Sudmeyer W, Schilling K: Klinische Erfahrungen mit der intravenösen Applikation der Beta-Rezeptoren-Blockers Propranolol in der Anasthesie und Intensivpflege. Z Prakt Anaesth Wiederbeleb 5:104, 1970

13. Valle R: Hysteroscopy in the evaluation of female infertility. Am J Obstet Gynecol 137:425, 1980

Hysteroscopy as an Outpatient Procedure ■ 19

Harry Van der Pas

The term *ambulant* or *outpatient* hysteroscopy means that the patient can leave immediately after the operation. Although the logic of looking into the trachea, the esophagus, and the intestine because of symptoms or signs of disease is accepted, women and many physicians are not convinced or aware of the possibility of observing the uterine cavity. Both must be alerted to the potential value of ambulant hysteroscopy. The uterine cavity can be examined by microcurettage, hysterosalpingography, and echography without the need to hospitalize the patient.

I performed hysteroscopic procedures with carbon dioxide distention and finished about 80% under local anesthesia. I am convinced that this method is safer than general anesthesia because the patient can breath spontaneously, and, should hypercarbia occur, she will automatically hyperventilate. If the patient seems disturbed, the procedure can be terminated.

If an additional intracavitary procedure is needed, a cervical dilatation becomes necessary to let the wider shaft through the cervical channel. Paracervical and intracervical blocks are used with a mixture of 7.5 ml of lidocaine 1% and epinephrine 1:100,000 with 22.5 ml of 1% mepivacaine (Scandicain, Carbocaine). The injection is given 5 ml to the left and to the right paracervically about 0.5-cm deep under the vaginal wall at an angle of 5 o'clock and 7 o'clock; this is followed by deep intracervical injections of 5 ml at each of four places while the injection needle is retracted slowly. Cervical dilatation can be done without causing pain with Hegar dilators, which succeed each other by half sizes. Why are gynecologists reluctant to use hysteroscopy? Is it a lack of familiarity with the technique, a concern with potential dangers from the procedure, concern about not being able to see, or the belief that manipulation within the cavity will cause unnecessary bleeding? The examiner with these prejudices will prefer to perform hysteroscopy under general anesthesia, believing that this way is more quiet and efficient. Experienced hysteroscopists prefer local anesthesia.

The instrument is composed of a cervical adaptor with a fixed shaft through which the hysteroscope is introduced. The shaft has a telescopic push-in mechanism that is operated with three fingers (Fig. 19-1). This involves two important advantages. First, the force normally starting from the shoulder and the elbow is now replaced by a sliding mechanism controlled with three fingers. Second, the telescopic shaft is constructed so that the hysteroscope cannot penetrate deeper than 7 cm into the uterine cavity. The danger of perforation is consequently minimized.

After seeing the cervix, the operator pushes

the hysteroscope about 1 cm outward through the cervical adaptor to be placed in the external os. The cup is directed correctly and fixed easily with the vacuum pump of the Metromat.* After the operator supplies light and carbon dioxide, the cervical channel unfolds. Without difficulty the thumb pushes the hysteroscope forward, keeping it under constant control, until a black spot suddenly appears. This is the internal os, to the center of which the scope must move to reach the cavity (Fig. 19-2). Moving the hysteroscope (which has a visual angle of 35 degrees) 45 degrees to the left and then to the right, both tubal ostia are located. As soon as the cavity has been inspected, the thumb slowly releases the pushed-in spring so that the hysteroscope slides backward. The cervical channel is inspected in all directions. It is not difficult to confirm the diagnosis photographically.

This ambulant procedure must be painless, and local analgesia must be given carefully. Hysteroscopic actions should be done slowly, with a light hand and good vision. The seal-tight system to distend the cavity is a prerequisite to good hysteroscopic examinations. Suspicious macroscopic lesions should be confirmed by a tissue diagnosis. Patients need not be hospitalized to have synechiae, polyps, small myomas, or "lost" intrauterine devices (IUDs) removed from the uterine cavity. Finally, effective and potentially reversible transcervical hysteroscopic sterilization through ambulant hysteroscopy may someday be possible.

* Metromat 2121 Insufflator. Richard Wolf Medical Instruments Corporation, Rosemont, IL.

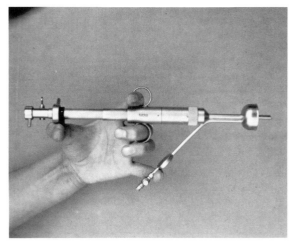

FIG. 19-1. The "three-finger" maneuver is used to introduce the hysteroscope and sheath through the cervical adapter.

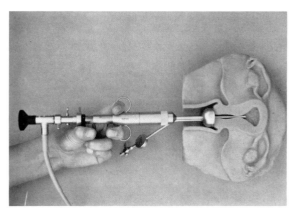

FIG. 19-2. Schematic representation shows the scope at the internal os.

Office Hysteroscopy

Bodo Karacz

MATERIALS AND METHODS

After I left the Elisabeth Hospital in Hamburg, West Germany, I performed 125 hysteroscopic examinations in my office. The indications were "missing," misplaced, or broken intrauterine devices (IUDs), abnormal uterine bleeding, infertility associated with malformations and adhesions, cervical polyps, and suspicious Papanicolaou (Pap) smears. Preoperatively a sedimentation rate, white blood cell (WBC) count, and cervical smear were done. For local anesthesia, a paracervical block with carticaine (Ultracain) was given. The usual disinfection was performed with isopovidone iodine (Isobetadine). All patients left the office within 15 min after hysteroscopy, possibly complaining of slight abdominal or typical shoulder pain. Occasionally spotting persisted for 1 or 2 days. When examinations were done at the end of the office routine, patients seemed to build up anxieties, making them prone to circulatory collapse. This occurred in 8% of the women.

RESULTS

All 25 "lost" IUDs or broken pieces were successfully removed without complications. A second hysteroscopy became necessary in one patient because of severe bleeding after dilatation and curettage.

Forty patients underwent hysteroscopy because of abnormal bleeding, and in 15 the findings were normal. Endometrial polyps (small, functional) were seen in 14, and 1 endometrial adenocarcinoma of pinhead size was found. Seven patients had large endometrial polyps, and two had had a previous dilatation and curettage with negative histologic findings. Submucous fibroids were discovered in three patients. Forty-five patients were examined hysteroscopically for infertility and sterility; of these, 17 were normal. A further 18 women had polyps in the cornual area without tubal occlusion. The others had the following abnormal findings: septate uteri (two), arcuate uteri (two), and Asherman's syndrome (three). Two of those last three became pregnant after treatment. Hysteroscopy done because of cervical polyps showed five additional endometrium polyps, two silent carcinomas, and seven normal uteri. An abnormal Pap smear could be caused by an occult endometrial carcinoma detectable by hysteroscopy.

COMMENT

Office hysteroscopy has not yet found the recognition it deserves. If the indications were widened by, for instance, a method for temporary sterilization, hysteroscopy would become more popular. In the meantime, this subject should not only be discussed in scientific journals but also in women's magazines and on television so that women would become informed and raise the subject with their gynecologists. The creation of workshops at as many universities and hospitals as possible would help disseminate information. Workshops can provide expert guidance to reduce the chance for failure, the usual cause for disinterest. The following factors would increase the use of hysteroscopy in private practice:

Enough patients with appropriate indications
Sufficient reliable, reasonably priced equipment and instruments
Cooperative colleagues
Specially trained nurses or assistants
A special room

Although patients know about cystoscopy, and endoscopes are commonly used for the digestive tract, women are normally not aware that an inspection of the uterus is possible, relatively painless, and not complicated.

More than two hysteroscopies a day are impracticable if one sees 50 patients daily. Hysteroscopy is too time consuming as a screening method, but it is valuable in high-risk patients and experimental studies. Although the operation takes no more than 10 min, a room is occupied for at least 30 min because of preparation and cleaning. The assistant is busy during this time and cannot attend to other matters. The instruments are expensive, and several weaknesses have not been eliminated, namely, an unreliable rubber seal and occasionally faulty welding in seams. Repairs can take up to 6 wk, and a spare set of instruments would also be ideal to overcome delays caused by cleaning and sterilization, which takes about 2 hr.

Adverse Effects ■ 21

Alvin M. Siegler

Hysteroscopy is generally a surgical procedure free of complications. Adverse effects resulting from diagnostic hysteroscopy will be fewer than those following its therapeutic use. Each stage of the procedure has particular hazards, any one of which can be increased by inexperience. However, reports of large series of hysteroscopic examinations and treatments under hysteroscopic control reveal comparatively few adverse reactions, and these are generally not serious. Schroeder, in 350 examinations with sterilized water, Marleschki, using a 5-mm instrument without any medium for uterine distention in over 300 patients, and Esposito, in 150 hysteroscopic studies with the balloon method, did not report any complications.[8,16,19] Faulty technique and selection of inappropriate patients are the most frequent causes of untoward sequelae.

TRAUMA

Cervical lacerations can result from tenacula, and manipulation must be gentle. Lacerations, as well as endometrial trauma, cause bleeding and obscure the view. Forceful cervical dilatation can provoke unnecessary bleeding, perforate the lower uterine segment, and create a false passage or tract. The physician should begin observing as the sheath and hysteroscope are inserted into the isthmic canal, without advancing the instrument except in a clear field of vision. A reddened or cloudy view may indicate juxtaposition to the uterine wall, inadequate uterine distention, or a lens with adherent blood or mucus. Additional force may result in uterine perforation, and the intestines quickly come into endoscopic view.[21] Lindemann reported only 6 fundal perforations in 5220 hysteroscopic examinations. If this accident occurs, remove the endoscope and observe the patient for symptoms and signs of shock. Bleeding from the uterine defect is usually minimal. I have seen this accident on two occasions during simultaneous laparoscopic examination; after withdrawal of the hysteroscope, minimal bleeding was detected in the peritoneal cavity from the uterine wound.[20] Neuwirth reported one uterine perforation that occurred during dissection of intrauterine adhesions and a partial perforation with myometrial penetration in another woman.[17]

I have seen a rupture of a hydrosalpinx during carbon dioxide hysteroscopy monitored by laparoscopy without any adverse effects.[20] The gas bubbled into the leaves of the broad ligament. Probes inserted into the tubal ostia can create a false passage and perforate the uterotubal junction. Electrocoagulation of this area for tubal sterilization is usually safe, but, as in laparoscopy, intestinal injury is possible. Several instances of thermointestinal accidents have been reported in the literature.[5] Any patient who complains of abdominal pain 3 or 4 days postoperatively should be examined promptly for signs of peritonitis. Procrastination can result in severe morbidity and even mortality. Laparotomy and appropriate resection of the injured intestine, drainage, and vigorous antibiotic therapy are necessary.

All specimens removed during a therapeutic hysteroscopy should be sent to the pathology department for study. Recently, during lysis of intrauterine adhesions, I sent a specimen to the laboratory for analysis. The report was "small fragment of intestinal mucosa." Immediate laparotomy revealed a 5-mm perforation of the ileum.[9] During an experimental study for cell-culturing techniques, Hahnemann failed to obtain adequate biopsy of extra-amniotic membranes and inadvertently punctured the amniotic membranes in eight instances. Although liquid media used for uterine distention enter the cul-de-sac in patients with patent tubes, this occurrence does not seem to cause any adverse effects. No evidence exists to suggest that displaced endometrial fragments cause endometriosis or that transported endometrial tumor cells metastasize.[12]

Slight uterine bleeding after hysteroscopy can last for a few days, but hemorrhage is unusual and instances of hemorrhagic shock have not been described.

INTRAVASATION

Unquestionably, venous intravasation of carbon dioxide and liquid media does occur. Bubbles of gas have been seen moving about the vessels of the infundibulopelvic ligament in patients having simultaneous laparoscopy. As in hysterosalpingography, certain conditions such as uterine tuberculosis, submucous tumors, a hypoplastic uterus, a recently traumatized uterine cavity, or proximal tubal obstruction predispose patients to this complication. Excessive pressure during instillation of medium and rapid introduction of large volumes are more likely to cause venous intravasation. Pulmonary embolism is a theoretical possibility, but the risk to the patient is minimal with the use of a controlled gas delivery system. Fatal and nonfatal accidents have occurred with imperfect gas flow monitors. With the flow rate, intrauterine pressure, and amount of carbon dioxide well controlled, the risk of gas embolism is nonexistent.[2] Lindemann reported no changes in electrocardiograms (ECGs), pco_2, or pH in 40 patients during carbon dioxide hysteroscopy.[13] Hulf and colleagues studied changes in arterial pco_2 during hysteroscopy when carbon dioxide was used as the insufflating gas.[11] The arterial pco_2 either fell or was unchanged in artificially ventilated patients. However, when nitrous oxide was used, arterial pco_2 rose, and in two patients this rise was significant. One of these patients, who apparently was in good health, developed a profound bradycardia some 8 min after hysteroscopy was started and required resuscitation.

The risks from intravasation of 50 ml of high-molecular-weight dextran are probably negligible, although Maddi and colleagues described anaphylactic reactions in seven patients who received intravenous (IV) high-molecular-weight dextran for therapy.[15] Treatment with epinephrine, vasopressors, and corticoids corrected the shocklike state. Even low-molecular-weight dextran can cause allergic manifestations. Obviously, intravasation is not a hazard in patients having contact hysteroscopy.[1]

INFECTION

The first occurrence of a tubal infection after hysteroscopy was reported by Bumm in 1885.[3] Frequency of infection after hysteroscopy may depend mainly on the type of patient studied. The procedure can exacerbate latent salpingitis, and susceptible patients should be excluded by a history and a pelvic examination before hysteroscopy. Postoperative salpingitis and peritonitis respond favorably to antibiotics. Febrile reactions following hysteroscopy should be treated with appropriate medication. Media currently used do not cause any aseptic reactions or granulomas in genital mucous membranes or peritoneum. Cohen and Dmowski reported that 1 of 34 infertile women developed symptoms and signs of pelvic inflammatory disease (PID) postoperatively, but the condition responded promptly to antibiotic therapy. Englund and associates had one patient who developed salpingitis and two others who had postoperative febrile reactions.[7]

MORTALITY

Duplay and Clado reported on one patient with a retained placenta who died of sepsis after hysteroscopy and curettage in 1898. A fatality occurred during hysteroscopy with carbon dioxide in which an inordinately large volume (30 liters to 50 liters) and a rapid rate of flow of carbon dioxide were employed. The carbon dioxide was instilled without volumetric controls or pressure manometers.[22] In another instance, 300 ml/min of carbon dioxide was instilled to create uterine distention, but the intrauterine pressure fell. The nurse was instructed to raise the flow rate to maintain the intrauterine pressure at 200 mm Hg. The cavity showed a submucous myoma; photographic equipment was attached; and the anesthesiologist reported a cardiac arrest 5 minutes after the procedure had begun.* Note that the insufflator for creating a pneumoperitoneum during laparoscopy should never be used to form the pneumometra in hysteroscopy because the uterus cannot safely tolerate 1 liter/min to 2 liter/min. Several types of carbon dioxide insufflators designed to limit the quantity of gas delivered each minute to 100 ml or less at the maximal intrauterine pressure of 200 mm Hg can obviate serious accidents and mortalities from careless introduction of gas for uterine distention. Porto cited reports of seven cardiac arrests during insufflation of the uterine cavity with carbon dioxide.[18] In each instance, either an unmonitored amount of the gas was used or the flow rate ex-

* Schomaker J: Personal communication, 1975.

ceeded 350 ml/min. Unrecognized intestinal injury after uterine cornual perforation during electrocoagulation for sterilization can cause severe peritonitis and death. The symptoms, signs, and management of this condition are the same as those for a thermal intestinal injury caused inadvertently during tubal coagulation at laparoscopy.

CONTRAINDICATIONS AND LIMITATIONS

Hysteroscopy can be dangerous or harmful when improperly or carelessly employed, as disclosed by deleterious effects previously described in the literature. Adnexal and endometrial infections contraindicate hysteroscopy, and the physician must proceed cautiously with women who have a history of PID.

Studies should be done, preferably in the postmenstrual and proliferative phase, for optimal observations, since a premenstrual endometrium limits the reliability of the examination. Menstruation and pregnancy are relative contraindications; however, recent uterine or tubal surgery and even pregnancy do not seem to predispose patients to complications. A cone biopsy or pelvic radiation may limit easy cervical dilatation or application of a cervical suction cup. As with all surgery, patients with cardiac or pulmonary disease are at increased risk. Laparoscopic control is essential in a woman who has a scarred uterus or in one with extensive intrauterine adhesions because it is easier to perforate these uteri.

REFERENCES

1. Baggish MS, Barbot J: Contact hysteroscopy for easier diagnosis. Contemp Obstet Gynecol 16:93, 1980
2. Bartisch EG, Dillon TF: Carbon dioxide hysteroscopy. Am J Obstet Gynecol 124:756, 1976
3. Bumm E: Diskussion über die Endometritis. In Chrobak R, Pfannenstiel J (eds): Verhandlungen der Deutschen Gesellschaft für Gynäkologie Kongress (Wien), p 524. Leipzig, Breitkopf and Härtel, 1895
4. Cohen MR, Dmowski WP: Modern hysteroscopy: Diagnostic and therapeutic potential. Fertil Steril 24:905, 1973

5. Darabi KF, Richart RM: Collaborative study on hysteroscopic sterilization procedures. Preliminary report. Obstet Gynecol 49:48, 1977

6. Duplay S, Clado S: Traité d'Hystéroscopie. Rennes, Simon, 1898

7. Englund S, Ingelman–Sundberg A, Westin B: Hysteroscopy in diagnosis and treatment of uterine bleeding. Gynaecologia 143:217, 1957

8. Esposito A: Une exploration gynécologique trop negligée: L'hystéroscopie. Gynecol Pract 19:165, 1968

9. Gentile GP, Siegler AM: Inadvertent intestinal biopsy during laparoscopy and hysteroscopy. A report of two cases. Fertil Steril 36:402, 1981

10. Hahnemann N: Early prenatal diagnosis: A study of biopsy techniques and cell culturing from extraembryonic membranes. Clin Genet 6:294, 1974

11. Hulf JA, Corall I, Strunin L, et al: Possible hazard of nitrous oxide for hysteroscopy. Br Med J 2:511, 1975

12. Joelsson I, Levine RU, Moberger G: Hysteroscopy as an adjunct in determining the extent of carcinoma of the endometrium. Am J Obstet Gynecol 111:696, 1971

13. Lindemann HJ: A symposium on advances in fiberoptic hysteroscopy. Contemp Obstet Gynecol 3:115, 1974

14. Lindemann HJ: Atlas der Hysteroskopie, p 39. Stuttgart, Gustav Fischer, 1980

15. Maddi VI, Wyso EM, Zinner EN: Dextran anaphylaxis. Angiology 20:243, 1969

16. Marleschki V: Hysteroskopische Feststellung der spontanen Perfusionsschwankungen am menschlichen Endometrium. Zentralbl Gynaekol 90:1094, 1968

17. Neuwirth RS: Hysteroscopy, pp 40–43. Philadelphia, W B Saunders, 1975

18. Porto R: Hystéroscopie. In Encyclopédie Médico-Chirurgie, Paris, 1974

19. Schroeder C: Über den Ausbau und die Leistungen der Hysteroskopie. Arch Gynaekol 156:407, 1934

20. Siegler AM, Kemmann EK: Hysteroscopy. Obstet Gynecol Surv 30:567, 1975

21. Wamsteker K: Hysteroscopie. Thesis. Women's Clinic of The University of Leiden, Holland, 1977

22. Obstetrician convicted in sterilization death; is placed on probation. Ob Gyn News 9:4, 1974

Complications from Microhysteroscopy ■ 22

Jacques Salat-Baroux
Jacques E. Hamou
Genevieve Maillard
Andre Chouraqui
Pierre Verges

MATERIALS AND METHODS

Anesthetic complications associated with hysteroscopy are of minor importance because 94% of patients who undergo these operative procedures do not require any anesthesia. From February 1979 until March 1980, local anesthesia was required for 12 patients and 41 received general anesthesia, 13 of whom had an associated surgical procedure done at the time of hysteroscopy. The remaining 949 examinations were performed without any anesthetic agents.[7] Since then, we have done 3000 hysteroscopic examinations under similar circumstances.

Most women have minimal discomfort, similar to that of menses and less than that from hysterosalpingography. Shoulder pain was noticed in 30 patients, especially when the procedure was prolonged, and 4 patients with syncope required a few minutes of rest. These 959 hysteroscopies were performed at an outpatient clinic. In 28 women the procedure was a failure, in 12 because of cervical atresia even when ethinyl estradiol, 10 μg/day, was given for 8 days. In 16 women the procedure was interrupted because of hemorrhage or obvious infection. For conventional hysteroscopy, local cervical anesthesia with procaine hydrochloride (Novacaine) is performed with a failure rate of 4% to 8%.[2-6] We even prefer hysteroscopy without anesthesia for lysis of adhesions because of the anesthetic risk from general anesthesia in prolonged operations.

A fixed retroverted uterus, cervical stenosis, and endometrial atrophy predispose patients to uterine perforation. We observed only 1 perforation in 615 women examined during synechiotomy under laparoscopic control.

Postoperative infection is rare. In our series, seven patients had mild infections. One severe infection resulted after an intratubal catheter was removed on the eighth postoperative day following a microsurgical repair.

Bacteriologic studies were done to evaluate our method of disinfection. The hysteroscope was kept overnight in a container with 2 tablets of trichloroethylene.

The cervix was cleaned with a cotton ball soaked with physiologic saline. The hysteroscope was rinsed with saline and 70% alcohol between operations. Two liquid culture media were used for aerobic and anaerobic organisms and one solid medium (blood gelose VF and TGY) was used (Tables 22-1 and 22-2).

Swab samples were taken from the box, the distal end of the hysteroscope, the carbon dioxide channel, and the cervix before and after cleaning. This procedure was repeated for each of six consecutive patients.

Table 22-1
RESULTS OF BACTERIOLOGIC CULTURES

PATIENTS	TIME OF CULTURE			
	Instrument Box	Hysteroscope Before Use	Cervix Before Examination	Hysteroscope After Use
Patient no. 1 (Nov. 5, 1981)	0	0	*Staphylococcus epidermidis, Micrococcus epidermidis*	*S. epidermidis, M. epidermidis*
Patient no. 2 (Nov. 26, 1981)	0	0	*Escherichea coli,* Enterococcus	0
Patient no. 3 (Nov. 26, 1981)	0	0	Enterococcus	Enterococcus

Table 22-2
RESULTS OF BACTERIOLOGIC CULTURES

PATIENTS	TIME OF EXAMINATION			
	Instrument Box	Hysteroscope Before Use	Cervix Before Examination	Hysteroscope After Use
Patient no. 4 (Dec. 3, 1981)	0	0	*Streptococcus* Group B, *Streptococcus hemolyticus*	*S.* Group B *S. hemolyticus*
Patient no. 5 (Dec. 3, 1981)	0	0	?	*S. faecalis*
Patient no. 6 (Dec. 3, 1981)	0	0	*Streptococcus faecalis, Staphylococcus epidermidis*	*S. faecalis S. epidermidis*

All cultures of the box and of the instrument before use were negative. Cultures of the instrument after use were positive for the organisms found on the cervix before hysteroscopy in all but one instance.

The hysteroscope was always sterilized before each procedure by careful alcohol washing. Microorganisms found were always present on the patient's cervix. No bacteria were transferred from one patient to another, and no infection occurred.

No infection was reported for the most recent 3000 hysteroscopies performed without any antibiotics. The major risk in hysteroscopy is related to the methods used for uterine distention.

Until 1973, 6 cardiac arrests occurring during hysteroscopy had been reported.[4] In each instance, the carbon dioxide insufflation was over 300 ml/min. Liquid media can cause complications, and an allergic reaction to high-molecular-weight dextran has even been described.[8]

Hulf reported on the chemical changes in the blood after the use of nitrous oxide and carbon dioxide for distending the uterus during hysteroscopy in 27 patients.[1] The poor solubility of nitrous oxide was noted, and one patient had a pulmonary embolism. Under normal temperatures and atmospheric pressure, 51.4 ml of carbon dioxide can be absorbed by 100 ml of blood because it is its natural vehicle.[2]

Hulf and colleagues revealed that in the nitrous oxide group, insufflation present at constant pressure with a variable flow altered the $PaCO_2$.[1] In the carbon dioxide group, the insuf-

Table 22-3

GROUP 1 ARTERIAL P_{CO_2} VALUES* DURING LAPAROSCOPY AND HYSTEROSCOPY USING CARBON DIOXIDE, NITROUS OXIDE, AND DEXTRAN 70 (GAS INSUFFLATED BY LAPAROFLATOR)

TIME OF SAMPLE	INSUFFLATING MEDIUM			
	Laparoscopy (control)	Hysteroscopy		
	Nitrous Oxide (N = 8)	*Carbon Dioxide (N = 10) (mm Hg)*	*Nitrous Oxide (N = 6)*	*Dextran 70 (N = 6)*
Before anesthesia	36 ± 2.25	39 ± 3.8	39.8 ± 6	36.8 ± 3.8
After 5 min of Ippv	30 ± 3	36 ± 3	37.5 ± 4.5	32.3 ± 3.8
Gas in uterus 3 min	30.8 ± 6.8	36 ± 4.5	39.8† ± 6.8	32.5 ± 3
Gas in uterus 6 min	29.3 ± 3.8	38.25 ± 3.8	42†† ± 6	33.8 ± 6
Gas out of uterus 5 min	29.3 ± 5.3	39 ± 3.8	39 ± 4.5	36.8 ± 6.8

* ± standard deviation.
† Compared with 5 minutes Ippv, P 0.05.
†† Compared with 5 minutes Ippv, P 0.005.
Ippv = intermittent positive pressure ventilation.

Table 22-4

GROUP 2 Pa_{CO_2} VALUES* DURING HYSTEROSCOPY USING CARBON DIOXIDE, NITROUS OXIDE, AND DEXTRAN 70 (GAS INTRODUCED BY ROCKET INSUFFLATOR)

TIME OF SAMPLE	INSUFFLATING MEDIUM		
	Nitrous Oxide (N = 8)	Carbon Dioxide (N = 8) (mm Hg)	Dextran 70 (N = 8)
After 5 min of Piv	35.3 ± 5.3	31.5 ± 4.5	29.3 ± 3.0
Gas in uterus 3 min	30.8 ± 5.3	30.8 ± 5.3	27.8 ± 2.8
Gas in uterus 6 min	32.3 ± 6.0	31.5 ± 1.28	27.8 ± 2.4
Gas out of uterus 5 min	30.0 ± 5.3	30.8 ± 6.8	27.8 ± 2.4

* ± standard deviation.

flator allowed a constant gas flow with a variable pressure (Hysteroflator), and no change in $PaCO_2$ was reported. Lindemann demonstrated that at a constant gas flow between 20 ml/min and 80 ml/min, cardiac rhythm, blood pH, $PaCO_2$, and bicarbonate were not changed either with general or local anesthesia or even with uterine bleeding.[2] No complications related to carbon dioxide distention were reported when pressure was maintained below 150 mm Hg for more than 5220 hysteroscopic examinations.

We performed a comparable study on three groups of patients with precise conditions of constant flow and variable pressure below 100 mm Hg. Nine patients received general anesthesia with controlled respirations, 10 patients had general anesthesia without such assistance, and 15 patients were examined without any anesthesia. The patients receiving general anesthesia also had a laparoscopy. They received premedication with atropine and diazepam; induction was performed with thiopental (1 ml/kg), curare, and respiratory assistance (frequency set at 14 mm Hg and flow at 6/min). Anesthesia was maintained by an equal mixture of nitrous oxide and oxygen. Four arterial blood samples were taken through a polytetrafluoroethylene (Teflon) catheter introduced in the radial artery before anesthesia, 5 min after anesthesia, 6 min after hysteroscopy, and during laparoscopy (Tables 22-3 and

Table 22-5
VARIATION OF pH, $PaCO_2$, PaO_2, AND CARBON DIOXIDE WITH GENERAL ANESTHESIA AND ASSISTED, CONTROLLED RESPIRATION

PATIENT	BASAL STATE				AFTER 5 MIN OF GENERAL ANESTHESIA				AFTER 6 MIN OF HYSTEROSCOPY				LAPAROSCOPY			
	pH	$PaCO_2$	Carbon Dioxide (T)	PaO_2	pH	$PaCO_2$	Carbon Dioxide (T)	PaO_2	pH	$PaCO_2$	Carbon Dioxide (T)	PaO_2	pH	$PaCO_2$	Carbon Dioxide (T)	PaO_2
1	7.407	36.8	23.9	66.6	7.353	38.3	21.9	9	7.485	27.3	21.2	142.3	7.433	33.7	23.2	111.3
2	7.416	39	25.8	84	7.428	32.5	22.1	293.3	7.444	30.8	21.8	251.9	7.413	34.3	22.6	269.8
3	7.409	30.3	19.8	96.2	7.401	31.7	20.3	185.8	7.454	28.5	20.6	169.2	7.388	33.2	20.6	160.7
4	7.46	39	28	93	7.439	31.6	22	246.8	7.457	29.5	21.5	164.3				
5	7.42	34.5	23.1	116	7.49	24	18.9	325	7.50	27.4	21.9	291.5	7.47	29	21.7	312
6	7.381	36.3	22.2	93.5	7.479	28.4	21.7	316.6	7.542	24.5	21.7	310.8	7.487	27.9	21.8	312.7
7	7.38	36.8	24	89.8	7.469	28.7	21.1	290	7.559	22.1	20.3	272	7.523	24.8	21	216.5
8	7.389	41.3	25.7	106.4	7.369	42	25	307.2	7.424	35.4	23.9	289.5	7.41	36.7	24	272.3
9	7.388	37.1	21.8	94.6	7.465	33	24.5	326	7.487	30.1	23.5	321.5	7.476	32.1	23.7	298
Average	7.41	36.79	23.81	93.4	7.432	32.2	22	267	7.483	28.4	21.8	245.8	7.450	31.5	22.3	244.1

T = total.

Table 22-6
VARIATION OF pH, $PaCO_2$, PaO_2, AND CARBON DIOXIDE DURING GENERAL ANESTHESIA AND SPONTANEOUS RESPIRATION

PATIENT	BASAL STATE				AFTER 5 MIN OF GENERAL ANESTHESIA				AFTER 6 MIN OF HYSTEROSCOPY				LAPAROSCOPY			
	pH	$PaCO_2$	Carbon Dioxide (T)	PaO_2	pH	$PaCO_2$	Carbon Dioxide (T)	PaO_2	pH	$PaCO_2$	Carbon Dioxide (T)	PaO_2	pH	$PaCO_2$	Carbon Dioxide (T)	PaO_2
1	7.381	39.8	23.5	93.5	7.345	42.6	24	89.6	7.311	47.9	25	88.5	7.412	37.3	22.9	160
2	7.405	38.5	22.1	98.2	7.445	38.5	27.3	92.6	7.373	44.7	26.8	87.8				
3	7.42	34.3	23.1	106.2	7.361	41.8	24.4	95.6	7.352	41.1	23.5	91.8	7.433	33.7	23.4	270
4					7.387	33	20.5	98.6	7.379	36.1	22	96.7				
5					7.381	33.1	20.3	97.8	7.39	36.3	22.7	95.3				
6					7.375	38.2	23	87.8	7.361	34	19.8	92.5				
7	7.407	31.3	20.2	97.3	7.371	39.5	23.6	90.6	7.38	40.3	24.6	95.8	7.410	36.7	24	272.4
8	7.391	32.5	21.8	96.8	7.385	35.2	21.2	94.8	7.383	34.4	21.1	93.8				
9	7.382	37.8	23.5	97.2	7.378	32	21.4	97.6	7.382	31.7	21.8	98.6	7.424	30.7	20.2	216.4
10	7.393	38.9	24.2	99.2	7.379	38.4	23.2	92.4	7.375	37.6	23.4	91.8	7.413	34.3	23.2	195.8
Average	7.397	36.1	22.62	98.3	7.380	36.23	22.89	93.7	7.368	38.31	23.07	93.2	7.419	34.5	22.74	222.92

T = total.

Table 22-7
VARIATION OF THE pH, Pa_{CO_2}, Pa_{O_2}, AND CARBON DIOXIDE DURING AMBULATORY HYSTEROSCOPY WITHOUT ANESTHESIA

PATIENT	BASAL STATE				DURING HYSTEROSCOPY			
	pH	Carbon Dioxide (T)	Pa_{CO_2}	Pa_{O_2}	pH	Carbon Dioxide (T)	Pa_{CO_2}	Pa_{O_2}
1	7.439	19.5	28	109.2	7.429	19.3	28.3	107
2	7.379	24.4	40.0	84.2	7.423	26.2	38.9	107.6
3	7.341	17.7	31.8	104.3	7.401	24.3	37.9	103.3
4	7.413	17.8	27.1	119.2	7.441	18.8	26.8	106.6
5	7.382	23.4	38.2	104.2	7.379	22	36.1	111.3
6	7.478	21.1	27.6	138.3	7.435	19.6	24.8	169.2
7	7.387	19.9	32.2	115	7.394	22.1	35.1	95.9
8	7.367	16.5	27.9	108.5	7.366	17.5	29.6	102
9	7.414	21.1	32	132.2	7.452	22.2	30.9	126
10	7.381	19.1	31.2	96.7	7.414	22.7	34.4	111.2
11	7.380	19.4	35.4	122	7.374	22.9	38.1	100.5
12	7.387	16.2	26.8	159	7.405	18.7	29.1	146
13	7.356	21.5	37.2	113.9	7.370	19.2	38.3	154.2
14	7.384	22.2	36	100.6	7.391	24.1	38.5	114.8
15	7.369	22.9	38.6	114.2	7.378	21.7	35.9	114.8
Average	7.390	20.18	32.667	114.76	7.403	21.486	33.51	117.98

T = total.

22-4). Between each sampling the catheter was rinsed with heparinized physiologic saline and the first 3 ml of blood was discarded for measurements of acid–base status to rule out any error caused by stagnant blood in the catheter. Transfer of the syringe was done in ice and protected from air.

RESULTS

In the first group of nine patients, blood pressure and hemodynamics were modified because of cyanosis secondary to intubation. Other measurements of $PaCO_2$, total carbon dioxide, and pH were modified in relation to hyperventilation; $PaCO_2$ and total carbon dioxide decreased, and pH increased (Table 22-5).

The results are similar in all stages of the menstrual cycle. In the second group of ten patients who received an anesthetic without controlled, assisted ventilation, half the group showed a pH with variation toward acidosis between the basal end point 5 min after general anesthesia. The changes increased during hysteroscopy and 6 min after hysteroscopy. The pH never reached a critical point except in one patient, whose average pH was 7.368 (Table 22-6). In the third group of 15 patients the operation lasted between 6 and 15 min. Most of them were hyperventilated, with an average blood pressure of 22 mm Hg and a rapid pulse rate (100 to 110). No detectable change in pH or $PaCO_2$ was noted (Table 22-7).

Severe complications may be expected if carbon dioxide flow and pressure are not strictly controlled. A laparoflator is connected, and high gas flow or pressure is used during the luteal phase if tubal obstruction or hemorrhage is present or if the procedure lasts more than 15 min. Under proper control, the danger to acid–base balance from either hysteroscopy or laparoscopy are minimal.

After 4 yr and 4000 hysteroscopic examinations, 90% of them performed in an office setting, we conclude that microhysteroscopy is a minor surgical procedure with minimal risk. With carbon dioxide for uterine insufflation at 30 ml/min and variable pressures, only 1 uterine perforation and 7 pelvic infections occurred. Bacteriologic studies revealed that no microorganisms were transmitted to patients, although the hysteroscope was used many times each day. Arterial blood gases were measured during different methods of anesthetic administrations and with three types of media to distend the uterus. The least alterations in blood gases resulted during carbon dioxide insufflation at a fixed rate of 30 ml/min, variable pressure, and without anesthesia.

REFERENCES

1. Hulf JA, Corall IM, Knights KM, et al: Blood carbon dioxide tension changes during hysteroscopy. Fertil Steril 32:193, 1979

2. Lindemann HJ: CO_2 hysteroscopy today. Endoscopy 11:94, 1979

3. March CM, Israel R, March AD: Hysteroscopic management of uterine adhesions. Am J Obstet Gynecol 130:633, 1978

4. Parent B, Barbot B, Doeufleu B, et al: Hystéroscopie de contact. Documentation scientifique. Paris, Laboratories Roland Marie S.A., 1976

5. Sciarra JJ, Valle RF: Hysteroscopy: A clinical experience with 320 patients. Am J Obstet Gynecol 127:340, 1977

6. Siegler AM, Kemmann EK, Gentile GP: Hysteroscopic procedures in 257 patients. Fertil Steril 25:1267, 1976

7. Sugimoto O: Diagnostic and therapeutic hysteroscopy for traumatic intrauterine adhesions. Am J Obstet Gynecol 131:539, 1978

8. Taylor PJ, Cumming DC: Hysteroscopy in 100 patients. Fertil Steril 31:301, 1979

9. Valle RF: Hysteroscopy: Diagnostic and therapetic applications. J Reprod Med 20:115, 1978

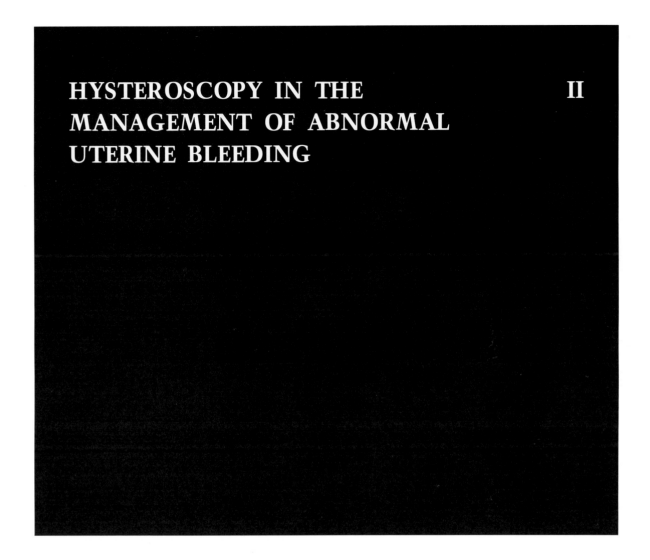

HYSTEROSCOPY IN THE MANAGEMENT OF ABNORMAL UTERINE BLEEDING

II

The authors in these seven chapters on abnormal uterine bleeding agree that hysteroscopy is not a substitute for tissue diagnosis, but hysteroscopic findings can augment the information available to the gynecologist. Hysteroscopy enables the physician to obtain a target or directed biopsy of a suspicious lesion, to remove clinically significant intrauterine tumors, and to repeat the hysteroscopic examination as a follow-up study of therapy. Curettage is indicated only if the hysteroscopic findings reveal an abnormality; otherwise, a simple random biopsy is probably sufficient.

All the authors (except Deutschmann and Lueken) use liquid media to distend the uterine cavity in patients selected for hysteroscopy. Even women 90 years of age tolerate the procedure without difficulty; general anesthesia is primarily used. Neuwirth and DeCherney decribe successful submucous myomectomy under hysteroscopic control without significant complications. Therapeutic hysteroscopy can be a difficult operation, and it is probably hazardous unless the physician is carefully trained and has had experience in diagnostic hysteroscopy. Patients must be carefully selected.

Hysteroscopic Diagnosis of Abnormal Uterine Bleeding: A Clinical Study ■

23

Mark W. Surrey
Sandra Aronberg

Abnormal uterine bleeding is a common problem, and an accurate diagnosis is essential because of the variety of causes, some of them serious. Dilatation and curettage has been used to evaluate this sign, but it finds the cause in less than 50% of patients, and many focal lesions are missed (see Chap. 26). Frequently the bleeding persists after curettage, so that a repeated curettage is required or eventually a hysterectomy, even in the absence of a definitive diagnosis. A better technique is needed to identify the cause of the bleeding. Hysteroscopy enables the physician to observe the endometrial cavity and to take a direct biopsy, thus improving accuracy of diagnosis.

MATERIALS AND METHODS

Over a 2-yr period, 110 hysteroscopies performed at the Cedars–Sinai Medical Center in Los Angeles were reviewed and represented 2% of the minor gynecologic operations done at the hospital. When hysteroscopy was initially performed at Cedars–Sinai the laparoscope was employed to see the uterine cavity. This technique did not allow adequate inspection. Then the cystoscope was used for resection and cauterization of endometrial polyps. Currently a standard hysteroscope is used. Most of the procedures were done using general anesthesia on an outpatient basis. Several distending media were used, including 5% and 10% dextrose and water, 32% dextran 70 (Hyskon), and, at present, carbon dioxide. Of the 110 hysteroscopies, 42 were performed for abnormal uterine bleeding and the remaining 68 for infertility.

RESULTS

The findings in the 42 patients who complained of abnormal uterine bleeding included endometrial polyps in 14, submucous myomas in 11, endometrial hyperplasia and endometrial adenocarcinoma in each of 2 patients, an intrauterine device (IUD) in 1 patient, and no abnormalities in 12 women. Five patients had major surgery immediately after the hysteroscopy, 3 had myomectomy, and 2 had hysterectomy; 68 operations were performed because of infertility, intrauterine adhesions were found in 3 patients, and 2 had submucous myomas. No complications occurred. The best observations were made using carbon dioxide.

COMMENT

Hysteroscopy can be performed in an office without discomfort to patients with a hysteroscope of small caliber, often without anesthesia. In this series, 70% of the patients who underwent hysteroscopy for abnormal uterine bleeding had intrauterine abnormalities seen with the hysteroscope. Curettage can miss even endometrial cancer in 10% of patients, and several studies have demonstrated the superiority of hysteroscopy over dilatation and curettage.[1-5] Nevertheless, a biopsy or directed curettage should be done with hysteroscopy if a lesion is suspected. Even if a standard hysteroscope is not available, the procedure can be performed with a cystoscope and provide important information. Less than 8% of hysteroscopies performed for infertility revealed a pathologic diagnosis. Therefore, hysteroscopy should be performed only in patients with a history of intrauterine instrumentation or infection as part of an infertility workup. In the evaluation of abnormal uterine bleeding, hysteroscopy is an important, underused aid. It should be performed in conjunction with curettage or biopsy for histopathologic diagnosis.

REFERENCES

1. Burnett JR Jr: Hysteroscopy-controlled curettage for endometrial polyps. Obstet Gynecol 24:621, 1964
2. Griff JJ: Hysteroscopy: An aid in gynecologic diagnosis. Obstet Gynecol 15:593, 1960
3. Mohr JW: Hysteroscopy as a diagnostic tool in postmenopausal bleeding. In Phillips JM (ed): Endoscopy in Gynecology, p 347. Downey, CA, American Association of Gynecologic Laparoscopists, 1977
4. Norment WB: The hysteroscope. Am J Obstet Gynecol 71:436, 1956
5. Valle RF: Hysteroscopic evaluation of patients with abnormal uterine bleeding. Surg Gynecol Obstet 153:521, 1981

Hysteroscopy in Abnormal Uterine Bleeding ■ 24

Santiago Dexeus
Ramon Labastida
Alfonso Arias

It should be unnecessary in 1982 to justify the importance of hysteroscopy for the gynecologist or the necessity for every well-equipped department of gynecology and obstetrics to have a hysteroscopic section. The aim of this chapter is to point out possibilities of that technique in metrorrhagia, the main indication for hysteroscopy.[1]

MATERIALS AND METHODS

We perform hysteroscopy on outpatients or on patients hospitalized for 1 day. General anesthesia is employed because hysteroscopy is followed by some surgical maneuver, generally curettage. The anesthesia is brief (always less than 30 min), and there is no need for prolonged postoperative medical supervision. Our hysteroscope was designed by Lindemann and Semm, with a 160-degree angle of vision. It is introduced with its sheath through the endocervical canal after previous aseptic precautions are observed. Initially 5% or 10% glucose solution was used, but we changed recently to a high-molecular-weight dextran 40. Its behavior is very similar to 32% dextran 70 (Hyskon). An assistant injects the solution slowly and continuously from a 50-ml syringe.

From April 1977 until July 1981, we performed 573 hysteroscopies. However, only the most recent 194 operations were analyzed because the previous procedures involved training to use the technique.

Abnormal uterine bleeding was the main indication (67.5%); 57.7% of patients had metrorrhagia (Table 24-1). Infertility was the next most frequent indication (20.6%). Sixty percent of patients examined for bleeding were over 46 yr, and the youngest woman was 28 yr. Menopausal patients constituted 65% of the explorations for bleeding, as shown in Table 24-2.

RESULTS

The hysteroscopic diagnosis was compared to the histologic findings from tissue obtained during the same exploration by direct curettage (Table 24-3). Only 8% of the women had normal cavities. Polyps were found at hysteroscopy in 22%, endometrial adenocarcinoma in 21%, and atrophic endometrium in 19%. The latter findings were confirmed histologically in 72% of patients. In one instance endometrial carcinoma was found in the curetting and missed at hysteroscopy because the endoscope could not be inserted into the cavity. Discrepancies between hysteroscopic and histologic findings occurred in 14 patients, as summarized in Table 24-4.

Table 24-1
HYSTEROSCOPIES ACCORDING TO INDICATIONS, 1980–1981 (18 MONTHS)

INDICATION	NO.	%
Intrauterine bleeding	131	67.51
Metrorrhagia*	112	57.73
Alterations of menstrual cycle	13	6.70
Diagnosis or control of hydatidiform mole	4	2.06
Postcoital bleeding	1	0.52
Bloody leukorrhea	1	0.52
Sterility and infertility of uterine origin	40	20.62
Sterility (primary and secondary)	20	10.31
Infertility (primary and secondary)	18	9.28
Sterility and metrorrhagia	2	1.03
Asymptomatic endometrial polyps (diagnosis and treatment)	13	6.70
Confirm doubtful myoma	4	2.06
"Lost" IUD	3	1.55
Dysmenorrhea	1	0.52
Hematometra	1	0.52
Secondary amenorrhea	1	0.52
Total	194	100

* Includes patients with adenocarcinoma, as much for study and classification as for control of nonsurgical treatment.

Table 24-2
AGE DISTRIBUTION* OF PATIENTS UNDERGOING HYSTEROSCOPY FOR METRORRHAGIA

AGE (YR)	NO.	%	CUMULATIVE
26–35	13	11.61	100
36–45	23	20.54	88.39
46–55	33	29.46	67.85
56–65	29	25.89	38.39
>66	14	12.50	12.50
Total	112	100	

* Youngest, 28 yr; eldest, 81 yr.

DISCUSSION

A rapid, correct diagnosis of the cause of uterine bleeding obviously results in earlier and better treatment. With cervical cytologic and colposcopic findings, the exocervical origin of any bleeding is eliminated.

The following diagnostic scheme is recommended (Fig. 24-1). If the patient is fertile, endometrial cytology is performed. If cytology is normal, the bleeding is ascribed to hormonal dysfunction, which may be treated hormonally or observed. If bleeding persists, hysteroscopy is performed. When hysteroscopy is normal, curettage is advisable; if hysteroscopy reveals atypical endometrial alterations, either fractionated or directed curettage is performed. In climacteric women with normal endometrial cytologic findings, we suggest a period of observation. If bleeding persists without clear medical cause, hysteroscopy is done, as is total direct and fractionated curettage, depending on hysteroscopic findings. If endometrial cytologic findings are abnormal, hysteroscopy is performed immediately.

Hysteroscopy is a visual method used to localize and to delineate macroscopic findings, but it never competes with a tissue diagnosis. On the contrary, these two techniques, one macroscopic and the other microscopic, are complementary and improve physicians' access to information. Hysteroscopy can locate abnormalities that are easily overlooked by conventional curettage or even by hysterosalpingography.

Direct observation of a submucous myoma is most helpful (Fig. 24-2). Even if a myoma is suspected during curettage, hysteroscopy establishes its localization and configuration and the possibility of removing it under endoscopic control. Likewise, hysteroscopy facilitates the diagnosis and removal of endometrial polyps using a modified Yglesias ureteral resector according to the technique developed by Neuwirth (Fig. 24-3).[2] It is not infrequent, in a patient who has had a cesarean section, to find small retention cysts in the uterine scar (Fig. 24-4). Atrophic endometrium should be suspected if endometrium is not obtained by curettage. Hysteroscopy can verify the existence of atrophy and also locate small proliferations in any area that could have been overlooked with simple curettage.

Hysteroscopy is invaluable for the study of the topography of endometrial carcinoma in ascertaining the origin, extension, uterine size, endocervical involvement, localization, and macroscopic or microscopic spread to the endocervix. Clinically, it is frequently impossible to ascertain the endocervical or endometrial

Table 24-3
HYSTEROSCOPIC AND HISTOLOGIC FINDINGS (112 EXPLORATIONS FOR UTERINE BLEEDING)

HYSTEROSCOPY \ HISTOLOGY	PROLIFERATIVE ENDOMETRIUM	SECRETORY ENDOMETRIUM	ENDOMETRIAL HYPOPLASIA	ATROPHY	ENDOMETRIAL HYPERPLASIA	ADENOCARCINOMA	BENIGN POLYP	MYOMA	INSUFFICIENT MATERIAL	INCOMPLETE ABORTIONS	TOTAL No.	%
Normal	6		2	1							9	8.04
Hypoplastic endometrium			5						1		6	5.36
Atrophic endometrium	2		9	10					1		22	19.64
Hyperplasic endometrium	2	3	1		16						22	19.64
Adenocarcinoma					1	23					24	21.43
Polyp					1		23	1			25	22.32
Intracavitary myoma							1	1			2	1.79
Incomplete abortion										1	1	0.89
Failed hysteroscopy					1						1	0.89
No.	10	3	17	11	18	24	24	2	2	1	112	100
Total %	8.93	2.68	15.18	9.82	16.07	21.43	21.43	1.79	1.79	0.89		

Table 24-4
DISCREPANCIES BETWEEN HISTEROSCOPIC AND HISTOLOGIC FINDINGS (112 EXPLORATIONS FOR UTERINE BLEEDING)

HYSTEROSCOPY \ HISTOLOGY	PROLIFERATIVE ENDOMETRIUM	SECRETORY ENDOMETRIUM	ENDOMETRIAL HYPOPLASIA	ATROPHY	ENDOMETRIAL HYPERPLASIA	BENIGN POLYP	MYOMA	TOTAL
Normal			2	1				3
Atrophic endometrium	2							2
Hyperplasic endometrium	2	2	1					5
Adenocarcinoma					1			1
Polyp					1		1	2
Intracavitary myoma						1		1
Total	4	2	3	1	2	1	1	14

origin of adenocarcinoma. Hysteroscopy either shows the entire uterine cavity free of neoplasia in endocervical tumors or its occupation in tumors of endometrial origin. When endometrial carcinoma is limited to a small area or where an endometrial polyp undergoes carcinomatous change, hysteroscopy enables an adequate classification. It locates the area in question for directed biopsy or curettage. According to the International Federation of Gynecology and Obstetrics (FIGO) classification stage II is an endometrial carcinoma affecting the endocervical canal, and until hysteroscopy was introduced, the correct classification was based on the findings from a fractioned curettage. Hysteroscopy represents a decisive aid in the study of the extension of endometrial carcinoma and offers the possibility of a directed biopsy in suspicious endocervical zones.[3,4] Many fractionated curettages tend to go beyond the canal, so that precise limits of the tumor cannot be delineated by histologic findings.[5]

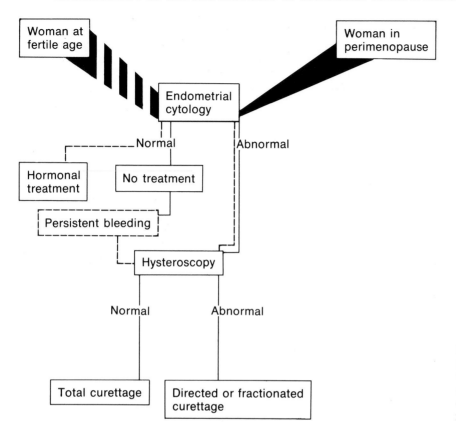

FIG. 24-1. Management of uterine bleeding for cervical cytology and colposcopy and for differential diagnosis of cervical abnormalities.

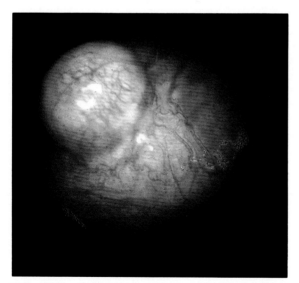

FIG. 24-2. Submucous myoma shows numerous fine vessels on its surface.

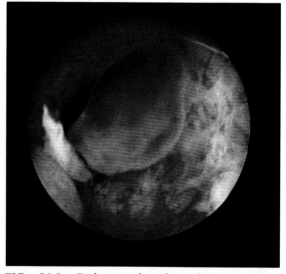

FIG. 24-3. Endometrial polyps being removed under hysteroscopic control.

The factors limiting the reliability of fractionated curettage are as follows:

It is not a routine procedure.

It is not always performed by an oncologic gynecologist.

It frequently passes the canal and confounds classification of the carcinoma.

The canal may be contaminated by intrauterine material.

Findings may vary considerably.

Curettage may not reach the cancer focus.

The size of the cavity (8 cm), which marks the dividing line between stage Ia and Ib of endometrial carcinoma, is measured by hysterometry. This simple procedure is subject to the following errors: intracavitary myomas, big submucous myomas, intrauterine adhesions, bicornuate or malformed uterus, marked retroflexion or anteflexion, forgotten bimanual exploration, and the operator's inexperience. All these mistakes are avoidable with hysteroscopy.

Hysteroscopy is useful for an intrauterine "second look" in patients with advanced carcinoma who cannot be treated surgically and undergo radiation therapy. It is also useful to extract radium capsules "lost" in the uterine cavity. With microcolpohysteroscopy at ×150 magnification, the cellular patterns can be studied *in situ*.

In comparing the tissue diagnosis and hysteroscopy (see Table 24-4), consider the false-positive diagnoses made by hysteroscopy. The configuration of an endometrial adenocarcinoma can be flat and have regular vascularization; it can thus be confused with endometrial "paving." Although it is possible to make a false-positive diagnosis, it is rare to miss a lesion on hysteroscopic examination. Confusion between endometrial polyposis and polypoid hyperplasia is an error of little importance and is difficult to avoid. Myomas should be readily distinguished from endometrial polyps because of the differences in consistency, color, and shape. With experience, the different physiologic stages of the endometrium can be recognized through the hysteroscope.

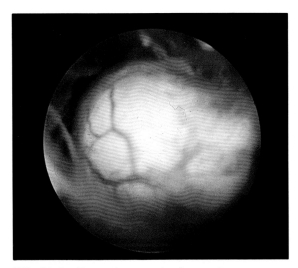

FIG. 24-4.   Retention cyst in the uterine scar.

CONCLUSION

Hysteroscopy is a perfected curettage and, in a certain way, a curettage that "sees and decides"—"sees" because the uterine cavity is observed and can be described, and "decides" because hysteroscopy can direct the biopsy or curettage to the area in question. Hysteroscopy is a simple and inexpensive technique with minimal risk and is accurate in 85% of observations. It adds to the findings of hysterosalpingograms and curettage and is indispensable in the differential diagnosis of metrorrhagia. It appears essential to the study and classification of endometrial carcinoma.

REFERENCES

1. Dexeus S, Labastida R, Galera L: Oncological indications of hysteroscopy. Eur J Gynaecol Oncol 2:61, 1981
2. Neuwirth RS: Hysteroscopy. Philadelphia, W B Saunders, 1975
3. Sugimoto O: Hysteroscopic diagnosis of endometrial carcinoma. A report of fifty-three cases examined at the Women's Clinic at the Kyoto University Hospital. Am J Obstet Gynecol 121:105, 1975
4. Valente S, Marcolin D: L'isteroscopia nella pratica clinica. Padua, SEMES, 1980
5. Word B, Gravlee LC, Wideman GL: The fallacy of simple uterine curettage. Obstet Gynecol 12:642, 1958

Hysteroscopy in the Management of Abnormal Uterine Bleeding in 199 Patients ■

25

Kees Wamsteker

Abnormal uterine bleeding is a frequent complaint of the gynecologic patient. Hysteroscopy in the management of that disorder has not been fully evaluated. From several studies it is clear that polyps and submucous fibroids are frequently undetected by curettage alone.[1-3,5,6] With hysteroscopy the entire uterine cavity can be seen, biopsies taken under visual control, and intrauterine tumors removed with special instruments. The results of hysteroscopy were compared with findings at dilatation and curettage in women who complained of abnormal uterine bleeding.

MATERIALS AND METHODS

At the Mariastichting in Haarlem and the Women's Clinic of the University Hospital in Leiden, The Netherlands, hysteroscopic examinations were attempted in 205 patients with abnormal uterine bleeding. Of these, 146 were premenopausal and 59 were postmenopausal. In 196 women dilatation and curettage was performed after the hysteroscopic procedure. In two patients only hysteroscopic biopsies were taken; in seven others who had normal findings at hysteroscopy, no tissue was removed for histologic examination. General anesthesia

was used in 177 operations, and in 28 others the procedure was performed under local anesthesia with a paracervical block (8 ml of 1% lidocaine in each uterosacral ligament). I used a 5-mm hysteroscope* with 32% dextran 70 (Hyskon) to distend the uterine cavity (Fig. 25-1). A rigid biopsy forceps could be introduced into the uterine cavity along the hysteroscope sheath. The 7-mm hysteroscope was also used but was unsatisfactory because of the too-easy flow of dextran 70 through the hysteroscope channel. When dextran 70 is used, the instruments must be washed in hot water with a detergent immediately after the procedure.

RESULTS

Intrauterine observation was accomplished easily in all but 6 women, and hysteroscopic diagnoses were made in the remaining 199 patients (Table 25-1). In 85 patients no abnormalities were seen; 20 patients had atrophic endometrium. Intrauterine tumors were found in 67 instances; endometrial hyperplasia, in 25 patients. In four patients the intrauterine lesion

* Storz, Tuttlingen, West Germany.

128

could not be classified. The hysteroscopic diagnosis was compared with histologic findings in 198 patients. There were few discrepancies among 80 patients whose uterine cavity and endometrium appeared normal on hysteroscopy; 1 had an atrophic endometrium histologically. Of 18 patients with hysteroscopic diagnoses of atrophic endometrium, 3 were found to have normal, irregular, or proliferative endometria on histologic examination. In 39, the hysteroscopic diagnosis of endometrial polyp (Figs. 25-2 to 25-4) was made, but these observations were not demonstrated histologically in 6 patients. Polyps were not always removed by curettage. After removal of polyps under visual control or reinspection of the uterine cavity after curettage to check for their removal, histologic examination showed polypoid tissue in all patients. Of 25 patients with hysteroscopic diagnoses of endometrial hyperplasia (Fig. 25-5), 7 showed proliferative endometrium histologically. Sixteen had hyperplastic endometrium, and two had focal endometrial adenocarcinoma. Endometrial adenocarcinoma was seen hysteroscopically in 12 and confirmed with histology in 9 instances. One patient had atypical adenomatous hyperplasia (Fig. 25-6), one had hyperplastic endometrium, and one had an endometrial polyp. The carcinoma was whitish or yellow with tortuous varicose vessels on the surface (Figs. 25-7 to 25-9). The extension of the carcinoma

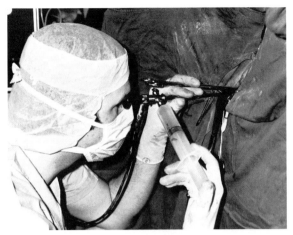

FIG. 25-1. Hysteroscopy in progress with the 5-mm Storz hysteroscope. Dextran 70 (Hyskon) is injected manually.

toward the internal os could be seen (Fig. 25-10). Submucous fibroids were seen with hysteroscopy in 16 patients, showing typical stretched vessels on the surface, but curettage missed them in 6 instances (Fig. 25-11).

CONCLUSION

Hysteroscopy is indispensable for the diagnosis of intrauterine tumors in women with abnormal uterine bleeding. Polyps and submucous fibroids are often missed by curettage alone. Moreover, the intrauterine extent of endometrial carcinoma can be delineated exactly.[4] It is a method for diagnosis and treatment of intrauterine abnormalities on an outpatient basis under local anesthesia. In case there is an intrauterine pathologic condition, histologic examination is always necessary to evaluate the hysteroscopic diagnosis. Endometrial polyps can be removed with a biopsy forceps under direct vision or with a curette after hysteroscopic localization. Reinspection of the uterine cavity is necessary to ensure complete removal. Without hysteroscopic verification, even very large polyps can be missed completely or removed only partially. For diagnosis of submucous fibroids, hysteroscopy is superior to other diagnostic methods.

Table 25-1
HYSTEROSCOPIC DIAGNOSIS IN 199 PATIENTS WITH ABNORMAL UTERINE BLEEDING

HYSTEROSCOPIC DIAGNOSIS	NO.	%
No abnormality	85	41.5
Endometrial polyp	39	19.0
Endometrial hyperplasia	25	12.2
Atrophic endometrium	20	9.8
Submucous fibroid	16	7.8
Endometrial adenocarcinoma	12	5.9
Adhesions	3	1.5
Placental remnants	1	0.4
No classification	4	1.9
Total	205*	100

* Six patients had two diagnoses.

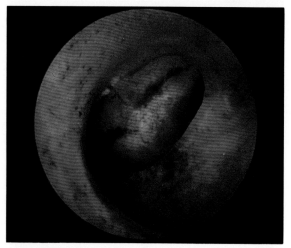

FIG. 25-2. Endometrial polyp.

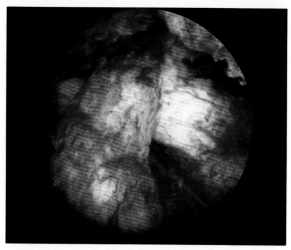

FIG. 25-5. Atypical adenomatous endometrial hyperplasia.

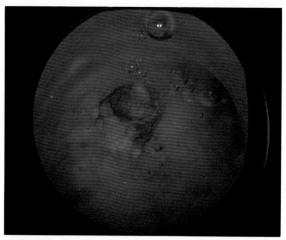

FIG. 25-3. Atypical endometrial polyp and atrophic endometrium.

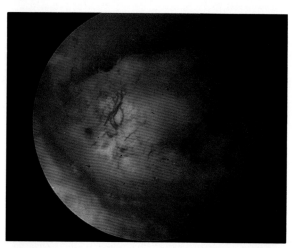

FIG. 25-6. Detail of atypical adenomatous endometrial hyperplasia mistaken for focal carcinoma.

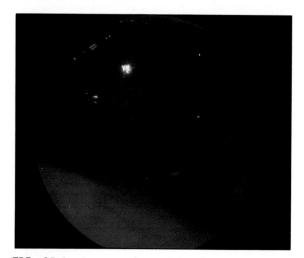

FIG. 25-4. Large endometrial polyp was missed with curettage.

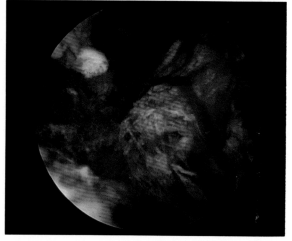

FIG. 25-7. Endometrial adenocarcinoma.

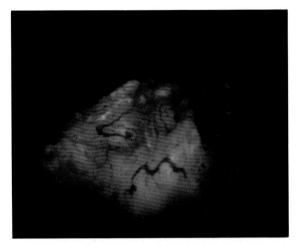

FIG. 25-8. Endometrial adenocarcinoma has typical whitish and yellow tissue with tortuous varicose vessels.

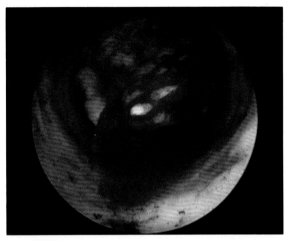

FIG. 25-10. Endometrial carcinoma. No extension to the internal cervical os is seen.

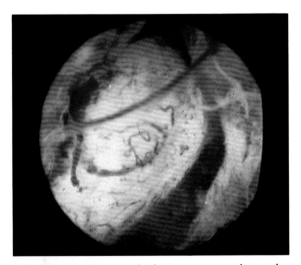

FIG. 25-9. Endometrial adenocarcinoma shows the typical tortuous vessels on the surface.

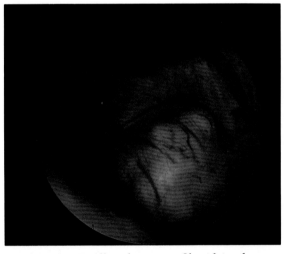

FIG. 25-11. Small, submucous fibroid in the cornual area with typical stretched vessels was missed with curettage.

REFERENCES

1. Burnett JE Jr: Hysteroscopy-controlled currettage for endometrial polyps. Obstet Gynecol 24:621, 1964
2. Englund F, Ingelmann-Sundberg A, Westin B: Hysteroscopy in diagnosis and treatment of uterine bleeding. Gynaecologia 143:217, 1957
3. Siegler AM, Kemmann EK, Gentile GP: Hysteroscopic procedures in 257 patients. Fertil Steril 27:1267, 1976
4. Sugimoto O: Hysteroscopic diagnosis of endometrial carcinoma. Am J Obstet Gynecol 121:105, 1975
5. Wamsteker K: Hysteroscopie. Thesis, Women's Clinic of the University Hospital, Leiden, Holland, 1977
6. Word B, Gravlee LC, Wideman GL: The fallacy of simple uterine curettage. Obstet Gynecol 12:642, 1958

26

Hysteroscopic Findings in Postmenopausal Bleeding ■

Christian Deutschmann
Rolf Peter Lueken

MATERIALS AND METHODS

From 1976 to 1981 we performed 853 hysteroscopic examinations because of perimenopausal and postmenopausal bleeding. Patients' ages ranged from 45 to 90 years. Carbon dioxide was used to distend the uterine cavity. Patients were referred because of persistent bleeding. Endoscopy was followed by curettage.[2,5] The combined operation is useful for making accurate diagnosis possible.[4,6,9] Even a trained gynecologist curettes at best 70% to 80% of the endometrium. Two of five possible endometrial areas remain unexplored, and an even greater failure rate of 36% has been described.[1] Hysteroscopic findings correlate highly with histologic results and are considered a basic method for further examination and diagnostic procedure.[7]

RESULTS

In 557 (65.3%) patients, no pathologic findings were noted. The hysteroscopic view of the normal cavity showed a proliferative or atrophic endometrium and bleeding vessels. The histologic findings correlated in all patients with these hysteroscopic findings and were taken from the proliferative stage in 34% of patients, secretory phase in 8%, disordered perimenopausal endometrium in 23.7%, insufficient luteal phase in 15.4%, nonspecific endometritis in 12.7%, and atrophy in 6.2%.

In 296 patients (34.7%), pathologic changes were obvious (Table 26-1). A polypoid endometrium was seen without evidence of solitary polyps in 118 women (40%). In each instance several biopsies were taken before curettage. In 54%, cystic hyperplasia was seen; it occurred most often in women aged 45 to 55 years (Table 26-2). An unphysiologic polypoid proliferation after hormonal treatment occurred with a frequency of 25.4% (mostly in women aged 55 to 90). Atypical hyperplasia (20%) occurred exclusively in the late postmenopausal phase. Atypical hyperplasia is considered precancerous, and hysterectomy was performed in each instance.

Polyps were observed in 29% of patients with abnormal hysteroscopic findings, recognized by their typical red yellow surface and tortuous vessels. Cervical and endometrial polyps occurred almost in the same frequency in each age group. We were able to cut and remove the polyps totally. Women aged 55 to 90 were affected 4 times more frequently. Cystic endometrial polyps (16 women) were described exclusively in the older age group.

In 67 women (23%) submucous myomas

were seen. Biopsy done before curettage confirmed the hysteroscopic diagnosis. Pedunculated myomas were cut and removed. In 25 patients (8.4%), hysteroscopic examination suggested endometrial adenocarcinoma. All the women except two belonged to the high-risk group and were aged 52 to 87 years. In 23 of the 25 women, biopsy and curettings confirmed the diagnosis. Curettings were negative, while biopsy specimens showed malignancy in one instance. In the other patient, the biopsy specimen showed cystic hyperplasia and the curettings revealed atypical hyperplasia. Hysterectomy revealed a small, circumscribed, endometrial adenocarcinoma without myometrial infiltration.

The high incidence of positive histologic findings has resulted from direct curettage after hysteroscopic detection of the areas in question.[3,8] Hysteroscopy is an improvement of diagnostic and therapeutic techniques in gynecology. Too often a dilatation and curettage fails to detect the source of bleeding, thus subjecting the patient to a disappointing diagnostic procedure. One such woman, aged 53 years, was transferred to us from another hospital because of heavy uterine bleeding. Two years previously she had been curetted twice,

Table 26-1

HYSTEROSCOPIC FINDINGS IN 853 PATIENTS WITH PERIMENOPAUSAL AND POSTMENOPAUSAL BLEEDING*

FINDING AND NO. OF PATIENTS	PATIENT AGE	
	Peri-menopausal, 45–55 yr	Post-menopausal, 55 yr and older
Normal (557)	405	152
Polyposis (118)	36	82
Polyps (86)	18	68
Myomas (67)	56	11
Possible carcinoma (25)	1	24

* Total number of pathologic findings was 296 (34.7%).

Table 26-2

HISTOLOGIC VERIFICATION IN 118 PATIENTS OF THE HYSTEROSCOPIC FINDING OF POLYPOSIS

HISTOLOGIC VERIFICATION	PATIENT AGE	
	45–55 yr	55 yr and older
Cystic hyperplasia	36	28
Polypoid proliferation	4	26
Atypical hyperplasia		24

FIG. 26-1. Hysterogram shows multiple defects that correspond with pedunculated submucous myomas.

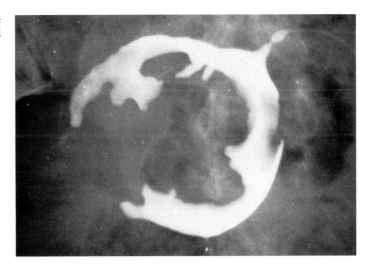

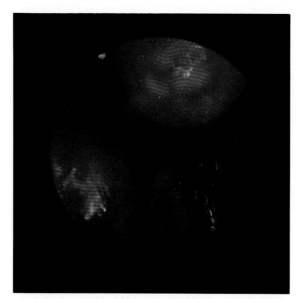

FIG. 26-2. Hysteroscopic view shows multiple pedunculated myomas in the uterine cavity.

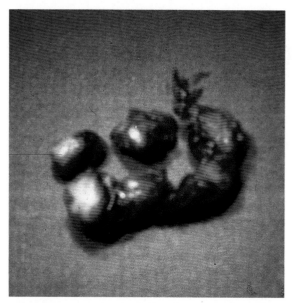

FIG. 26-3. Some pedunculated myomas have been cut and removed from the uterine cavity.

and metrorrhagia had reappeared. In January 1981 another curettage was performed, followed by hormonal treatment. After weeks of remission, abnormal bleeding recurred. Another curettage was performed, and 3 liters of blood were transfused because of severe anemia. Histologic examination revealed some fibromuscular tissue. Hysterosalpingography was done 2 wk later (Fig. 26-1). Hysteroscopic investigation revealed multiple, pedunculated myomas (Fig. 26-2). The myomas were cut and removed entirely, and histologic examination confirmed the diagnosis (Fig. 26-3). A Lippes loop was inserted, and 10 mg of estradiol (Progynon) was given intramuscularly. No more abnormal bleeding occurred, and the patient was instructed to return for "second-look" hysteroscopy.

REFERENCES

1. Englund F, Ingelman-Sundberg A, Westin B: Hysteroscopy in diagnosis and treatment of uterine bleeding. Gynaecologia 143:217, 1957
2. Hepp H: Diagnostics in hysteroscopy. Endoscoy 10:232, 1978
3. Joelsson I, Levine RU, Moberger G: Hysteroscopy as an adjunct in determining the extent of carcinoma of the endometrium. Am J Obstet Gynecol 111:696, 1971
4. Lindemann HJ, Mohr J: CO_2 hysteroscopy: Diagnosis and treatment. Am J Obstet Gynecol 124:129, 1976
5. Lübke F: Über den diagnostischen Wert der Hysteroskopie. Arch Gynaekol 219:255, 1975
6. Mohr J: Hysteroscopy as a diagnostic tool in postmenopausal bleeding. In Phillips JM (ed): Endoscopy in Gynecology. Downey, CA, American Association of Gynecologic Laparoscopists, 1977
7. Mohr J, Lindemann HJ: Vergleichende Resultate zwischen CO_2-Hysteroskopie, Hysterosalpingographie und Histologie. Arch Gynaekol 219:256, 1975
8. Sugimoto O: Hysteroscopic diagnosis of endometrial carcinoma. A report of fifty-three cases examined at the Women's Clinic of Kyoto University Hospital. Am J Obstet Gynecol 121:105, 1975
9. Valle RF, Sciarra JJ: Hysteroscopy: A useful diagnostic adjunct in gynecology. Am J Obstet Gynecol 122:230, 1975

Hysteroscopic Resection of Submucous Fibroids ■ 27

Robert S. Neuwirth

The submucous fibroid is a debilitating manifestation of the most frequent pelvic tumor of women, leiomyoma uteri. Although not all submucous fibroids cause menorrhagia, they are a common finding in a woman with a myomatous uterus who is complaining of a progressively heavy menstrual flow. Indeed, the tumor often produces secondary anemia. Traditionally the diagnosis is established by hysterography or curettage. Both of these techniques give false-positive and false-negative results. The hysterogram and curet may miss a submucous fibroid. The classic management of this lesion is myomectomy or hysterectomy by the abdominal or vaginal route. Rarely, transvaginal or transcervical myomectomy is performed.

Hysteroscopy introduces a more precise diagnostic technique and provides the visual control for a transcervical, total excision of the pedunculated variety and partial resection of the sessile type of fibroid. This chapter will outline methods, equipment, indications, contraindications, risks, and experiences with the hysteroscopic approach to submucous fibroids.

INDICATIONS AND CONTRAINDICATIONS

The indications for submucous myomectomy by hysteroscopic resection include menorrhagia, normal ovarian function or failure of progestins to correct bleeding associated with anovulation in the presence of a submucous fibroid, and the patient's desire to preserve the uterus. The contraindications are a large pelvic mass or an adnexal tumor, a uterine cavity 10 cm or more, malignant or premalignant endometrial tissue, and the patient's refusal to accept possible hysterectomy. The diagnosis may be suspected by history, curettage, or hysterogram but must be confirmed at hysteroscopy.

MATERIALS AND METHODS

To proceed, inject dextran 70 (Hyskon) from 50-ml syringes into the hysteroscope cannula. The use of sterile, plastic blood bags preloaded with dextran 70 in the operating room avoids the interruption of flow that occurs with the 50-ml syringe is changed. Use the standard foroblique telescope in a urologic resectoscope sheath (Fig. 27-1). Use an electrosurgical current of 50 watts for the cutting loop.

Once the fibroid is located, define its margins. If it is pedunculated, concomitant laparoscopy may be avoided. However, if the pedicle is broad or the tumor is sessile, perform laparoscopy for visual control and to separate the intestine from the uterus by pneumoperitoneum or instrumental manipulation.

Perform the resection in an orderly, progressive fashion (Fig. 27-2). If the tumor is

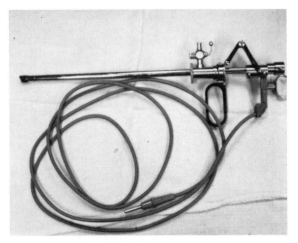

FIG. 27-1. Instrument used for submucous myomectomy.

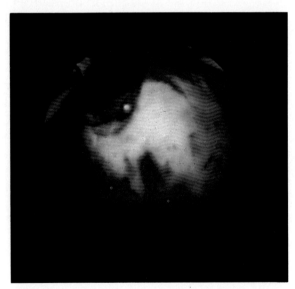

FIG. 27-2. Submucous myoma being resected.

pedunculated, reduce the mass so that it can pass through the cervix and then cut or twist off the pedicle. If the tumor is sessile, shave down the mass as close as possible to the level of the adjacent endometrial cavity. Remove fragments of tissue during the procedure to maintain a good view. Once the procedure is completed (Fig. 27-3), a Silastic rubber balloon

is usually inserted into the uterus and inflated to tamponade the raw surface (Fig. 27-4). Remove the balloon on the second postoperative morning; if there is no bleeding, discharge the patient on that day or on the following morning with advice to avoid coitus for 1 mo and to increase activities and diet as tolerated. A 24-hr antibiotic course is used prophylactically in the perioperative period, and estrogens are given for 10 days postoperatively.

The risks of the procedure are infection, hemorrhage, and uterine perforation. I have had no cases of perforation. A patient with an infection that occurred 1 mo postoperatively was treated with antibiotics for several days. One patient developed a hemorrhage 2 wk later and underwent a hysterectomy elsewhere because of an incompletely excised submucous fibroid.

RESULTS

I have used the technique described above for 4 yr. Twenty-eight patients have had the procedure. The longest hospitalization was 3 days. Two patients were lost to follow-up study. Five patients underwent subsequent hysterectomy, but in two women no submucous tumors were found. Two patients had repeat hysteroscopic

Table 27-1
RESULTS OF HYSTEROSCOPIC SUBMUCOUS MYOMECTOMY IN 28 PATIENTS

OUTCOME	NO. OF PATIENTS
Followed and cured	19
Not followed	2
Underwent subsequent hysterectomy	5
2 wk	(1)
5 mo	(1)
2 yr	(2)
3 yr	(1)
Underwent repeat hysteroscopic submucous myomectomy	2
3 yr	(1)
4 yr	(1)

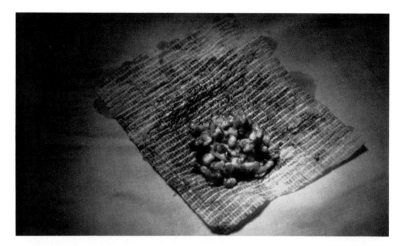

FIG. 27-3.   Morcellated specimen.

FIG. 27-4.   Intrauterine balloon.

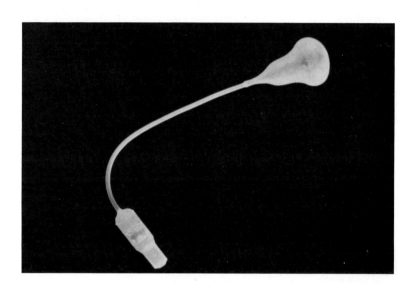

myomectomies and are doing well. Therefore, 80% of the patients have retained their uterus and are doing well (Table 27-1). Most of the patients were over 35 years of age.

Patients with pedunculated myomas have become pregnant after operation, and they have had vaginal deliveries. One patient became pregnant after partial resection of a sessile fibroid but underwent a voluntary termination of the pregnancy.

COMMENT

Although the overall results with this technique have been satisfactory, the procedure must be evaluated further before its general use can be assessed. It is not an operation for the neophyte endoscopist, but physicians with experience in hysteroscopy and laparoscopy can use the procedure in properly selected situations.

Treatment of Irregular Menstrual Bleeding by Hysteroscopic Resection of Submucous Myomas and Polyps ■

28

Alan H. DeCherney

Treatment of the reproductive-aged patient with irregular menses is a challenge to the gynecologist. Empirical therapy with gonadal steroids has been employed, and, if unsuccessful, then diagnostic and therapeutic procedures such as dilatation and curettage were used. With the advent of new technology, the cause of abnormal uterine bleeding can be more precisely ascertained and selectivity treated.[7]

MATERIALS AND METHODS

Fourteen patients with abnormal, nonendocrinologic uterine bleeding for more than 4 mo were evaluated at the Yale–New Haven Hospital. No patients with postmenopausal bleeding or endometrial hyperplasia were included; ages ranged from 31 to 44 years. Patients underwent a preoperative endometrial biopsy, hysterosalpingogram, and hysteroscopy.

Under general anesthesia, laparoscopic and concomitant hysteroscopic examinations were performed. Less than 100 ml of dextran 70 (Hyskon) was used for hysteroscopy. A nonmodified urologic cystoscope, 24 French (8 mm) with only 1 valve and a 70-degree lens system, was used in conjunction with an Aspen electrocautery unit* with approximately 30 watts

* Aspen Laboratories, Littleton, CO.

of cutting current and a wire loop (Fig. 28-1). Patients were managed in the ambulatory surgical unit and discharged approximately 4 to 6 hr after surgery. Curettage was done on all patients after endoscopic evaluation and treatment. Patients were given ampicillin, 500 mg 4 times a day, 24 hr preoperatively and 4 hr postoperatively. Conjugated estrogen, 5 mg, was prescribed daily for 30 days postoperatively.

RESULTS

On preoperative endometrial biopsy, nine patients had secretory endometrium, and five others had the proliferative type. At surgery, eight patients had submucous myomas (six solitary and two multiple) and six others had polyps. All lesions were removed with the cystoscopic–resectoscope without any significant sequelae. Biopsies were obtained on all lesions to rule out malignancy. Four patients required an intrauterine 5-ml Foley catheter for less than 6 hr to control bleeding.

Hysterographic findings of an intracavitary defect were confirmed in all 14 women by hysteroscopy, although it was impossible to ascertain whether the lesion was a submucous myoma or a polyp from the radiologic study. No patient had a postoperative hysterosalpin-

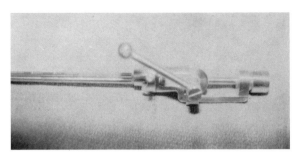

FIG. 28-1. Aspen electrocautery unit.

gogram or hysteroscopy, because irregular uterine bleeding did not recur after a minimum of 1 yr of follow-up study. No postoperative complications were noted.

DISCUSSION

The occurrence of irregular menses in women with normal-sized uteri can be a perplexing problem. Is the uterus dysfunctional or anovulatory? Is there an intracavitary lesion? After excluding endocrinologic causes, hysterosalpingography is indicated to search for intracavitary defects; suspicious findings should be followed by hysteroscopy. Should all patients with irregular menses have hysteroscopy? Although all the women mentioned above had radiographic defects confirmed by hysteroscopy, other workers have not made similar observations.[1,5,8] Valle and Sciarra noted that approximately 57% of their patients with abnormal findings on hysterograms showed abnormalities at hysteroscopy, and approximately 50% of patients evaluated for infertility had pathologic findings on endoscopy.[6,9] In addition, Valle and Sciarra found that 31% of premenopausal women evaluated hysteroscopically for abnormal bleeding had an intracavitary lesion.[8]

Neuwirth treated patients with submucous myomas under hysteroscopic control with good results, his technique being similar to mine.[4] He avoided sessile lesions, and on follow-up hysteroscopy he found excellent healing. Goldrath and co-workers suggested a neodymium-Yag laser for treating such patients.[2] Other authors attempted removal of intrauterine lesions with the resectoscope and reported good results.[1,3,5,8,9]

REFERENCES

1. Edström KGB: Intrauterine surgical procedures during hysteroscopy. Endoscopy 6:175, 1974
2. Goldrath MH, Fuller TA, Segal S: Laser photovaporization of endometrium for the treatment of menorrhagia. Am J Obstet Gynecol 140:14, 1981
3. Haning RV Jr, Harkins PG, Uehling DT: Preservation of fertility by transcervical resection of a benign mesodermal uterine tumor with a resectoscope and glycine distending medium. Fertil Steril 33:209, 1980
4. Neuwirth RS: A new technique for and additional experience with hysteroscopic resection of submucous fibroids. Am J Obstet Gynecol 131:91, 1978
5. Siegler AM, Kemmann EK: Hysteroscopy. Obstet Gynecol Surv 30:567, 1975
6. Valle RF: Hysteroscopy in the evaluation of female infertility. Am J Obstet Gynecol 137:425, 1980
7. Valle RF: Hysteroscopic evaluation of patients with abnormal uterine bleeding. Surg Gynecol Obstet 153:521, 1981
8. Valle RF, Sciarra JJ: Hysteroscopy: A useful adjunct in gynecology. Am J Obstet Gynecol 122:230, 1975
9. Valle RF, Sciarra JJ: Current status of hysteroscopy in gynecologic practice. Fertil Steril 32:619, 1979

The Management of Intractable Uterine Bleeding 29
Utilizing the Cystoscopic Resectoscope ∎

Alan H. DeCherney
Ina Cholst
Frederick Naftolin

Patients with intractable uterine bleeding present a challenge to the physician that has been met in the past with various techniques, including the use of gonadal steroids, intravenous (IV) conjugated estrogens, radiation therapy, cryosurgery, selective arterial embolization, chemical agents, and recently the neodymium-Yag Laser.[1-3,5-8] All these techniques have variable success. Some are dangerous, others are temporarily helpful, and most require prolonged, repeated treatments. To solve the problem, we have successfully used the cystoscopic resectoscope* in hysteroscopy to control intractable uterine bleeding.

MATERIALS AND METHODS

Eleven patients were evaluated at the Yale–New Haven Hospital for intractable uterine bleeding during 18 mo ending August 1981. None responded to IV conjugated estrogen therapy (25 mg) or to sequential gonadal steroids. Three patients had leukemia, six patients were extreme anesthestic risks, and two patients refused hysterectomy. The patients with leukemia had profound coagulation defects. The six patients who were poor anesthestic risks included four severe alcoholics and

two drug addicts. No malignancy was found in preoperative endometrial biopsy specimens. An unmodified American Cystoscope urologic resectoscope, 24 French and 8 mm, was inserted to the level of the cervical os. Dextran 70 (Hyskon) was used to distend the uterine cavity, and in no patient was more than 100 ml instilled. The entire endometrium was cauterized with a coagulating electric current at 30 watts from an Aspen electrocoagulation apparatus.† Satisfactory cauterization was obtained by moving the resectoscope in addition to the wire loop and its handle mechanism. Diazepam or ketamine and occasionally supplemental nitrous oxide and oxygen were used for analgesia. Patients' ages ranged from 14 to 39 years. Vaginal bleeding had persisted for as long as 1 mo or as short as 48 hr before the procedure, and it varied in severity. Preoperatively, patients had hematocrits between 27% and 33%, but all the women required blood transfusions before the procedure. None had specific intrauterine lesions at hysteroscopy; endometria appeared pink to yellow. Preoperative biopsies showed nine proliferative, one atrophic, and one secretory endometrium and no evidence of endometrial hyperplasia. The procedure was not done within 72 hr of any exogenous hormonal therapy.

---

* American Cystoscope Maker, Inc. Stamford, CT.

† Aspen Laboratories, Littleton, CO.

RESULTS

The procedure required 30 min or less. Three patients needed a temporary (≤6 hr) tamponade with a 5 ml intrauterine Foley catheter bag. There were no long- or short-term sequelae. Follow-up study was done on all patients. Two of the three patients with leukemia died within 3 mo after surgery but no longer had severe uterine bleeding. Postmortem examination of the uterus showed endometrial hyalinization and fibrosis. The remaining nine patients were followed from 6 to 18 mo; 6 remained amenorrheic and 3 had occasional, light spotting. No postoperative hysterosalpingograms were obtained.

DISCUSSION

Refractory uterine bleeding presents patients and their physicians with a distinct quandary. Because these women are often critically ill, they do not respond to usual hormonal treatment, and often no specific or localized lesion is present. Resectoscopic desiccation of the entire endometrium represents a safe solution to this problem.

Experimental efforts have been made in both laboratory animals and women to ablate the entire endometrium. Droegemuller and colleagues used a freon probe in 16 women.[2] In 10 patients amenorrhea persisted until hysterectomy, 8 wk after treatment. Examination of the extirpated uteri showed regeneration of endometrial tissue in the cornua. During the freezing process, cramping occurred but no untoward effects were noted. In a subsequent study, the same authors reported on the effects of nitrous oxide with a freezing point of −88.5 C as opposed to −39.8 C for freon.[1] It caused more widespread endometrial destruction in 11 patients. Schenker and Polishuk treated rabbits similarly but found endometrial regeneration 21 to 30 days postoperatively.[5] They reported endometrial ablation in rabbits treated with 10% formalin.

Schwartz and associates performed selective arterial embolization to control refractory uterine bleeding, but the procedure was prolonged and required experienced personnel.[7] Recent work by Goldrath and coauthors showed the feasibility of endometrial photocoagulation with the neodymium-Yag laser.[3] The uterus is ideal for this technique because of the protective effect of the relatively thick myometrium. Their patients were sterilized before the procedure to decrease the amount of dextran 70 introduced into the peritoneal cavity. The patients also received perioperative danazol to reduce endometrial thickness and debris. The resectoscopic technique has been used to treat submucous myomas successfully under laparoscopic control.[8] No concomitant laparoscopy was used in this series because of severe illness in these women.

CONCLUSION

Resectoscopic endometrial ablation by coagulation is a safe, effective alternative to other treatment of intractable uterine bleeding. Its main advantages include the readily available equipment and the speed and safety that this treatment affords. The procedure could perhaps be done under local, paracervical block and analgesia in those patients with a parous cervical os.

REFERENCES

1. Droegemuller W, Greer B, Makowski E: Cryosurgery in patients with dysfunctional uterine bleeding. Obstet Gynecol 38:256, 1971
2. Droegemuller W, Makowski E, Macsalka R: Destruction of the endometrium by cryosurgery. Am J Obstet Gynecol 110:467, 1971
3. Goldrath MH, Fuller TA, Segal S: Laser photovaporization of endometrium for the treatment of menorrhagia. Am J Obstet Gynecol 140:14, 1981
4. Neuwirth RS: A new technique for and additional experience with hysteroscopic resection of submucous fibroids. Am J Obstet Gynecol 131:91, 1978
5. Schenker JG, Polishuk WZ: Regeneration of rabbit endometrium after cryosurgery. Obstet Gynecol 40:638, 1972
6. Schenker JG, Polishuk WZ: Regeneration of rabbit endometrium following intrauterine instillation of chemical agents. Gynecol Invest 4:1, 1973

7. Schwartz PE, Goldstein HM, Wallace S, et al: Control of arterial hemorrhage using percutaneous arterial catheter techniques in patients with gynecologic malignancies. Gynecol Oncol 3:276, 1975

8. Speroff L, Glass RH, Kase NG: Clinical Gynecologic Endocrinology and Infertility, 2d ed, pp 161–164. Baltimore, Williams & Wilkins, 1978

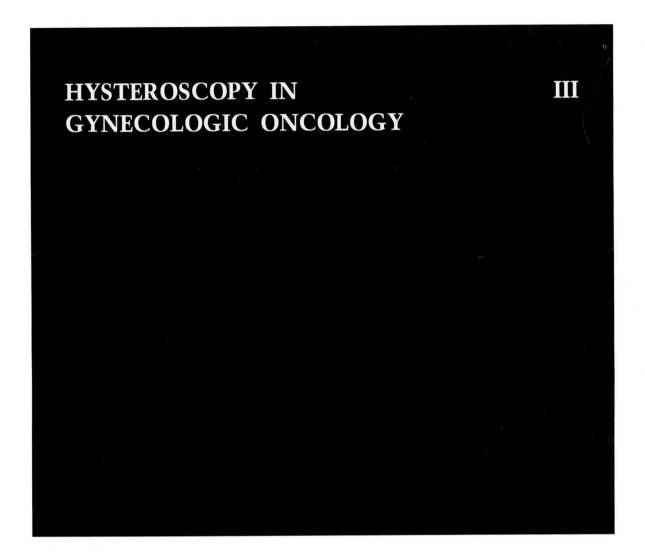

HYSTEROSCOPY IN GYNECOLOGIC ONCOLOGY

III

Nagel and coauthors found endometrial tissue in the cul-de-sac after hysteroscopy in over 50% of women. Does this tissue implant? Will it predispose to endometriosis? Do malignant cells transported in this manner from an endometrial adenocarcinoma involve or invade the peritoneal cavity? Thus far, no positive evidence has been forthcoming to answer any of these questions affirmatively. Based on the use of hysterography and the more recent use of hysteroscopy in patients with adenocarci-noma, no increase in either endometriosis or pelvic metastases from an endometrial adeno-carcinoma has been observed.

Hysteroscopy can play a valuable role in the detection and subsequent management of endometrial adenocarcinoma. Precursor lesions are described by Cittadini and associates and by Scarselli and co-workers. Although ade-nomatous hyperplasia shows a characteristic pattern according to these authors, a tissue diagnosis is always essential. The morphology and surface extension of endometrial adenocarcinoma are detectable; appropriate therapy should be devised accordingly.

All the authors except Baggish seem to prefer a panoramic type of endoscope to locate the suspicious areas. Descriptions of contact hysteroscopy, like colposcopy, evaluate the lesions for their color, contour, consistency, and vascular pattern. Joelsson and Sugimoto and coworkers probably have had the greatest amount of experience using hysteroscopy for the detection, localization, and evaluation of endometrial adenocarcinoma. They believe that hysteroscopy should improve the clinical management of this tumor because it can find the lesion at an early stage and allow the physician to observe surface endocervical involvement and in some instances follow the results after intracavitary radium insertion. Joelsson noted that hysteroscopy failed to detect the lower extent of the lesion in only 3% of 80 patients who had had a hysterectomy.

Tubal Reflux of Endometrial Tissue During Hysteroscopy ■ 30

Theodore C. Nagel
Richard A. Kopher
George E. Tagatz
Takashi Okagaki
Doris C. Brooker

When hysteroscopy is performed using a liquid medium to distend the endometrial cavity, fluid is passed through the tubal ostia.[2] This fluid may carry endometrial cells or tissue through the tubes into the peritoneal cavity. The study described in this chapter was undertaken to assess the risk of contaminating the peritoneal cavity with endometrial tissue as a result of hysteroscopy. Existing endometrial and pelvic abnormalities and the presence or absence of tissue in the peritoneal fluid were compared.

MATERIALS AND METHODS

Thirty-five premenopausal patients underwent hysteroscopy followed by diagnostic laparoscopy and curettage. Hysteroscopy was done in 33 as part of an infertility evaluation; 1 patient was evaluated for dysfunctional bleeding and another for pelvic pain. Six additional patients had laparoscopy not preceded by hysteroscopy, and curettage was done in four; five were infertile, and another had had tubal ligation.

Hysteroscopy was done using a Semm–Lindemann hysteroscope.* In 30 patients lactated

* Richard Wolf Medical Instruments Corporation, Rosemont, IL.

Ringer's (LR) solution was used to distend the uterine cavity. A 32% dextran 70 solution (Hyskon) was used in the other five patients. In the six patients in whom hysteroscopy was not done, fluid found in the cul-de-sac was aspirated at laparoscopy.

The fluid obtained from the cul-de-sac was passed through a millipore filter with a pore size of 8 μm. The filter was cleared with chloroform, and the slide was stained with Papanicolaou (Pap) polychromatic stain. The slides were examined microscopically for endometrial tissue (Fig. 30-1).

RESULTS

Seventeen of the 30 patients (57%) in whom LR was used had endometrial tissue present in the fluid aspirated from the cul-de-sac. Endometrial tissue was found in the fluid in the five patients in whom dextran 70 was used, but tissue was not found in peritoneal fluids from patients who did not undergo hysteroscopy.

Endometriosis was noted in 17 patients at laparoscopy. In the 14 women with endometriosis in whom LR was used for hysteroscopy, 7 had endometrial tissue or cells present in the fluid aspirated from the cul-de-sac. This was

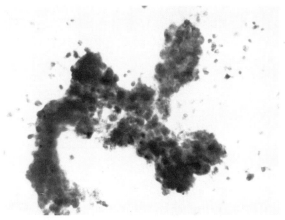

FIG. 30-1. An endometrial gland found in peritoneal fluid (P stain, original magnification × 130).

true in three of the five patients in whom dextran 70 was used. None of the patients who did not have hysteroscopy had demonstrable endometriosis (Table 30-1).

An attempt was made to correlate the presence of endometrial tissue in peritoneal fluid with hysteroscopic and pathologic diagnoses (see Table 30-1). In the 30 patients in whom LR was used, uterine abnormalities were found in 10, which may have contributed to reflux of endometrial tissue through the tubes. Five of 17 patients with positive peritoneal fluids had endometrial polypys (3), hyperplasia (1), or submucous myoma (1). Similar uterine findings were noted in 5 of the 13 patients with negative fluid. Additionally, one patient in this group had an endocervical polyp, and two had synechiae. In the five patients in whom dextran 70 was used, two had endometrial polyps, one had hyperplasia, and one had a septate uterus.

The phase of the menstrual cycle and the contents of the peritoneal fluid (Table 30-2) were compared. Of the patients in whom LR was used, the endometrium was proliferative in 12 of 17 with a positive fluid and in 10 of 13 with negative cytologic findings. It was proliferative in four of the five patients in whom dextran 70 was used. In four patients undergoing laparoscopy without hysteroscopy in whom a curettage was done, the endometrium was in the secretory phase. It was hyperplastic in one patient and normal in the other three.

DISCUSSION

Our findings indicate that during hysteroscopy, endometrial tissue frequently passes through the fallopian tubes into the peritoneal cavity when liquid media are used to distend the cavity. The reflux seems greater when dextran 70 is used, possibly because greater pressure is employed. Since dextran 70 was used in only a few patients, it is difficult to evaluate these results compared with those seen when LR solution was used.

Endometrial abnormalities did not predispose patients to tubal transfer of endometrial tissue. Uterine abnormalities were present in 5 of 17 patients with endometrial tissue in the peritoneal fluid and in 5 of 13 patients with no endometrial cells in cul-de-sac fluid. There was no correlation with the phase of the menstrual cycle either. However, 22 of 30 patients (73%) in the LR group and 4 of 5 in the dextran 70 group had hysteroscopy done during the proliferative phase.

Pelvic endometriosis was not consistently associated with the presence of endometrial tissue in the peritoneal fluid. Seventeen patients had established pelvic endometriosis. In ten patients (three dextran 70, seven LR) the fluid was positive, and in seven (all LR) it was negative. In those patients with positive fluid, endometriosis was mild in two, moderate in three, and severe in two. In those with negative fluid it was mild in four, moderate in one, and severe in two. Examination of cul-de-sac fluid is not a satisfactory finding for the diagnosis of endometriosis, nor is it a sensitive method for making that diagnosis.

The potential for the tissue introduced into the peritoneal cavity to initiate endometriosis is unclear. It is classically accepted that the retrograde passage of endometrial cells, either spontaneous or iatrogenic, may be a significant factor in causing endometriosis.[3] Other factors, such as a genetic predisposition to endometriosis or an altered immune state, may play a role.[1,4] Whether the phase of the menstrual cycle or the medium used for hysteroscopy affects the risk of endometriosis is unknown.

Table 30-1

PRESENCE OF ENDOMETRIAL TISSUE IN PERITONEAL FLUID IN 35 PATIENTS UNDERGOING HYSTEROSCOPY

DIAGNOSIS	ENDOMETRIAL TISSUE			
	Present		Absent	
	Dextran 70 (N = 5)	*Ringer's (N = 17)*	*Ringer's (N = 13)*	*None (N = 4)*
Endometriosis	3	7	7	0
Endometrial polyp, hyperplasia, or myoma	3	5	5	1*
Total	6	12	12	1

* N = patients in whom dilatation and curettage was done.

Table 30-2

PHASE OF THE MENSTRUAL CYCLE IN PATIENTS WITH ENDOMETRIAL TISSUE IN PERITONEAL FLUID

ENDOMETRIUM	ENDOMETRIAL TISSUE			
	Present		Absent	
	Dextran 70	*Ringer's*	*Ringer's*	*None*
Proliferative	4	12	10	0
Secretory	1	5	3	4
Total	5	17	13	4

We have begun aspirating peritoneal fluid before and after hysteroscopy to ascertain the validity of the above findings and after chromopertubation to separate the hydrodynamic role of fluid regurgitation from any mechanical effect resulting from endometrial trauma at hysteroscopy. If chromopertubation results in transtubal passage of fluid, it may be advisable to lavage the pelvis and aspirate the fluid whenever this procedure is done.

REFERENCES

1. Dmowski WP, Steele RW, Baker GF: Deficient cellular immunity in endometriosis. Am J Obstet Gynecol 141:377, 1981
2. Levine RU, Neuwirth RS: Evaluation of a method of hysteroscopy with the use of thirty percent dextran. Am J Obstet Gynecol 113:696, 1972
3. Sampson JA: Heterotopic or misplaced endometrial tissue. Am J Obstet Gynecol 10:649, 1925
4. Simpson JL, Elias S, Malinak LR, et al: Heritable aspects of endometriosis. I. Genetic studies. Am J Obstet Gynecol 137:327, 1980

Ettore Cittadini
Antonio Perino
Domenico Gullo

Valid epidemiologic and clinical arguments exist for stating that women receiving replacement therapy with estrogens because of menopausal symptoms have a greater risk of developing endometrial carcinoma.[1,5,6,9] Unopposed estrogen therapy can cause endometrial cystic hyperplasia and its possible progression toward adenomatous hyperplasia and endometrial adenocarcinoma in patients with risk factors; it may happen with prolonged hormonal stimulation.[3] Replacement therapy in postmenopausal women should be carefully programmed to avoid the development of endometrial hyperplasia. Scientific interest in this problem has led to a deeper knowledge of the risk factors involved and a clearer definition of the biologic precursors of endometrial adenocarcinoma.

New intrauterine diagnostic techniques are becoming more accurate and easy to use.[4] With microhysteroscopy, a new, simple, atraumatic method of examination, the gynecologist can make an immediate *in situ* diagnosis, thus avoiding other techniques used in the examination of the uterine cavity.[2]

This chapter will discuss a hysteroscopic and histologic study made on the endometria of a group of postmenopausal women who received cyclic therapy with conjugated estrogens.

MATERIALS AND METHODS

Twenty-three patients who had replacement hormonal treatment with conjugated estrogens for menopausal symptoms came to a gynecologic outpatient department during the last 2 yr. Hysteroscopies were performed with the Hamou microcolpohysteroscope, which has a diameter of 4 mm. A cold light of 150 watts was the source of illumination. A hysteroinsufflator giving a steady flow of 30 ml/min to 50 ml/min of carbon dioxide was used to distend the uterine cavity for panoramic vision. Hysteroscopic examinations were done without cervical dilatation or anesthesia.

Histologic examinations of the endometrial biopsies were performed in all patients. When endometrial hyperplasia was found, estrogen therapy was stopped and norethisterone acetate was prescribed, 5 mg daily, for 2 cycles of 21 days between menstrual periods. A hysteroscopic examination and repeated endometrial biopsy were performed after the second cycle of progestin therapy; if the endometrium contin-

Table 31-1
ENDOMETRIAL MORPHOLOGIC FINDINGS IN 23 TREATED PATIENTS

FINDING	NO. OF PATIENTS	CONJUGATED ESTROGENS (mg)	
		0.625	1.25
Atrophic endometrium	5	3	2
Proliferative endometrium	11	4	7
Cystic hyperplasia	4	2	2
Adenomatous hyperplasia	2	0	2
Adenocarcinoma	1	0	1
Total	23	9	14

ued to show abnormal morphologic aspects, progestin was continued until surgery.

RESULTS

Hysteroscopic endometrial findings were classified as follows:

1. Functioning endometrium (proliferative and secretory phases). The hysteroscopic image of the normal uterine cavity is typical. The mucosa of the anterior and posterior walls, and of the uterine fundus with the tubal orifices, is homogenous; its vascularization cannot be seen. In the proliferative phase the endometrium is pink, compact, and smooth; there may be menstrual residue. In the secretory phase the endometrium is homogenous but softer, expanded, shiny, and yellowish.
2. Atrophic endometrium. The endometrium appears whitish, smooth, and thin with submucosal vascularization. Hemorrhagic petechiae may be linked to the spotting that occurs in some of these patients.
3. Hyperplastic endometrial patterns. An increase in the volume of a proliferative type of endometrium that is not compatible with the patient's age is present. Histologically some abnormalities appear in the glands.

Excessive stimulation from estrogens results in cystic and atypical endometrial hyperplasia. Welch and Scully noted three different forms: a mild type showing architectural atypia, an intermediate form with architectural atypia and modest cytologic atypia, and a serious form with severe architectural and cytologic atypia.[8]

The hysteroscopic view of cystic hyperplasia and atypical endometrial hyperplasia is polymorphous. The mucosa has widespread or circumscribed mamillations with regular surfaces that stick out in the lumen, reducing the size of uterine cavity. In complex types of hyperplasia, necrotic and hemorrhagic phenomena are found, and the excessive endometrial growth may lead to interparietal bridging.

Finally, hysteroscopy can be used to diagnose endometrial adenocarcinoma. This tumor shows a considerable increase of tissue, having an encephaloid or crateriform appearance and necrotic and hemorrhagic areas that distort the uterine cavity. The different morphologic findings are shown in Table 31-1. Hormonal treatment varied from 4 mo to 8 yr; 9 women were treated with 0.625 mg of conjugated estrogens, and the remaining 14 were treated with 1.25 mg.

Cystic hyperplasia was found in 4 women; all the patients showed a secretory endometrium after 2 cycles of progestins for 21 days. There were two instances of adenomatous hyperplasia, one mild and one severe; the patients had been treated with higher doses without the addition of progestins. For 2 cycles the first patient showed a normal endometrium after 21 days of norethisterone acetate, but in the other patient an abnormal endometrium persisted despite 2 cycles of therapy. Endometrial adeno-

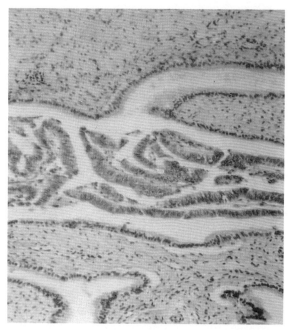

FIG. 31-1. Microphotograph of a tubal section in endometrial adenocarcinoma. Note the endometrial neoplastic tissue in the tubal lumen.

carcinoma was found in a patient treated continually with 1.25 mg of conjugated estrogens for more than 4 yr. Hysteroscopy performed before definitive surgery showed abnormal proliferation with encephaloid, necrotic, and hemorrhagic areas. The hysterectomy revealed an adenocarcinoma, stage I, grade I.

DISCUSSION

Estrogen therapy, even in small doses, can cause cystic endometrial hyperplasia, and, if stimulation is prolonged, it may lead to atypical hyperplasia, a precursor of adenocarcinoma.[1,3,5,6,9] Some authors reported that progestins can prevent or correct hyperplasia, and cyclic therapy of small doses of estrogens given with progestins from 7 to 12 days/mo minimizes the risk.[7]

Microhysteroscopy proved extremely useful in the control of menopausal patients receiving replacement hormonal treatment. The possibility exists of neoplastic dissemination after carbon dioxide insufflation (Fig. 31-1). The biologic significance of this possibility has yet to be evaluated, but it is advisable to prescribe long-term progestin therapy for patients with endometrial carcinoma and also for patients with a borderline diagnosis in whom a hysteroscopy has been performed.

REFERENCES

1. Autunes CMF, Stolley PD, Rosenheim NB, et al: Endometrial cancer and estrogen use. N Engl J Med 300:9, 1979
2. Cittadini E, Quartararo P, Perino A: Prospective diagnostiche di una nuova tecnica endoscopia: La colpomicroisteroscopia. Contracep Fertil Sem 8:19, 1981
3. Gusberg SB, Kaplan AL: Precursors of corpus carcinoma. Am J Obstet Gynecol 87:662, 1963
4. Hamou JE: Hysteroscopy and microhysteroscopy with a new instrument: The microhysteroscope. Acta Eur Fertil 10:29, 1981
5. Mack TM, Pike MC, Henderson BE, et al: Estrogens and endometrial cancer in a retirement community. N Engl J Med 294:1262, 1976
6. Smith DC, Prentice R, Thompson DJ, et al: Association of exogenous estrogens and endometrial carcinoma. N Engl J Med 293:1164, 1975
7. Thom MH, White PJ, Williams RM, et al: Prevention and treatment of endometrial disease in climacteric women receiving estrogen therapy. Lancet 2:455, 1979
8. Welch WR, Scully RE: Precancerous lesions of the endometrium. Hum Pathol 8:503, 1977
9. Ziel HK, Finkle WD: Increased risk of endometrial carcinoma among users of conjugated estrogens. N Engl J Med 293:1167, 1975

The Standardization of Morphologic Precursors of Endometrial Adenocarcinoma by Microhysteroscopy ■

32

Gianfranco Scarselli
Luca Mencaglia
Maurizio Colafranceschi
Gianluca Taddei
Francesco Branconi
Carlo Tantini

Endometrial carcinoma may represent the last stage of progressive endometrial hyperplasia in about 20% of patients.[4] Theoretically, three methods can be used to identify patients who will develop endometrial carcinoma:

Prospective study of patients affected by lesions suspected as precursors of endometrial carcinoma

Retrospective study of patients who had curettage or endometrial biopsy before they developed endometrial carcinoma

Study of morphologic lesions associated with endometrial carcinoma in extirpated specimens

MATERIALS AND METHODS

A study of endometrial carcinoma in extirpated specimens was done to identify possible morphologic precursors.[5] Atypical endometrial hyperplasia was present in 25% of patients, and endometrial atrophy was found in an equal number.

Endometrial carcinoma has often been associated with the most severe grade of atypical hyperplasia, and 59% of carcinomas showed high differentiation. In our experience, atypical hyperplasia represents the most frequent morphologic lesion associated with endometrial carcinoma in women under 55 years of age. Our research was directed to standardize endometrial lesions and to identify their evolution with the microhysteroscope of Hamou.[1] With this method a prospective study of endometrial lesions becomes possible, although conventional hysteroscopy poses some technical difficulties. In the endoscopy center of the Obstetric and Gynecologic Department of the University of Florence, Italy, 850 patients were examined microhysteroscopically, and 450 of these women were at risk for endometrial cancer based on their age.[2] One or more clinical risk factors for endometrial carcinoma were found in 90% of patients.

The main contribution of the microhysteroscopic technique is the possibility of a very clear view of the endometrium. No anesthesia

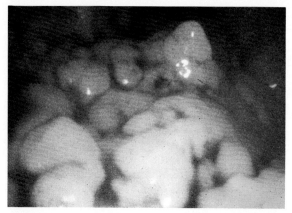

FIG. 32-1. Hysteroscopic view shows endometrial adenocarcinoma.

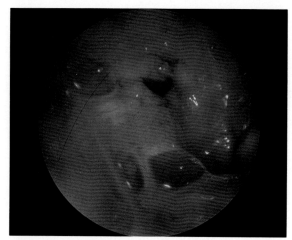

FIG. 32-2. Cystic endometrial hyperplasia reveals "bubbles" in the endometrium.

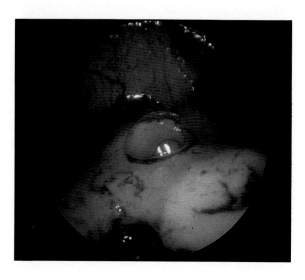

or cervical dilatation is needed. Hospitalization and anesthesia were required in 3% of patients. A remarkable agreement was noted between hysteroscopic and histologic diagnoses. Histologic agreement was found in 93% of patients with functional or atrophic endometrium and in 100% of patients with carcinoma (Fig. 32-1).[3]

RESULTS

The main problem with microhysteroscopy is the classification of the various endometrial hyperplastic changes. The extreme sensitivity of endometrium to exogenous or endogenous hormones explains the difficulty in evaluating endometrial hyperplasia with microhysteroscopy. Endometrial hyperplasia results from estrogenic overstimulation (various grades of atypical hyperplasia, cystic hyperplasia) or from progestational overstimulation (secretory hyperplasia, irregular shedding). Mild forms of endometrial atypical hyperplasia are hardly differentiable by microhysteroscopy from other pictures of endometrial overstimulation. However, the basic feature of endometrial atypical hyperplasia is the presence of regular mammillary projections or digitations or, sometimes, small mucosal excavations. In cystic hyperplasia, cystic glands form translucent, hemispheric "bubbles" of various sizes (Fig. 32-2).

In progestational overstimulation, the endometrium shows the same features as in the secretory phase, but it becomes almost a puffy mucosa, often with increased size and number of vessels, and sometimes with umbilicated plaques (Fig. 32-3). An endometrium in patients receiving oral (PO) contraceptives shows no characteristic picture besides a hyperplasia (Fig. 32-4).

In severe, atypical hyperplasia, the uterine cavity is often intensely hemorrhagic with ne-

FIG. 32-3. After 6 months of therapy with progestins, the endometrium is puffy with increased vascularization.

crotic areas, whitish digitations, polypoid or papillar formations, interparietal bridges, and excavations of the mucosa, testifying to the irregular endometrial growth.

CONCLUSION

Microhysteroscopy can help identify neoplastic lesions and functional or atrophic endometrium. Curettage can be avoided, and focal lesions can be recognized (Fig. 32-5). This technique allows physicians to recognize, in most patients, the morphologic precursors of endometrial adenocarcinoma and to select patients at risk. A further effort is required to differentiate among the various hyperplastic features; the ability to perform a divided biopsy under microhysteroscopic vision will clarify this problem (Fig. 32-6).

REFERENCES

1. Hamou J: Hysteroscopie et microhysteroscopie avec un instrument nouveau: Le microhysteroscope. In Albano V, Cittadini E, Quartararo P (eds): Endoscopia Ginecologica, p 131. Palermo, Sicily, CoFeSe 1980
2. Scarselli G, Mencaglia L, Hamou J: Atlante di Microcolposteroscopia. Palermo, Sicily, Co Fe Se 1981
3. Scarselli G, Mencaglia L, Colafranceschi M, et al: Microhysteroscopy: The reliability of a new hysteroscopic technique in the diagnosis of endometrial hyperplasia. Presented at the Tenth Annual Meeting of American Association of Gynecologic Laparoscopists, Phoenix, 1981
4. Welch WR, Scully RE: Precancerous lesions of the endometrium. Hum Pathol 8:503, 1977
5. Zampi G, Colafranceschi M, Taddei G: Morfologia delle lesioni preneoplastiche dell'endometrio. In Zampi G (ed): Apporto Alla Ricerca di Base al Controllo Della Crescita Neoplastia, p 429. Napoli, Idelson, 1981

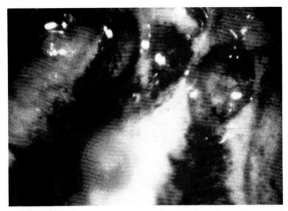

FIG. 32-4. Endometrium of patient who takes oral contraceptives.

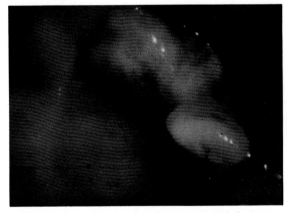

FIG. 32-5. Endometrial polyps cover tubal ostium.

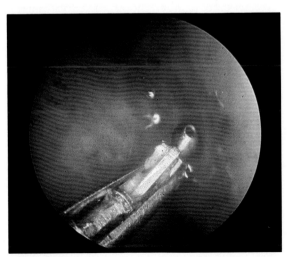

FIG. 32-6. Endometrial biopsy performed under hysteroscopic control.

Hysteroscopy for Delineating the Intrauterine Extent of Endometrial Carcinoma ■

33

Ingemar S. Joelsson

Hysteroscopy is a reliable method for achieving the correct diagnosis of intrauterine diseases. The differential diagnosis between the causes of uterine bleeding, polyps, or submucous myomas is easily made despite bleeding.[4] Intrauterine adhesions can be seen and fragmented; sometimes partly embedded intrauterine devices (IUDs) can be localized and removed with the help of instruments inserted through a separate channel in the sheath.[1] Likewise, biopsies from suspicious lesions can be excised with forceps under visual control.[6,9] Hysteroscopy can be recommended for detecting the anatomic extent of endometrial carcinoma.[5,10,11] Although attempts in this direction have been accepted in some countries, many physicians have criticized them.

MATERIALS AND METHODS

The diameter of the instrument can cause some difficulty in the small uterine cavity. Apposition of the anterior and posterior uterine walls, dilatation of the internal os, and insertion of the hysteroscope can make it difficult to avoid bleeding. This difficulty is particularly evident with proliferative types of endometrial carcinoma. Blood is drained from the cavity by rinsing with various liquids, usually water or saline. The liquid is either sucked from the cavity or flushed through it under pressure. The choice between these two methods is based on the knowledge that the uterine cavity must be distended for proper visibility and tempered by the anticipated risk that fluid and malignant tissue will penetrate the fallopian tubes, ultimately entering the abdomen. Several authors have studied the correlation between the presence of fluid in the abdominal cavity after hysteroscopy and intrauterine pressure during the procedure. With pressures of about 50 mm Hg to 65 mm Hg, fluid does not pass through the tubes. On the other hand, the use of 90 mm Hg pressure is advocated by some investigators to distend the uterine cavity adequately. Rinsing the uterine cavity with water or saline did not solve the problem of bleeding because blood mixed easily; the resultant, diffuse, red color rendered the medium between the optical lens and the uterine wall almost opaque. Norment and Silander modified these techniques by placing the optical device in a thin-walled rubber balloon filled with fluid, but even this improvement was not sufficient.[12,17,18] Viscous liquids of the polyvinylpyrrolidine type were used but had to be abandoned because of their physicochemical properties. The use of carbon dioxide for insufflation and hysteroscopy was introduced by

Rubin in 1925, and the technique has been fully developed by Lindemann, by Semm, and by Porto.[8,13–16] It has limitations in patients with endometrial carcinoma, who sometimes bleed excessively during hysteroscopy.

The use of dextran as a medium for draining and distending the uterine cavity during hysteroscopy was described by Edström and Fernström in 1970.[3] A 35% solution of dextran (average molecular weight 70,000) in glucose is used. This solution is colorless, has excellent optical properties, and renders the image very bright, giving clear contrasts between light and dark areas. The dextran solution has such a high viscosity (260 cp at room temperature) that it must be injected into the uterus under pressure through the channel in the sheath of the hysteroscope. A continuous flow of dextran through the cavity is necessary to avoid an accumulation of blood and tissue fragments, which would obscure the view. Dextran has the additional advantage of being immiscible with blood.

Having tested several possibilities, I consider that a slow outflow of dextran from the uterus along the sheath of the hysteroscope is more efficient than drainage through the outflow channel in the hysteroscope or through a separate catheter. If the cervical canal is dilated up to a diameter 1 mm larger than that of the hysteroscope, an adequate intrauterine pressure is easily created. In about 50% of the women examined with this technique, dextran was observed to pass through the fallopian tubes. The solution was recovered from the cul-de-sac during laparotomy performed on the same day or on the day after hysteroscopy. Dextran has a minimal irritant effect on the tissues. This may be a result of electrical phenomena associated with the coating of tissue surfaces with dextran. In nonhuman experimental surgery, dextran prevents the formation of peritoneal adhesions.[2]

The extent and the malignancy grade of endometrial carcinoma are the main factors on which to base the therapeutic plan for these patients: surgery, radiotherapy, or a combination. The importance of the extent of the carcinoma for prognosis is evident from statistics collected by numerous institutions.[7] In such statistics from Radiumhemmet in Stockholm, Sweden, the corrected 5-yr survival rate for 714 patients with stage I disease was 85.2%, while the corresponding figure for 146 patients with stage II disease was 60.9%. In the latter group the endocervix was involved in the carcinoma. The difference in the natural history of the disease when it is limited to the endometrium as opposed to involvement of the cervix is indicated by the occasional growth in the pelvic lymph nodes in the patients with cervical involvement. This makes it desirable to evaluate the isthmus and endocervix carefully for the presence of carcinoma before deciding on treatment.

RESULTS

Hysteroscopy with dextran in over 100 patients with endometrial carcinoma did not lead to any complications more serious than uterine perforation. No instance of endometritis, salpingitis, or fever was caused by hysteroscopy. The objective was to delineate the intrauterine extent of carcinoma. The hysteroscopic finding of the distal border of the tumor correlated with a histologic verification of cancer in tissue obtained by fractional curettage. More convincing evidence of the efficacy of hysteroscopy was obtained through histologic examination of hysterectomy specimens. Hysteroscopy failed to detect the distal border of the carcinoma correctly in only 3% of patients, but in these patients' uteri the malignant growth had reached the cervix through submucosal extension within the myometrium. The figure is based on observations of 80 patients examined with hysteroscopy before hysterectomy. The uterus was carefully examined microscopically. Although hysteroscopy in endometrial carcinoma points to a possibility of diagnosing the grade of malignancy, the accuracy of such a diagnosis has not been evaluated. Because I believe that both the diagnosis and the grade of malignancy must be confirmed histologically, I did not attempt to ascertain malignancy grade by hysteroscopy.

The use of hysteroscopy for examining patients with endometrial carcinoma has been questioned on the grounds of the risk of spreading cancer through the tubes into the abdominal cavity. One or two cases have been described where spread of tumor to the fallopian tubes was thought to be caused by hysterosalpingography. Several medical centers use hysterosalpingography routinely in the preoperative work-up of patients without reporting increases in the risk of intra-abdominal or distant metastases. Experience with hysterosalpingography is similar to hysteroscopy: in about 50% of patients with endometrial carcinoma, contrast medium or dextran passes through the tubes. In the others, the tubes are not patent; growth of carcinoma deep in the myometrium around the intramural segment is verified histologically in the majority. Distant metastases will become manifest early in such patients even though the surface spread of the carcinoma is limited. Contrast medium in the tubes during hysterosalpingography was seen less often in patients who developed metastases than in those who did not. The difference was statistically significant.

REFERENCES

1. Borell U, Fernström I, Ohlson L: Membrane-like structures in the uterine cavity. A hysterographic study. Acta Obstet Gynecol Scand 49:185, 1970
2. Choate WH, Just−Viera JO, Yeager GH: Prevention of experimental peritoneal adhesions by dextran. Arch Surg 88:249, 1964
3. Edström K, Fernström I: The diagnostic possibilities of a modified hysteroscopic technique. Acta Obstet Gynecol Scand 49:327, 1970
4. Englund F, Ingelman−Sundberg A, Westin B: Hysteroscopy in diagnosis and treatment of uterine bleeding. Gynaecologia 143:217, 1957
5. Joelsson I, Levine RU, Moberger G: Hysteroscopy as an adjunct in determining the extent of carcinoma of the endometrium. Am J Obstet Gynecol 111:696, 1971
6. Johnsson JE: Hysterography and diagnostic curettage in carcinoma of the uterine body. Acta Radiol (Suppl) 326:1, 1973
7. Kottmeier HL (ed): Annual Report on the Results of Treatment in Carcinoma of the Uterus and Vagina, Vol 16. Stockholm, International Federation of Gynecology and Obstetrics, 1976
8. Lindemann HJ: Eine neue Untersuchungsmethode für die Hysteroskopie. Endoscopy 4:194, 1971
9. Neuwirth RS: Hysteroscopy. Philadelphia, WB Saunders, 1975
10. Norman O: Hysterography in cancer of the corpus of the uterus. Acta Radiol (Suppl) 79, 1950
11. Norman O: Hysterography in cancer of the uterus. Semin Roentgenol 4:244, 1969
12. Norment WB: Hysteroscopy in diagnosis of pathological conditions of uterine canal. JAMA 148:917, 1952
13. Porto R: Une nouvelle méthode d'hystéroscopie. Marseille, Thèse, 1972
14. Rubin IC: Uterine endoscopy, endometroscopy with the aid of uterine insufflation. Am J Obstet Gynecol 10:313, 1925
15. Semm K: Die Laparoskopie in der Gynäkologie. Geburtshilfe Frauenheilkd 27:1029, 1967
16. Semm K: Pelviskopie und Hysteroskopie. Farbatlas und Lehrbuch. Stuttgart, FK Schattauer, 1976
17. Silander T: Hysteroscopy through a transparent rubber balloon. Surg Gynecol Obstet 114:125, 1962
18. Silander T: Hysteroscopy through a transparent rubber balloon in patients with carcinoma of the uterine endometrium. Acta Obstet Gynecol Scand 42:284, 1963

Diagnostic Hysteroscopy for Endometrial Carcinoma ■

34

Osamu Sugimoto
Takahisa Ushiroyama
Yoshihiko Fukuda

Although curettage has been the most reliable method for diagnosis of endometrial cancer, it can miss some localized lesions. Hysteroscopy can confirm the existence, location, and extent of endometrial carcinoma, and a biopsy of the suspicious area is feasible under direct vision.[1-3] The initial sign in women with endometrial cancer is abnormal bleeding, and hysteroscopy is done before curettage to search for the bleeding area.

This study reports 182 cases of endometrial carcinoma in a series of over 10,500 patients who had suspected intrauterine abnormalities and who were examined by hysteroscopy in the Women's Clinic of the Kyoto University Hospital and Osaka Medical College Hospital from 1968 to 1977.

MATERIALS AND METHODS

Of 7800 patients with abnormal uterine bleeding, 182 were found to have endometrial carcinoma at hysteroscopy (Table 34-1). Their ages ranged from 37 to 83 yr. The first phase of the examination begins in the cervical canal without mechanical dilation, especially in postmenopausal women. The hysteroscope is applied to the external os, and the physician looks into the cervical canal, which is dilated by gradual rinsing with saline. Intracervical carcinoma or cervical invasion of endometrial carcinoma can be detected. Then the uterine cavity is explored after the cervix is dilated by Hegar's dilators up to no. 7; the outer sleeve with obturator is inserted in the cervix, and the hysteroscope is introduced in place of the obturator. Observation begins near the internal os and moves gradually upward to the fundus and the tubal cornua.

RESULTS

Hysteroscopy can identify an endometrial carcinoma in detail depending on the morphologic characteristics of the superficial components of the neoplastic tissue. It is either diffuse or circumscribed, and it may show an exophytic or endophytic pattern of growth. Of 182 patients with endometrial carcinoma, 167 had circumscribed, exophytic growths with polypoid, nodular, or papillary processes, often accompanied by ulceration, necrosis, and infection (see Table 34-1).

POLYPOID CARCINOMA

A polypoid appearance noted in 19 patients consisted of several projections (Fig. 34-1). The surface is light gray, rough, and uneven with engorged superficial vessels. Histologically,

157

Table 34-1
ENDOMETRIAL CARCINOMA: RELATIONSHIP BETWEEN HYSTEROSCOPIC AND HISTOPATHOLOGIC FINDINGS

HYSTEROSCOPIC MORPHOLOGY	HISTOPATHOLOGY				TOTAL
	Differentiated (adenocarcinoma)			Undifferentiated	
	Tubular	*Adenomatous*	*Papillary*		
Circumscribed					
Polypoid	12	7			19 ⎤
Nodular	15	23	4		42 ⎥ 167
Papillary			71		71 ⎥
Ulcerated	4	13	9	9	35 ⎦
Diffuse			11	4	15
Total	31	43	95	13	182

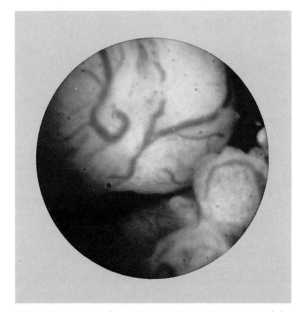

FIG. 34-1. A polypoid growth is characterized by undulated lining with dilated vessels. Histologic studies disclosed tubular adenocarcinoma.

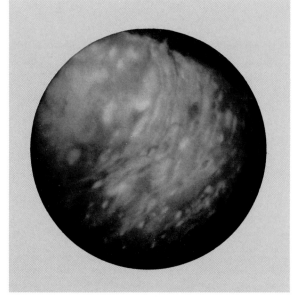

FIG. 34-2. Adenomatous endometrial polyp shows sporadically distributed glandular openings on the ragged surface, but few vessels.

the carcinoma usually has a well-differentiated glandular or tubular pattern. The tubular variety (12 patients) is pale blue or yellowish gray with gentle undulations, and its surface is sporadically pierced with glandular openings that have yellowish indentations. Adenomatous adenocarcinoma also has a fine, uneven surface with dense and wide glandular openings. It must be differentiated from a benign endometrial adenomatous polyp (Fig. 34-2), in which the surface sometimes has a fine network of regular, thin blood vessels.

NODULAR CARCINOMA

A nodular type of carcinoma found in 42 patients had bulges with a fairly sessile base (Fig. 34-3). The adenomatous type occurs more frequently than polypoid carcinoma. Dilated superficial blood vessels may form tortuous vari-

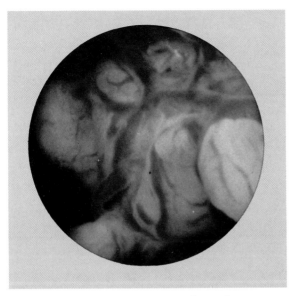

FIG. 34-3. Nodular carcinoma shows knotty protrusions of neoplastic tissue with engorged, irregularly distributed vessels.

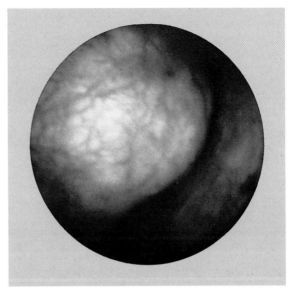

FIG. 34-4. Submucous leiomyoma has vessels on its surface that are regularly arranged and not dilated.

cosities. Ulceration and infection occur more frequently in nodular than in polypoid carcinoma. A submucous fibroid (Fig. 34-4) also shows nodular protrusion into the cavity, and the covering endometrium is thin; subepithelial blood vessels are regularly arranged and not engorged.

PAPILLARY CARCINOMA

A papillary carcinoma with numerous dendritic projections is the most common pattern seen on hysteroscopy. It was found in 71 of the 182 patients. The surface is covered with numerous projections of the tissues, which quiver in the rinsing saline. These tentacles, some long and others short, gather and form a dendritic mass (Fig. 34-5). They look light pink because numerous cancer cells proliferate around the blood vessels, as noted on histologic examination. Short tentacles look like clusters of grapes; long ones, interlocking with each other, appear as balls of yarn.

ULCERATED CARCINOMA

Ulceration was seen hysteroscopically in 35 women; 19 were diffusely infected and had a

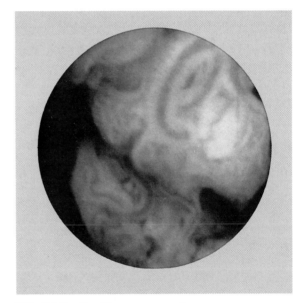

FIG. 34-5. Papillary pattern shows numerous projections forming a dendritic mass.

uterus covered with pus. Ulceration seemed to increase as the tumors became less differentiated. The ulcerated surface appears rough, fragile, and dull; infection alters the characteristic features because of pus and debris (Fig. 34-6). It is difficult to estimate the morphology

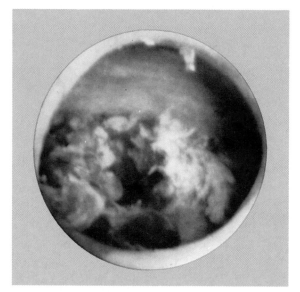

FIG. 34-6. A stage I ulcerated endometrial carcinoma appears rough and fragile, and the cervix and internal os are normal. Blood clots and pus covering the surface of the lesions were washed out by rinsing saline.

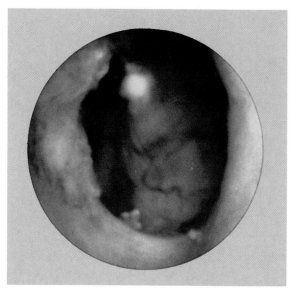

FIG. 34-8. Nodular carcinoma invading the cervical canal. The left upper quarter of the internal os is affected by ulcerated carcinoma, while the main tumor is in the uterine cavity.

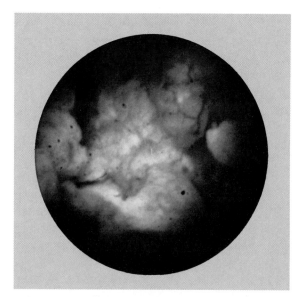

FIG. 34-7. Diffuse carcinoma involves almost the entire uterine lining, and irregularly arranged vessels also are seen on the rugged surface.

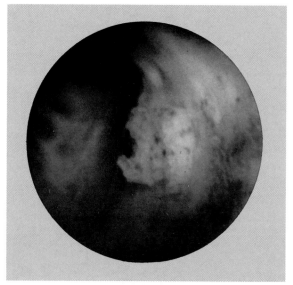

FIG. 34-9. A small carcinoma under the left cornu.

on hysteroscopy, but histologic examination in these 35 women revealed 13 adenomatous, 9 papillary, 9 undifferentiated, and 4 tubular patterns.

DIFFUSE CARCINOMA

Diffuse carcinoma was encountered in 11 patients, and it involved almost the entire uterine lining (Fig. 34-7). The surface is irregular, ragged, and friable. The appearance is probably caused by necrosis, ulceration, and infection. The ulceration makes it difficult to estimate the precise morphology at hysteroscopy. It may be similar to endometrial polypoid hyperplasia, which looks light pink, smooth, and velvety. Diffuse carcinoma has engorged blood vessels somewhere on the ragged surface.

CERVICAL INVASION

Cervical extension of endometrial carcinoma, detected in 22 patients at hysteroscopy, showed rough, fragile neoplastic tissue involving the endometrial canal beyond the internal os (Fig. 34-8). These patients were treated as clinical stage II or higher and underwent radical hysterectomy and pelvic lymphadenectomy.

CANCER IN VERY EARLY STAGE

Tiny circumscribed carcinomas, 2 mm to 5 mm in diameter, were found in 5 instances by hysteroscopy (Fig. 34-9). All patients had postmenopausal bleeding, a previous endometrial cavity cell sampling, and fractional curettage. Only two were suspected of having endometrial carcinoma. The tumors, polypoid or nodular, were biopsied under visual control because it was difficult to differentiate them from focal hyperplasia (Fig. 34-10) or a benign endometrial polyp.

COMMENT

Hysteroscopy is an indispensable procedure for accurate, prompt diagnosis of intrauterine ma-

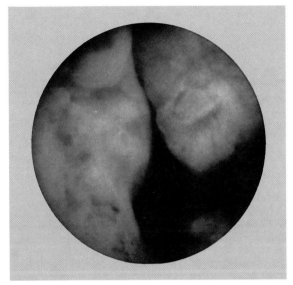

FIG. 34-10. Polypoid and focal endometrial hyperplasia do not show any engorged vessels on the surface.

lignancy. It is simple to locate small lesions and to detect the extension of cancer to the cervix. Consequently, prompt diagnosis can lead to suitable treatment with minimal delay. The risks of uterine perforation, hemorrhage, dissemination of cancer cells, and pelvic infection can be avoided if the procedure is done carefully. Since many endometrial carcinomas have a specific gross appearance, most are readily diagnosed by hysteroscopy. Endometrial carcinoma at hysteroscopy is characterized by roughness, ulceration, elevation or protrusion of the surface, bleeding spots, and engorged vessels. Suspected lesions can be biopsied with special forceps under visual control.

REFERENCES

1. Shih–Chiu C, Sugimoto O: Diagnostic hysteroscopy for postmenopausal uterine bleeding. Acta Obstet Gynecol Jpn 30:1737, 1978
2. Sugimoto O: Hysteroscopic diagnosis of endometrial carcinoma. Am J Obstet Gynecol 121:105, 1975
3. Sugimoto O: Diagnostic and Therapeutic Hysteroscopy. Tokyo, Igaku–Shoin, 1978

Contact Endoscopy for Evaluation of Endometrial Adenocarcinoma ■

35

Michael S. Baggish

Contact hysteroscopy is an old endoscopic technique resurrected by Barbot and by Baggish.[1,2] Although the indications and applications of the contact hysteroscope are numerous, this chapter will only describe its uses for the diagnosis and staging of endometrial and endocervical neoplasia. Compared to conventional hysteroscopy, the contact method does not require distention of the uterine cavity or a special light source, and blood or other liquids will not obstruct vision. The technique is simple, and examinations can be made in any office or outpatient facility. It is ideally suited for investigative oncology because there is no risk of translocating endometrial cancer cells through the oviducts into the peritoneal cavity, and despite bleeding in malignant lesions, this instrument is reliable for direct observation of endometrial carcinoma. As with colposcopy, observation of the lesion and directed sampling offer substantial advantages to the oncologist.

MATERIALS AND METHODS

The MTO 6-mm and 8-mm diameter ($\times 1.6$) contact hysteroscopes* were used in this study. These models have an overall length of

*Advanced Biomedical Instruments.

200 mm and a focal length of 5 mm to contact surface. A focusing magnifier ($\times 2$) was usually attached to the eyepiece of the hysteroscope. Ambient room light was focused on the light trapping cylinder; occasionally more intense light sources were used (e.g., a 250-W halogen lamp when photography was desired). An operating room or examining room light provides excellent illumination. All patients' cervices and vaginas were prepared with povidone-iodine (Betadine) after a Papanicolaou (Pap) smear had been obtained. The anterior lip of the cervix was grasped with a single-tooth tenaculum, and the cervix was dilated between 27 and 29 French (with the 8-mm instrument). When the 6-mm scope was used, dilatation varied from none in multiparous women to 21 French in nulliparous patients. Dilatation was frequently accomplished after a paracervical block, either in the office or clinic. The hysteroscope was inserted through the external os of the cervix, and the endocervical canal was examined visually. The junction of the endometrial and endocervical cavities was clearly seen as the instrument passed through the internal os. The endometrium was inspected in an organized fashion so the entire cavity could be seen; this was followed by biopsy or dilatation and curettage. Postcurettage inspection proved valuable to ascertain the amount of tissue left behind and to decide whether further

Table 35-1

COMPARISON OF HYSTEROSCOPIC AND HISTOLOGIC DIAGNOSES IN 33 PATIENTS WITH ENDOMETRIAL AND ENDOCERVICAL MALIGNANCIES

HYSTEROSCOPY	HISTOLOGY	PATIENTS	
		No.	%
Polypoid endometrium with hyperplasia	Mixed mesodermal tumor	1	3
Atypical endometrial hyperplasia	Adenocarcinoma, endometrium	2	6
Adenocarcinoma, endometrium	Adenocarcinoma, endometrium	27	82
* Adenocarcinoma, endometrium and endocervix	Primary adenocarcinoma, endocervix	3	9
Total		33	100

* One carcinoma metastasized to the endocervix.

sampling was necessary. After every dilatation and curettage, hysteroscopic inspection revealed that approximately one third of the endometrium remained.

Thirty-three women ranging from 35 to 75 yr of age were examined by contact hysteroscopy because of suspected malignancy, and all were subsequently found to have either endocervical or endometrial tumors as corroborated by histopathologic examination. All hysteroscopic diagnoses were transcribed before pathologic diagnoses on the patient's chart. Five patterns were associated with the contact hysteroscopic diagnosis of adenocarcinoma: white epithelium, grey flocculence, luminescence, brainlike vessels, and abnormal vessels.

RESULTS

The types of malignancies are shown in Table 35-1. Three primary endocervical adenocarcinomas were found; the remainder were endometrial cancers. Hysteroscopic diagnoses were correct in 30 of 33 instances (91%). Two patients had adenocarcinoma, although on hysteroscopy it seemed like atypical hyperplasia. A mixed mesodermal sarcoma was thought to be polypoid endometrial hyperplasia at hysteroscopy. No patient had a normal endometrium; all were associated with bleeding, and in 20 the bleeding was brisk. This condition probably would have precluded conventional hysteroscopic techniques employing water,

Table 35-2

SPREAD OF TUMOR BASED ON HYSTEROSCOPIC EVALUATION OF 33 PATIENTS

HYSTEROSCOPY	TUMOR TYPE	NO. OF PATIENTS
Diffuse spread	Mixed mesodermal	1
	Adenocarcinoma	2
Right fundus–corpus	Adenocarcinoma	18
Left fundus–corpus	Adenocarcinoma	8
Corpus only	Adenocarcinoma	1
Fundus only	Adenocarcinoma	1
Endocervical spread	Adenocarcinoma, endometrium and endocervix	2
Total		33

dextran, or carbon dioxide as the distending medium.

DISCUSSION

Contact hysteroscopy is analogous to colposcopy because the close examination of the endometrium allows precise localization of the cancer and enables the gynecologist to direct a biopsy to the site in question. Accurate visual appraisal for staging and ultimate prognosis are added advantages. Endocervical curettage remains a "blind" procedure with limitations. Direct observation of endocervical tumor by hysteroscopy is the best method to stage the disease, since the view of the endocervical canal is good. As with colposcopy, this procedure is learned by observing lesions for color, contour, pattern, and consistency. The contact hysteroscope adds the sense of "feeling" lesions: are they firm, soft, fixed, or mobile? By correlating the physical findings with the histologic diagnosis, the physician can form a composite picture and differentiate one lesion from another (Table 35-2).

REFERENCES

1. Baggish MS: Contact hysteroscopy: A new technique to explore the uterine cavity. Obstet Gynecol 54:350, 1979
2. Barbot J: L'hystéroscopie de contact. Paris, Thèse, 1975

Selective Use of Hysteroscopy in Gynecologic Oncology ∎

36

Kunio Miyazawa

Although hysteroscopy was introduced by Pantaleoni in 1869, it has only recently become a widely investigated procedure in gynecologic practice.[15,19] The discovery of new media such as 32% dextran 70 (Hyskon) by Edström and Fernström and carbon dioxide gas insufflation by Lindemann has opened a new era for a detailed evaluation of the uterine cavity.[6,8,9]

The evaluation and staging of endometrial carcinoma have been reported through the use of hysteroscopy, but most of its use has remained in the area of benign endometrial conditions.[8,13,18] Recent advances in optical technology have also brought about new instruments such as the contact hysteroscope by Baggish[1] and by Barbot[3] and the microhysteroscope by Hamou that have made it possible to evaluate more detailed endometrial and endocervical abnormalities.[1,3,7] This chapter presents several selective uses of hysteroscopy in gynecologic oncology.

MATERIALS AND METHODS

From July 1980 to December 1981, hysteroscopy was selectively used to evaluate and manage patients with gynecologic malignancy by the Gynecologic Oncology Service of Tripler Army Medical Center, Honolulu, Hawaii. From my past experience with dextran 70, I prefer to use the Wolf–Lindemann–Semm hysteroscope. A recently acquired contact hysteroscope has broadened the selective use of hysteroscopy in gynecologic oncology. All patients were carefully investigated preoperatively and counselled. I performed all hysteroscopic procedures with the aid of a resident staff member. All patients involved in this study were diagnosed as having uterine or vaginal invasive carcinoma or preinvasive neoplasia.

RESULTS

The following five types of cases were encountered, and I currently use hysteroscopy for similar types of gynecologic malignancy.

APPLICATION I

Hysteroscopy was used for vaginal examination of infants and children with suspected pelvic malignancy and to monitor their response to treatment. A female infant aged 2 yr had been vaginally spotting for 3 mo, and sarcoma botryoides was suspected. Pelvic examination was very difficult even under general anesthesia. Biopsy from the outer third of vagina confirmed sarcoma botryoides. Dextran 70 and a hysteroscope were used during vaginoscopy to inspect the vagina and cervix. A visible cluster of tumor in the mid-vagina after 3 mo of vincristine, actinomycin D, and cyclophosphamide (Cytoxan) chemotherapy was seen. Vag-

165

inoscopic and pelvic examination revealed a very good response to the treatment. The small diameter of the hysteroscope is ideal for inspecting the vaginal canal and ectocervix. Dextran 70 drained vaginally without any adverse effect.

APPLICATION II

The hysteroscope was used for vaginal examination of adults with stenotic introitus who had received radiation therapy for gynecologic carcinoma or who presented with suspected vaginal or cervical malignancy. A woman aged 81 yr, gravida 1 para 1, was previously treated with external radiation to the whole pelvis and intracavitary radiation for Stage IIB squamous cell cervical carcinoma. Follow-up pelvic examination had been very difficult because of a stenotic introitus and vagina despite local estrogen treatment. Because of vaginal spotting and discharge, a contact hysteroscope was used in the office to inspect the vagina and cervix. A hemorrhagic, necrotic area was noted in the obliterated vaginal apex. Pelvic examination under anesthesia was not remarkable, and cytologic and biopsy specimens were negative for tumor.

APPLICATION III

Hysteroscopy was used to detect endometrial extension of cervical carcinoma and to monitor patients' response to radiation treatment. A woman aged 54 yr, gravida 15 para 11 abortus 4, had Stage IB squamous cell cervical carcinoma. Fractional dilatation and curettage showed endocervical and endometrial curettings with squamous carcinoma. Biopsy of the ulcerated cervical lesion showed the same tumor. She was treated by 4500 rad of external radiation to the whole pelvis and was then admitted for intracavitary cesium treatment. Before applicator insertion, the uterine cavity revealed tumor in the posterior wall of the lower uterine segment and corpus, which responded to radiotherapy. Less than 30 ml of dextran 70 was instilled at a very low pressure. No attempt was made to seal the cervical canal or to distend the uterine cavity forcefully.

In the International Federation of Gynecology and Obstetrics (FIGO) staging system, Stage I includes carcinoma strictly confined to the cervix, but extension to the corpus is disregarded. Extension of squamous cell cervical carcinoma into the uterine cavity is known to influence the result significantly.[16] This identification ensures planned treatment for adequate dose distribution over the uterus. Radiobiologic behavior observed on hysteroscopic examination will provide necessary information for subsequent radiotherapy.

APPLICATION IV

Hysteroscopy was used to differentiate between endocervical adenocarcinoma and downward extension of endometrial adenocarcinoma. A woman aged 62 yr, gravida 6 para 4 abortus 2, had been spotting for 3 mo. A biopsy of a small ulcerated lesion at the external cervical os showed adenocarcinoma, probably of endometrial origin, but the pathologist could not rule out endocervical origin. Endocervical and endometrial curettings showed the same pathologic picture. Dextran 70 hysteroscopy revealed a normal endometrial cavity, but the endocervical canal showed a tumor. The patient subsequently underwent a radical hysterectomy and bilateral pelvic lymphadenectomy for Stage IB adenocarcinoma of the endocervix. Peritoneal washings did not reveal tumor cells. Well-differentiated adenocarcinoma was found in the endocervix, and the endometrium was of the proliferative type.

When the adenocarcinoma is a papillary or ulcerative lesion at the external cervical os, it is sometimes difficult to differentiate between endocervical origin and endocervical extension from endometrial carcinoma. Microscopic differentiation is not always certain unless sufficient tissue is obtained from the endometrial cavity and from the endocervix.[4,14] Hysteroscopy has been used to ascertain the extent of endometrial carcinoma, but it has the potential of spreading tumor cells through the fallopian tubes or into the uterine vessels.[10] However, it has been reported that almost all patients who undergo dilatation and curettage, hysterectomy, or pelvic examination could have tumor cells spread in the venous circulation, but few will develop distant metastases.[12,17] Carefully conducted hysteroscopy will result in less trauma than dilatation and curettage. Although hysteroscopy is not indicated routinely for evaluation of endometrial adenocarcinoma, it becomes useful when a pathologic diagnosis is questionable and endocervical evaluation is not conclusive.

APPLICATION V

Hysteroscopy was used to evaluate suspected endometrial malignancy not detected by conventional dilatation and curettage or recurrent abnormal uterine bleeding after previous treatment by dilatation and curettage. A woman aged 48 years, gravida 3 para 3, had had a fractional dilatation and curettage for perimenopausal bleeding that showed benign endocervical tissue and proliferative endometrium. She was readmitted for recurrent bleeding. Dextran 70 hysteroscopy showed a polypoid lesion on the posterior wall of the uterine body. Directed curettage showed an endometrial polyp with moderate adenomatous hyperplasia, and subsequent hysterectomy confirmed the diagnosis. A single curettage will not fully remove all the surface endometrium from the uterine cavity even if performed by an experienced gynecologist.[11] Hysteroscopically directed curettage will prevent unnecessary hysterectomy in some patients if applied properly with a good clinical evaluation.

DISCUSSION

The following three applications are examples of hysteroscopy considered for investigational research.

APPLICATION VI

Hysteroscopy can be used to define the extent of the transformation zone in the endocervical canal. In the presence of abnormal cervical cytologic findings, an unsatisfactory colposcopic examination (without full observation of the transformation zone extending into cervical canal) calls for further investigation of the endocervix by endocervical curettage and cervical conization. If a contact hysteroscope or microhysteroscope is able to locate the transformation zone, and results of endocervical curettage, cytology, colposcopy, and colposcopically directed biopsy agree, the patient (if she desires further pregnancy) can be followed closely without conization but by office treatment.

APPLICATION VII

Hysteroscopy can be used to investigate the uterine cavity and endometrium in women exposed as fetuses to diethylstilbestrol (DES). These women have degrees of epithelial and structural abnormalities such as vaginal adenosis, cervical collar, cockscomb, and abnormality of the uterine cavity.[5] Further investigation with the contact hysteroscope or microhysteroscope can detect possible uterine malformations.

APPLICATION VIII

Hysteroscopy can be used to localize abnormal endometrial areas and destroy them by modified laser ray. Laser rays can be precisely delivered under the direction of a hysteroscope, enabling the normal tissue to be preserved.

COMMENT

Proficiency with the contact hysteroscope depends on experience, and approximately 50 patients are required to reach great accuracy.[2] With proper clinical evaluation of the patient and expert usage of these techniques, the physician's diagnostic acumen appears enhanced.

REFERENCES

1. Baggish MS: Contact hysteroscopy: A new technique to explore the uterine cavity. Obstet Gynecol 54:350, 1979
2. Baggish MS, Barbot J: Contact hysteroscopy for easier diagnosis. Contemp Obstet Gynecol 16:93, 1980
3. Barbot J: Contact hysteroscopy: Another method of endoscopic examination of the uterine cavity. Am J Obstet Gynecol 136:721, 1980

4. Blaustein AU: Pathology of The Female Genital Tract, pp 189–195. New York, Springer–Verlag, 1977

5. DiSaia PJ, Creaseman WT: Clinical Gynecologic Oncology, pp 38–49. St. Louis, C V Mosby, 1981

6. Edström K, Fernström I: The diagnostic possibilities of a modified hysteroscopic technique. Acta Obstet Gynecol Scand 49:327, 1970

7. Hamou J: Microhysteroscopy. A new procedure and its original application in gynecology. J Reprod Med 26:375, 1981

8. Lindemann HJ: The use of CO_2 in the uterine cavity for hysteroscopy. Int J Fertil 17:221, 1972

9. Lindemann HJ, Mohr J: CO_2 hysteroscopy: Diagnosis and treatment. Am J Obstet Gynecol 124:129, 1976

10. Morrow CP, Townsend DE: Synopsis of Gynecologic Oncology, pp 153–155. New York, John Wiley & Sons, 1981

11. Mattingly RF: TeLinde's Operative Gynecology, pp 420–425. Philadelphia, J B Lippincott, 1977

12. Merrill JA: Dissemination of cancer cells during surgical curettage. Am J Surg 29:206, 1963

13. Neuwirth RS: Hysteroscopy. Philadelphia, W B Saunders, 1975

14. Novak ER, Woodruff JD: Novak's Gynecologic & Obstetric Pathology, pp 140–142. Philadelphia, W B Saunders, 1979

15. Pantaleoni D: On endoscopic examination of the cavity of the womb. Med Press Circ 8:26, 1869

16. Perez CA, Zivnuska F, Askin F, et al: Prognostic significance of endometrial extension from primary carcinoma of the uterine cervix. Cancer 35:1493, 1975

17. Roberts S, Long L, Janasson O, et al: The isolation of cancer cells from the blood stream during uterine curettage. Surg Gynecol Obstet 111:3, 1960

18. Siegler AM, Kemmann, EK: Location and removal of misplaced or embedded intrauterine devices by hysteroscopy. J Reprod Med 16:139, 1976

19. Valle RF: Clinical application of hysteroscopy. In Phillips JM (ed): Endoscopy in Gynecology, pp 327–333. Downey, CA, American Association of Gynecologic Laparoscopists, 1978

Hysteroscopy in a Case of Hydatidiform Mole ■

37

Wilhelm Braendle
Albrecht Schulz-Classen
Hans-Egon Stegner

Hysteroscopy is an endoscopic method for observing the uterine cavity. Intrauterine synechiae and submucous fibroids are detectable and treatable under hysteroscopic control. The following case exemplifies another indication for hysteroscopy and its possible therapeutic value.

A patient 25 yr of age was admitted to the hospital because of a positive pregnancy test after curettage for hydatidiform mole. Serum human chorionic gonadotropin (hCG) levels ranged between 7000 and 8000 IU 10 days after curettage. After ectopic pregnancy was excluded by laparoscopy, hysteroscopy was performed. A submucous 5-mm tumor was seen in the posterior uterine wall and removed. Histologically the myoma included trophoblastic cells without signs of malignancy (Fig. 37-1). Postoperatively, serum hCG levels fell but remained between 5 and 15 IU, although regular menses occurred (Fig. 37-2). After regular menses and ovulatory cycles for 5 mo, amenorrhea occurred, with a rise in serum hCG levels. An early pregnancy was suspected, but ultrasonography, laparoscopy, and hysteroscopy could not detect it. Curettage did not reveal any trophoblastic tissue. Chemotherapy was instituted, and serum hCG levels became undetectable after the third course of treatment (Fig. 37-3).

This case demonstrates that hysteroscopic observation and excision of a small tumor was possible, an unlikely result with curettage. The levels of hCG immediately fell, although the excision did not succeed in completely removing all cells producing hCG. Serum hCG levels persisted and, after 10 mo, were exacerbated; the patient was then treated with chemotherapy.

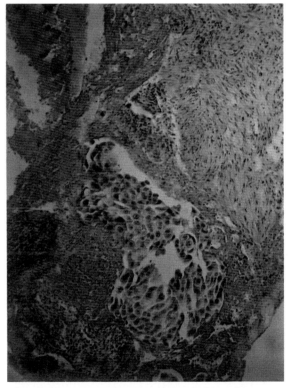

FIG. 37-1. A photomicrograph of the submucous tumor, which is partly a myoma with enclosed trophoblastic cells.

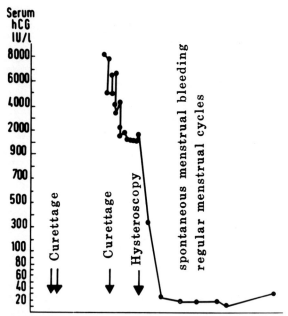

FIG. 37-2.   Serum hCG levels are shown after curettage and hysteroscopic removal of the submucous tumor.

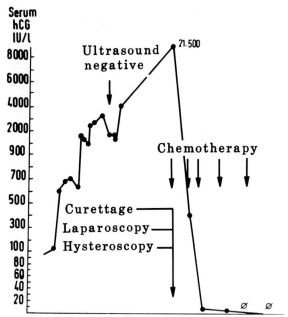

FIG. 37-3.   Serum hCG levels after 5 months of regular menses followed by subsequent amenorrhea.

HYSTEROSCOPY IN INFERTILITY AND STERILITY IV

The management of intrauterine adhesions under hysteroscopic control is described by Valle and Sciarra, by Sugimoto and co-workers, and by Wamsteker. All these authors use hysterography and hysteroscopy to classify or grade this disease, but they use different media to distend the uterine cavity. Lysis of adhesions is monitored by laparoscopy in almost half the patients. Postoperatively, most of the women receive antibiotics, intrauterine devices (IUDs), estrogens, and progestins. Patients who have severe adhesions (amenorrhea, severely distorted uteri on hysterography, and fibromuscular adhesions at hysteroscopy) are generally not cured. Although menses return, most women never achieve term pregnancies.

Gallinat, Labastida and colleagues, and Lübke and Hindenburg support the usefulness of hysteroscopy in selected infertile women. The procedure seems of limited value in patients having a normal hysterogram, but hysteroscopy often discloses the cause of abnormal shadows seen on x-ray film. Polyps, myomas, adhesions, and artifacts can be differentiated from one another more precisely by hysteroscopy. Taylor and colleagues combine hysteroscopy and laparoscopy, and they note minimal risk in 602 ovulatory women. Although in one third of normal infertile women some intrauterine abnormality was seen at hysteroscopy, the clinical significance of these findings is yet to be ascertained.

Dolff describes a procedure he calls *salpingocatheterization*, in which the intramural segment is probed with a Charrière (no. 3) catheter. He was able to locate proximal tubal obstruction and differentiate it from spasm, but the maneuver is not simple and has a risk of uterine perforation. DeCherney reports results on resection of 15 arcuate and septate uteri under laparoscopic control using a modified resectoscope for patients who have had repeated abortions. The advantages of being able to form a normal uterine cavity in this manner include obviating the need for a laparotomy or for automatic cesarean section.

Hysteroscopy as an Examination Method in Sterility ■

38

Friedhelm Lübke
Hans-Joachim Hindenburg

Up until now, physicians could only obtain incomplete information on the intrauterine causes of sterility. Total or partial uterine atresia, endometrial atrophy, and intramural tubal occlusion are recognizable. The hypoplastic uterus and uterine synechiae cause infertility, depending on their severity. Uterine malformations such as septate and bicornuate uteri and deformities such as submucous myoma and cervical insufficiency may be responsible for infertility by causing habitual abortions. The accuracy in diagnosis of these pathologic changes has been improved by radiologic examination, namely, hysterosalpingography. Since the development of hysteroscopy by Lindemann, the uterine cavity can be assessed visually.[1] With this method physicians can assess the endocervical canal, the internal os, the shape of the uterine cavity, the endometrium, and the intramural tubal ostia.

Although ruptures, scars, and excessive dilatation of the internal os can cause infertility, it is doubtful that a submucous myoma can cause sterility. Submucous and intramural myomas can cause implantation difficulties, but successful pregnancies have been observed despite such findings. Neither Asherman's syndrome nor severe synechiae necessarily cause sterility or infertility. The hypoplastic and malformed uterus can hinder implantation, but some normal pregnancies have been

observed in these women. Therefore, a complete evaluation is indicated before uterine defects are surgically corrected.

The endometrium can be easily examined by hysteroscopy. Polyps and polypoid changes (diffuse or isolated) can be detected, although the tubal ostia are not always identifiable. Endometrial synechiae can be delineated in sterile patients more frequently than can other abnormalities. It is uncertain whether these findings cause sterility. After Lindemann described the use of hysteroscopy in infertility during the Seventh World Congress for Fertility and Sterility, I was able to confirm its value in two subsequent studies.[2,4,5]

MATERIALS AND METHODS

Laparoscopy and hysteroscopy were performed together in 236 patients. Primary sterility occurred in 156 women (66%), and 80 women (34%) had secondary sterility.

RESULTS

Nine patients had congenital deformities, and six women had submucous myomas. In 221 examinations, normal findings resulted (Table 38-1). Normal endometrial findings were seen

Table 38-1
RESULTS OF HYSTEROSCOPIC EXAMINATIONS IN 236
INFERTILE WOMEN

HYSTEROSCOPY	PATIENTS	
	No.	%
Normal	221	93.7
Uterine malformations	9	3.8
Arcuate	(2)	
Subseptate	(5)	
Septate	(1)	
Bicornuate	(1)	
Submucous myoma	6	2.5
Total	236	100

Table 38-2
CORRELATIONS BETWEEN HYSTEROSCOPIC AND
PATHOLOGIC DIAGNOSES IN 160 PATIENTS

HYSTEROSCOPY	NO. OF PATIENTS	HISTO-PATHOLOGY	NO. OF PATIENTS
Myoma	6	Normal	5
		Myoma	1
Polypoid changes	134	Normal	131
		Polyps	3
		Myoma	1
Polyps	9	Normal	7
		Polyps	2
Synechiae	11	Normal	11
Total	160		160

Table 38-3
EVALUATION OF 102 TUBAL OSTIA

OSTIUM	LEFT		RIGHT	
	No.	%	No.	%
Normal	16	6.8	20	8.5
Polypoid	21	8.9	29	12.3
Not seen	2	0.8		
Obstruction	6	2.5	8	3.4
Total	45		57	

in 87 women (34.7%), while polypoid changes were found in 134 (56.8%). Nine polyps and 11 synechiae were observed.

Hysteroscopic diagnoses were not confirmed by histopathologic studies in many instances (Table 38-2). Direct observation of the endometrium permits detection of local findings, which is not possible with histologic examination. In comparison, Lindemann observed 413 uteri of infertile women and noted abnormalities in 48.6%.[2] I discovered even more changes. This difference emphasizes the subjective interpretation of the hysteroscopic findings.[3] The difference between normal endometrial structures and superficial polypoid changes is minimal. Lindemann believes that such changes need not necessarily be classified as pathologic, since they are discharged with the endometrium during menstruation.

Hysteroscopic evaluation of the tubal openings is easy when they are circular. Gas bubbles that flow through these apertures suggest that the internal tubal orifices are patent. Probing them is possible. In 102 observations (43.2%), changes in one or both of the tubal apertures were seen (Table 38-3). Although pathologic significance has not been proved, the high percentage of sterile patients with such findings is remarkable. Changes in the tubal orifices were seen in only 25% of patients during hysteroscopy that was being done for other reasons (e.g., sterilization). It is not clear whether these structural alterations affect sperm migration. Tubal patency can be judged through the controlled gas flow and the Rubin insufflation test, but these results must be evaluated with caution.[6] Despite minimal passage of the gas, tubes appeared patent at laparoscopy.

REFERENCES

1. Lindemann HJ: Eine neue Untersuchungsmethode für die Hysteroskopie. Endoscopy 4:194, 1971
2. Lindemann HJ: Hysteroscopy for the diagnosis of intrauterine causes of sterility. Presented at the Eighth World Congress on Fertility and Sterility, Tokyo and Kyoto, October 17–23, 1971
3. Lindemann HJ: Atlas der Hysteroskopie. Stuttgart, Gustav Fischer, 1980
4. Lübke F: The diagnostic value of intrauterine causes for sterility and infertility, using hysteroscopy. Presented at the Ninth World Congress on Fertility and Sterility, Buenos Aires, November 3–9, 1974
5. Lübke F: Über den diagnostischen Wert der Hysteroskopie. Arch Gynaekol 219:255, 1975
6. Rubin IC: Uterotubal Insufflation. St. Louis, C V Mosby, 1947

Infertility and Hysteroscopy ■ 39

Ramon Labastida
Santiago Dexeus
Alfonso Arias

Diagnosis of uterine abnormalities responsible for sterility and infertility usually is made by indirect methods. However, the improvement of endoscopic equipment has made hysteroscopy valuable for diagnosis and treatment of these uterine abnormalities. This chapter will evaluate the usefulness of hysteroscopy in the infertile patient and compare these findings with hysterographic findings. Any endometrial tissue obtained was reviewed, and the results of surgical therapy were analyzed by hysteroscopic observation.

HYSTEROGRAPHY AND HYSTEROSCOPY

Hysterography is an important procedure for the indirect study of the uterine cavity. In many instances radiologic findings are misleading, as demonstrated subsequently during hysteroscopy. False-negative diagnoses on hysterography are uncommon, although functional intrauterine abnormalities and endometritis are not detectable radiographically. In the cornual region the hysterogram can show linear shadows suggesting a sphincter or valve. The cause of this picture is probably a fold of endometrium at the uterotubal junction, sometimes visible at hysteroscopy. Poor technique in taking hysterograms causes multiple errors in interpretation of the x-ray films (e.g., pseudodefects from air bubbles or intravasation from poor placement of the cannula).

Hysteroscopic and hysterographic examinations were performed on 91 infertile patients, and the diagnoses obtained from each technique were compared (Table 39-1). Hysteroscopic and hysterographic findings differed in 36 (39.5%). Hysteroscopy revealed a normal cavity in 14 patients (15.4%) who had abnormal hysterograms, but only 5 instances of false-negative hysterograms were found. In 17 women both techniques revealed abnormalities but of different types (Tables 39-2 to 39-4). Abnormal hysterograms seen in 75 women were reinterpreted after the endoscopic procedure in 31 instances (Figs. 39-1 to 39-4).

ENDOMETRIAL BIOPSY AND HYSTEROSCOPY

The hysteroscope enables the gynecologist to view the endometrial surfaces of the uterine

Table 39-1

COMPARISON BETWEEN HYSTEROGRAPHIC AND
HYSTEROSCOPIC FINDINGS IN 91 PATIENTS

HYSTER-OGRAPHY	HYSTEROSCOPY		
	Normal	Abnormal	
		Agree	*Divergent*
Normal	11 (12%)		5 (5.4%)
Abnormal	14 (15.3%)	44 (48.3%)	17 (18.6%)

Table 39-2

FINDINGS ABNORMAL ON HYSTEROGRAPHY AND
NORMAL ON HYSTEROSCOPY

HYSTEROGRAPHY	HYSTEROSCOPY
Endometrial abnormalities	
Endometritis (suspected)	2
Endometriosis (suspected)	1
Asherman's syndrome	1
Submucous myoma	1
Polyps or papilloma	3
Imprecise diagnosis	
Filling defect	4
Cornual blockage	2
Total	14

cavity, but it should not replace histologic study. Some endometrial samples are difficult to interpret because of insufficient tissue or because specimens are inadvertently taken from the lower uterine segment. Sometimes focal lesions are missed, and an unsuspected early pregnancy can be interrupted. Material obtained by endometrial biopsy constitutes less than 1% of the total volume of the endometrium.[2] Consequently, representative samples must be correctly taken from the uterine fundus. The amount of material obtained in biopsies after hysteroscopy was 40% greater than that from the most recent 91 biopsies for sterility, secured by curettage or aspiration. Endometrial samples obtained in patients with Asherman's syndrome were normal in 32%.

Table 39-3

FINDINGS NORMAL ON HYSTEROGRAPHY AND
ABNORMAL ON HYSTEROSCOPY

HYSTEROSCOPY	HYSTEROGRAPHY
Asherman's syndrome	1
Polyps	1
Endometrial hyperplasia	3
Total	5

Table 39-4

DIVERGENT ABNORMAL FINDINGS ON HYSTEROGRAPHY AND HYSTEROSCOPY IN 17 PATIENTS

HYSTEROGRAPHY \ HYSTEROSCOPY	Endometrial Hyperplasia	Asherman's Syndrome	Submucous Myoma	Polyps	Uterine Septum	Endometritis	Endometriosis	Adenocarcinoma	Postcesarean Retention Cysts	TOTAL
Endometriosis						1		1		2
Endometritis	1						1			2
Asherman's syndrome					1					1
Uterine septum		2								2
Submucous myoma	1			3					1	5
Polyps	3		2							5
Total	5	2	2	3	1	1	1	1	1	17

Focal, small endometrial lesions require direct biopsy, either with the operating hysteroscope or after cervical dilatation with a grasping forceps placed alongside the hysteroscope. An atrophic endometrium or endometrial hyperplasia has a characteristic hysteroscopic appearance. Chronic endometritis can result from retention of products of conception, submucous myomas, polyps, foreign intrauterine bodies, cervical stenosis after conization, or cervical amputation; hysteroscopic findings can ascertain the probable cause of the infection.

The colpomicrohysteroscope may allow the physician to differentiate among the types of endometritis and also to detect alterations in the normal menstrual cycle. Can infertility result from a nonuniformly reacting endometrium? Are there areas of local endometritis that prevent implantation? Are these factors in unexplained infertility? Can hysteroscopy with magnification answer these questions?

TREATMENT OF INTRAUTERINE ABNORMALITIES WITH HYSTEROSCOPY

A more accurate diagnosis generally leads to more successful and appropriate therapy. Studies by Barbot and colleagues, Edström and Fernström, Sugimoto, and Porto have compared the findings of hysteroscopy with hysterography.[1,3,5,7] Valle, and Sciarra and Valle, reported on failures in the treatment of patients with selected intrauterine defects because of the lack of visual control.[6,8] Lysis of significant intrauterine adhesions is difficult without hysteroscopic control, and even with such monitoring some patients cannot be cured. Resection of polyps and pedunculated myomas without hysteroscopic control is difficult and wider caliber curets are needed, increasing the occurrence of Asherman's syndrome. Removal of these tumors under hysteroscopic control, according to the technique developed by Neuwirth and Amin, represents a notable improvement in treatment.[4] The removal or resection of an intrauterine septum with the aid of hysteroscopy requires, in addition, a very precise technique, special instruments, and laparoscopic surveillance. We anticipate good results with this technique in the future. The removal of intrauterine devices after myomectomy or tubal microsurgery or of other kinds of foreign bodies is easy with hysteroscopy, and unnecessary surgical manipulation is avoided.

POSTSURGICAL HYSTEROSCOPIC CONTROL

Hysteroscopic exploration of the uterine cavity has been used after myomectomy to assess the configuration of the repaired uterus and the uterotubal junctions. Hysteroscopy enables the physician to see the anatomic results of cerclage, cesarean section scars, and metroplasty, and, after a tubal implantation, the new orifice can be examined directly and catheterized as indicated.

REFERENCES

1. Barbot J, Parent B, Dubuisson JB: Contact hysteroscopy: Another method of endoscopic examination of the uterine cavity. Am J Obstet Gynecol 136:721, 1980
2. Behrman SJ, Kistner RW: Progress In Fertility, 2d ed, pp 91–115. Boston, Little, Brown & Co, 1968
3. Edström K, Fernström I: The diagnostic possibilities of a modified hysteroscopic technique. Acta Obstet Gynecol Scand 49:327, 1970
4. Neuwirth RS, Amin HK: Excision of submucous fibroids with hysteroscopic control. Am J Obstet Gynecol 126:95, 1976
5. Porto R: Hystéroscopie. Travail de la Clinique Obstétricale et Gynécologique de la Faculté de Médicine de Marseille. Paris, Searle, 1975
6. Sciarra JJ, Valle RF: Hysteroscopy: A clinical experience with 320 patients. Am J Obstet Gynecol 127:340, 1977
7. Sugimoto O: Diagnostic and Therapeutic Hysteroscopy. Tokyo, Igaku–Shoin, 1978
8. Valle RF: Hysteroscopy in the evaluation of female infertility. Am J Obstet Gynecol 137:425, 1980

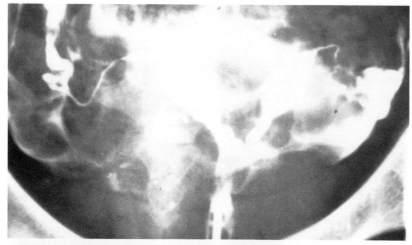

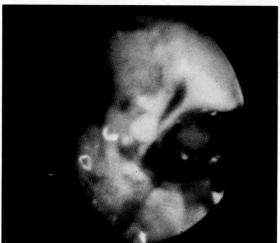

A

B

FIG. 39-1. Results of hysterography and hysteroscopy. (*A*) Hysterogram suggests a septate uterus. (*B*) Hysteroscopy reveals a thick intrauterine adhesion.

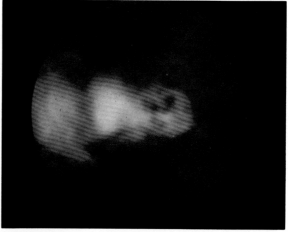

A *B*

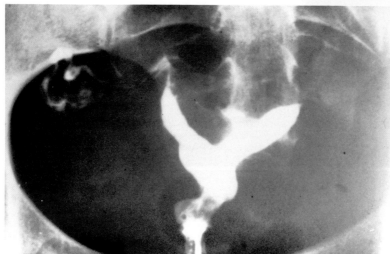

FIG. 39-2. Results of hysterography and hysteroscopy. (*A*) Hysterogram interpreted as an arcuate uterus. (*B*) Uterine synechiae seen on the hysteroscopic view.

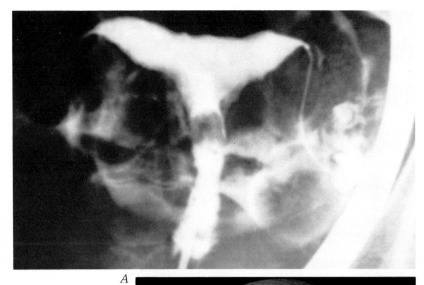

FIG. 39-3. Results of hysterography and hysteroscopy. (A) Hysterogram clearly delineates an oval defect in the lower uterine segment. (B) At hysteroscopy, the lesions seemed like a pedunculated growth.

A
B

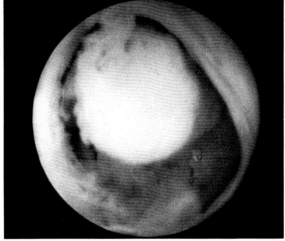

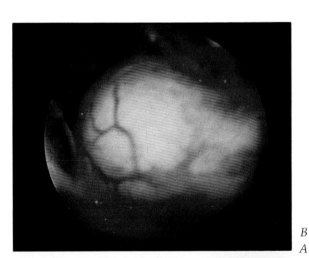

B
A

FIG. 39-4. Results of hysterography and hysteroscopy. (A) Hysterogram shows persistent filling defect in the lower uterine segment. (B) A cyst was present in this area at hysteroscopy.

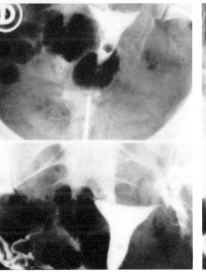
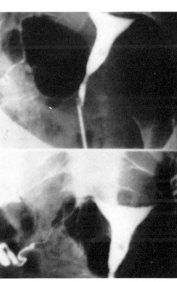

Hysteroscopy as a Diagnostic and Therapeutic Procedure in Sterility ∎

40

Adolf Gallinat

Hysteroscopy is an important diagnostic procedure in the study of infertility. Before endoscopy, ovulation is confirmed by basal body temperature (BBT), and a Sims−Huhner test is done. Hysteroscopy enables the examiner to localize and diagnose abnormal changes in the uterine cavity and cervical canal. Tubal patency can be measured by reading the manometer for pressure and flow, as in the Rubin test (Fig. 40-1).[4] After hysteroscopy, the scope is left in place and used as an elevator and for chromopertubation during laparoscopy.

Intrauterine abnormalities (Figs. 40-2 to 40-5) were recorded in 19% to 62% of infertile women in various studies.[1,7,11,12] Most often polyps and polyposis are seen. Small polyps are frequently located in the cornual area and possibly simulate a tubal occlusion (Fig. 40-6).[9,10] After nidation in the vicinity of a myoma, a disturbed placentation leads to abortion.[9,10] Pedunculated fibroids and polyps protruding into the cavity have effects similar to those of an intrauterine device (IUD). Malformations, such as septate or subseptate uteri, are easily recognized (Fig. 40-7). To exclude tubal spasm, it is desirable to catheterize the tubes under controlled hysteroscopy and laparoscopy.[5]

In 1980, 210 women complaining of sterility were examined. Intrauterine abnormalities were found in 34.3% (Table 40-1). Only 3% had adhesions, whereas Sciarra and Valle,

Taylor and colleagues, and Lindemann and Gallinat noted an incidence of 11% to 35%.[5,8,11] Endometrial strands or filaments are not classified as adhesions. In 15% of infertile women, no causes are found; they have the so-called unexplained infertility. The extended sperm migration test has been done since 1976 in 134 women. In the preovulatory phase, 2 to 5 hr after coitus, the Sims−Huhner test is done, and then fluid is aspirated out of the cul-de-sac at laparoscopy. During carbon dioxide hysteroscopy, mucus is suctioned out of the uterine cavity and tubal ostia (Fig. 40-8). In the uterine cavity, thin, watery, and transparent mucus is similar to the type found in the cervix at this time. Of 134 tests, 98 patients showed mobile and 36 patients showed immobile sperm (Fig. 40-9). In the latter group, no sperm were seen in the upper genital tract in 17 women. Surprisingly, mobile sperm were detected in tubal mucus in four. In the 98 women with positive cervical mucus, the number and motility of sperm were reduced proportionally as samples were retrieved from higher in the genital tract. In one patient, mobile sperm were detected in the fallopian tubes 4 days after coitus. If no sperm are found in the higher regions of the genital tract, the prognosis for conception is not good.[3] If only immobile sperm are discovered by the Sims−Huhner test, it does not mean that no sperm migration

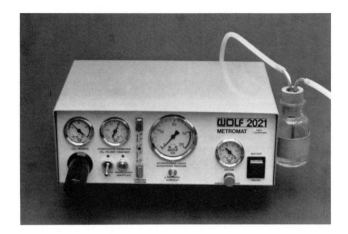

FIG. 40-1. Metromat is used for carbon dioxide hysteroscopy.

will take place. The decreasing number of sperm in higher regions could indicate an endometrial barrier.[5]

The hysteroscope can play an equally important role as a therapeutic instrument. Through targeted biopsies, histologic confirmation can be obtained (Fig. 40-10). If synechiae or polyps are discovered, they can be resected. Pedunculated polyps cannot always be removed by curettage because they slip away; they are thus ideal for hysteroscopic resection. The cornual areas especially cannot be curetted completely, and hysteroscopic observation and treatment of lesions in this region is particularly valuable. Here small polyps are most often found. Resecting synechiae is no problem, and submucous myomas up to 2 cm can be resected (Fig. 40-11).[2,5] A special hysteroscope with a straight working tunnel is necessary (Fig. 40-12), as are rigid instruments such as hook scissors and a strong biopsy forceps (Fig. 40-13). Neuwirth described another technique using a resectoscope.[6]

Of malformations, only the septate and subseptate uterus can be treated under hysteroscopic control, provided that prior laparoscopy excluded a bicornuate uterus (Fig. 40-14). These malformations do not cause infertility, but the septum should be removed in patients having repeated abortions. Resections were done on 12 septae in the last 3 yr, and 5 patients conceived; 4 of them delivered vaginally without complications. One is still pregnant. Postoperatively, insertion of a Lippes loop is indicated for a few

Table 40-1

INTRAUTERINE CHANGES AMONG 210 STERILE PATIENTS

Polyps	35
Polyposis	16
Synechiae	7
Submucous fibroids	5
Uterus septus	3
Uterus subseptus	2
Uterus arcuatus	1
Cervical stenosis	3
(Forgotten IUD	1)
Total	72 = 34.3%

weeks after resection of myomas, synechiae, and septae.[2] Simultaneously, the endometrium should be stimulated with exogenous gonadal steroids to prevent adhesions, as discussed below. One patient, aged 34 yr, had had four spontaneous abortions; the hysteroscopic diagnosis was a septate uterus. Hysteroscopic resection of the septum was controlled laparoscopically. A Lippes loop was inserted for 4 wk, and after its removal conception occurred, followed by an uncomplicated pregnancy. A second woman, aged 32, had had primary sterility for 6 yr; a subseptate uterus was discovered on hysterosalpingography. Hysteroscopic resection was done, and a Lippes loop was inserted for 4 wk and was followed by conception. Twelve weeks later the patient aborted, but she conceived again and has entered her 35th week of gestation.

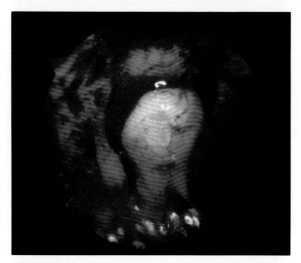

FIG. 40-2. Endometrial polyp is clearly visible at the fundus.

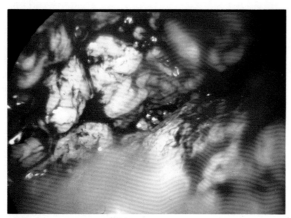

FIG. 40-3. Multiple small polyps.

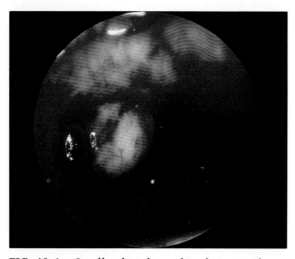

FIG. 40-4. Small polyps located in the cornual area can cause tubal occlusion.

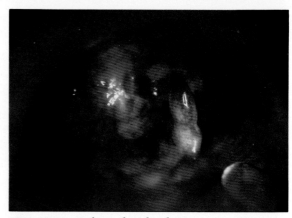

FIG. 40-5. Pedunculated polyp.

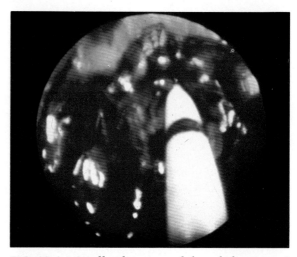

FIG. 40-6. Small polyps around the tubal ostium. A tubal occlusion can be excluded by sounding.

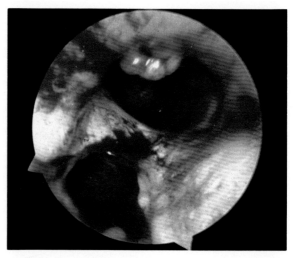

FIG. 40-7. Malformations such as a septate or subseptate uterus are easily recognized.

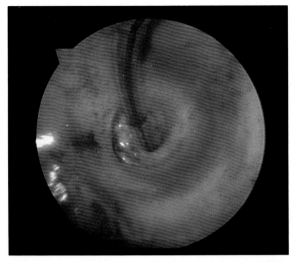

FIG. 40-8. Carbon dioxide hysteroscopy enables mucus to be suctioned out of the cavity and the tubal ostia.

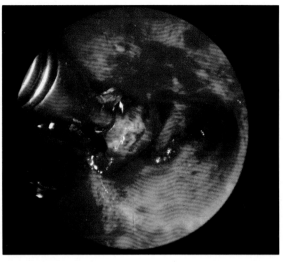

FIG. 40-10. Histologic confirmation can be obtained with target biopsies.

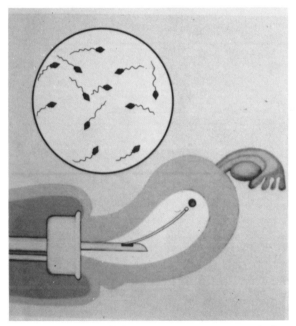

FIG. 40-9. Extended sperm migration test (schematic representation). ms = mobile sperm; is = immobile sperm.

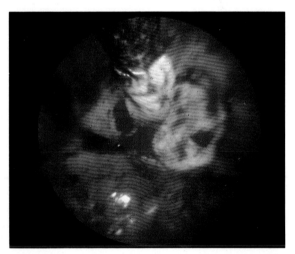

FIG. 40-11. Submucous myomas up to 2 cm can be resected.

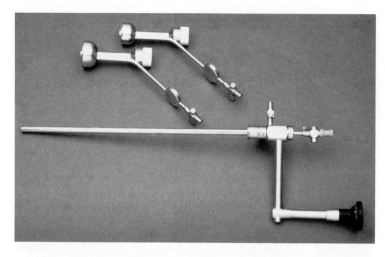

FIG. 40-12. Hysteroscope has a straight working channel.

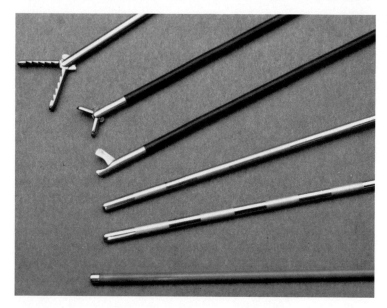

FIG. 40-13. Hook scissors and a strong biopsy forceps.

FIG. 40-14. Uterine malformation (schematic). (*A*) Uterus subseptus. (*B*) Bicornuate uterus.

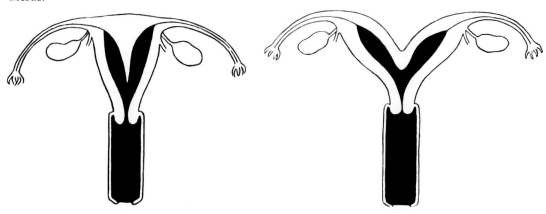

REFERENCES

1. Cohen MR, Dmowski WP: Modern hysteroscopy: Diagnostic and therapeutic potential. Fertil Steril 24:905, 1973
2. Edström KGB: Intrauterine surgical procedures during hysteroscopy. Endoscopy 6:175, 1974
3. Koch UJ; Sperm migration in the human female genital tract with and without intrauterine devices. Acta Eur Fertil 11:33, 1980
4. Lindemann HJ, Gallinat A: Physikalische und physiologische Grundlagen der CO_2–Hysteroskopie. Geburtshilfe Frauenheilkd 36:729, 1976
5. Lindemann HJ: Atlas der Hysteroskopie. Stuttgart, Gustav Fischer, 1980
6. Neuwirth RS: A new way to manage submucous fibroids. Contemp Obstet Gynecol 12:101, 1978
7. Rosenfeld DL: A study of hysteroscopy as an adjunct to laparoscopy in the evaluation of the infertile woman. In Phillips JM (ed): Endoscopy in Gynecology, p 337. Downey, CA, American Association of Gynecologic Laparoscopists, 1977
8. Sciarra JJ, Valle RF: Hysteroscopy: A clinical experience with 320 patients. Am J Obstet Gynecol 127:340, 1977
9. Siegler AM, Kemmann EK: Hysteroscopy. Obstet Gynecol Surv 30:567, 1975
10. Sugimoto O: Diagnostic and Therapeutic Hysteroscopy. Tokyo, Igaku–Shoin, 1978
11. Taylor, PJ, Cumming DC, Hill PJ: Significance of intrauterine adhesions detected hysteroscopically in eumenorrheic infertile women and role of antecedent curettage in their formation. Am J Obstet Gynecol 139:239, 1981
12. Valle RF: Hysteroscopy in the evaluation of female infertility. Am J Obstet Gynecol 137:425, 1980

Diagnostic and Therapeutic Hysteroscopy for Traumatic Intrauterine Adhesions ■

41

Osamu Sugimoto
Takahisa Ushiroyama
Yoshihiko Fukuda

The diagnosis of intrauterine adhesions has been made from irregular, ragged contours of filling defects on the hysterogram (Figs. 41-1 and 41-2). Nevertheless, the hysterogram may not reveal the existence or the extent of some of these adhesions. Hysteroscopy has improved the diagnosis and management of intrauterine adhesion.[1,2]

MATERIALS AND METHODS

Diagnostic hysteroscopy was performed in the Women's Clinic of Osaka Medical College Hospital from 1968 to 1977. Intrauterine adhesions were found in 258 patients; 221 of them showed irregular filling defects on the hysterogram (see Figs. 41-1 and 41-2), and 37 had had unexplained causes of sterility.

All 258 patients had had a previous intrauterine operation, and 83 had had postoperative infectious morbidity. Most patients had had a pregnancy-related curettage for various reasons: bleeding following a postpartum hemorrhage in 44, incomplete abortion in 98, induced abortion in 82, and molar pregnancy in 18 (Table 41-1). The chief complaints were amenorrhea in 34, hypomenorrhea in 131, dysmenorrhea in 28, repeated abortion in 75, and sterility in 183. Primary sterility was noted in only eight patients; seven had had a previous myomectomy, eight had had a cesarean section, and diagnostic curettage was the only uterine operation one patient had undergone.

A Machida rigid hysteroscope was used with saline irrigation or a viscous dextran solution. A clear image of the adhesions could be obtained when the uterine cavity was moderately dilated by the rinsing saline. The adhesions were bluntly removed when the tip of the outer sleeve of the hysteroscope was pushed against them (Fig. 41-3). Central adhesions were readily dissected by this method, however dense they might be. On the other hand, some of the severe marginal adhesions proved to be difficult to separate with the metal sleeve. In these cases, blunt lysis by Kelly forceps was successfully done by inserting them toward the adhesions in place of the hysteroscope. As the tip of the forceps was opened near the adhesions, the anterior and posterior walls of the uterus gradually separated from each other, allowing blunt removal of adhesions (Fig. 41-4). No scissors or electrocautery probe was used in our series. Whether the lysis had been done well was judged by a repeat hysteroscopy. Most of the firm marginal adhesions of connective tissue could not be eliminated by a single procedure; they required sharp dissection by abdominal hysterotomy. To prevent re-

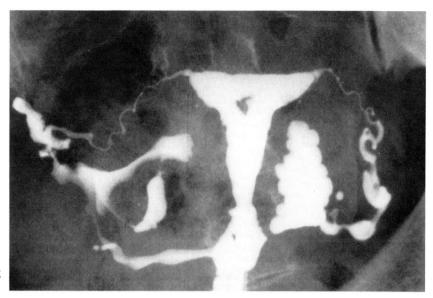

FIG. 41-1. Irregular filling caused by a central adhesion.

FIG. 41-2. A marginal adhesion caused this filling defect.

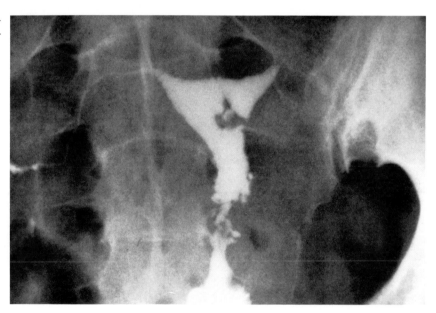

currence after lysis, the Ota ring was inserted for three to four menstrual cycles until cure was ascertained by subsequent hysteroscopy.

RESULTS

Most adhesions showed a bridgelike connection between the uterine walls, although some projected from the side walls of the cavity. The former were defined as central adhesions (Figs. 41-5 and 41-6) and the latter as marginal ones (Fig. 41-7). Extensive adhesions were mostly mixed with central and marginal; they were termed *multiple adhesions* (Fig. 41-8). Adhesions were central in 181 patients, marginal in 58, and multiple in 19. All adhesions except those 19 multiple ones were successfully re-

Table 41-1

CAUSE AND SYMPTOMS IN 258 PATIENTS WITH ASHERMAN'S SYNDROME

ETIOLOGY	NO. OF PATIENTS	MENSTRUAL DISORDERS			PAST CONCEPTION	
		Amenorrhea	Hypomenorrhea	Dysmenorrhea	Repeated Abortion	Sterility
Puerperal curettage	44 (14)*	12	26	7	15	29
Incomplete abortion	98 (35)*	14	56	7	30	68
Induced abortion	82 (24)*	2	41	11	25	57
Molar pregnancy	18 (6)*	4	7	1	4	14
Diagnostic curettage	1 (0)*	0	1	0	0	1
Myomectomy	7 (2)*	0	2	2	0	7
Cesarean section	8 (2)*	2	4	0	1	7
Total	258 (83)*	34	137	28	75	183
			199			

* Patients with postoperative infectious morbidity.

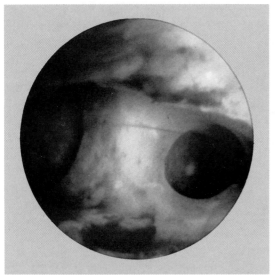
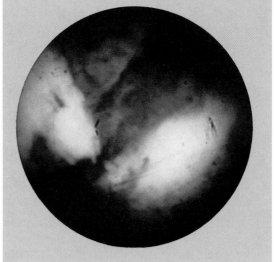
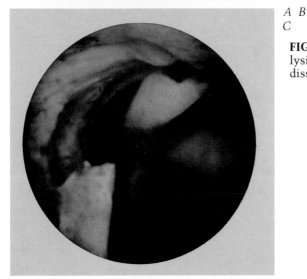

A B
C

FIG. 41-3. Myofibrous central adhesion. (*A*) Before lysis. (*B*) Adhesiotomy done by hysteroscopic blunt dissection. (*C*) Adhesion was completely disrupted.

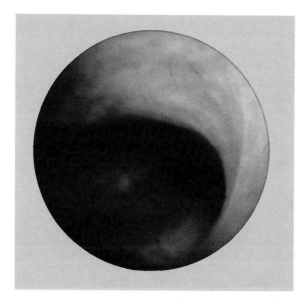

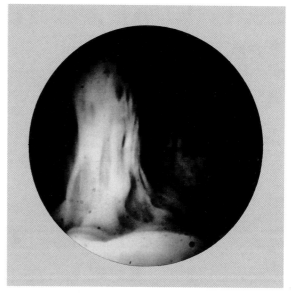

FIG. 41-5.   Central adhesion shows bridgelike connection between the anterior and posterior walls of the uterus. This is a myofibrous adhesion.

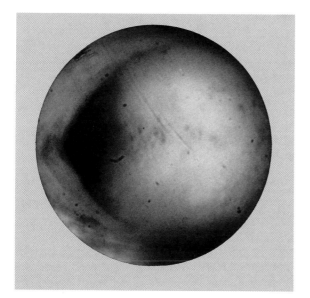

FIG. 41-4.   Myofibrous marginal adhesions. (A) Before adhesiotomy. (B) Kelly forceps has broken adhesions.

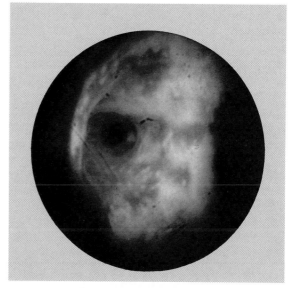

FIG. 41-6.   This central adhesion consists of endometrium with decidual change.

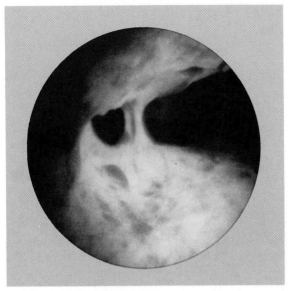

FIG. 41-7. Multiple adhesions combined central and marginal adhesion of the right uterine wall.

moved under visual control of hysteroscopy. Six of the 19 patients with dense adhesions underwent abdominal synechiotomy. An Ota ring was inserted in those patients who had had adhesiotomy, and two to three menstrual cycles later it was removed. All the central adhesions and most of the marginal ones were bluntly dissected with the tip of the outer sleeve under hysteroscopic observation. The composition and severity of the adhesions could be estimated from the superficial appearance on hysteroscopy before and after dissection and from the force needed to remove them. Hysteroscopy could classify the adhesions into three types according to tissue component: endometrial, myofibrous, or connective (Table 41-2).

Endometrial adhesions in 71 patients appeared quite similar to the surrounding endometrium. They were usually so fragile, whether central or marginal, that they could be easily removed by slight force. Fragments of the separated adhesions, swaying in the rinsing saline, formed soft, white, ciliary projections. Bleeding was hardly visible during the separation.

Myofibrous adhesions in 148 patients had a thin covering of endometrium with many glandular openings visible by hysteroscopy. Re-

moval of such adhesions needed slightly more force than endometrial adhesiotomy. The fragments were rough and reddish with oozing hemorrhage. Central myofibrous adhesions in 100 patients were easily separated by manipulating the outer sleeve. On the other hand, in 9 of 48 patients with marginal or multiple adhesions, lysis under visual control was difficult.

The most resistant adhesions, made of connective tissue, were found in 39 patients. The surface, without a lining endometrium, appeared glossy and ischemic. The denuded surface, after lysis of cicatrized central adhesions, was jagged like the stump of a snapped tree trunk and appeared pale because of minimal bleeding. Central connective tissue adhesions in 24 patients were removed vaginally, although 2 of 15 patients with marginal or multiple adhesions required abdominal synechiotomy.

The endometrium not involved in adhesions usually did not differ much from normal endometrium. In some patients after extensive firm adhesions were broken, only partial, poor regrowth of the endometrium occurred without cyclic changes. Superficial unevenness became more conspicuous after healing. This focal endometrial hypoplasia or scarring was

Table 41-2

TYPE, LOCATION, AND TREATMENT OF INTRAUTERINE ADHESIONS IN 258 PATIENTS

HISTOLOGY	NO. OF PATIENTS	LOCATION OF ADHESION			TREATMENT		
		Central	Marginal	Multiple	Vaginal	Abdominal	Pseudopregnancy Therapy
Endometrial tissue	71	57	10	4	71 (40)*	0	4
Myofibrous tissue	148	100	36	12	139 (112)*	4 (4)*	31
Connective tissue	39	24	12	3	33 (31)*	2 (2)*	16
Total	258	181	58	19	243 (210)*	6 (6)*	51

* Patients who had an IUD inserted.

Table 41-3

MENSTRUAL PATTERNS BEFORE AND AFTER THERAPY IN 258 PATIENTS

MENSTRUATION PREOPERATIVELY		MENSTRUATION POSTOPERATIVELY			
		Eumenorrhea	Hypomenorrhea	Amenorrhea	Dysmenorrhea
Eumenorrhea	93	93			
Hypomenorrhea	131	75	56		
Amenorrhea	34	12	22		
Dysmenorrhea	28				20
Total	258	180	78		20

Table 41-4

FERTILITY BEFORE AND AFTER LYSIS OF INTRAUTERINE ADHESIONS

FERTILITY BEFORE THERAPY		FERTILITY AFTER THERAPY				
		Sterility	Abortion	Premature Delivery	Full-term Delivery	Stillbirth
Repeated abortion	75	22	18	4	29	2
Sterility	183	129	19	3	30	2
Total	258	151	37	7	59	4
				107		

not reversible, even after insertion of an intrauterine device (IUD) and pseudopregnancy.

All 34 patients with amenorrhea before treatment regained regular menstruation; 12 patients became eumenorrheic, and 22 had hypomenorrhea (Table 41-3). Dysmenorrhea was not related to the degree or location of the adhesions. Pseudopregnancy was not as effective in restoring endometrial function, as evaluated by an increase in the amount of menstrual flow or the pregnancy rate.

Almost all 258 patients finished treatment before 1978, and 107 became pregnant (41.4%); 4 conceived twice or more (Table 41-4). Early spontaneous abortion occurred in 37 patients, and premature delivery occurred in 7 patients. As a result, 64 patients (24.8%) achieved viable delivery; 59 were full term and 5 premature. Among them, 11 needed manual removal of the placenta or curettage because of placental retention or adhesion. Postpartum observation showed three patients with persistent bleeding, and, at hysteroscopy, newly developed adhesions and retained placental fragments were seen.

COMMENT

Most intrauterine adhesions follow puerperal curettage or instrumental abortion, and in our series a previous operation and a recent pregnancy were noted in all but 8 of the 258 patients with intrauterine adhesions. Intrauterine synechiae cause filling defects of the uterine shadow on hysterogram, but these can also be caused by endometrial polyps, submucous fibroids, or air bubbles. Hysteroscopy can locate adhesions and delineate the presence, extent, and degree of the adhesions. Moreover, hysteroscopy detected adhesions even in patients with unknown causes of sterility or repeated abortion.

Hysteroscopy can roughly estimate the degree and composition of the adhesions from their superficial appearance before and after dissection. It is important to know whether endometrial, myofibrous, or connective tissues form the adhesions. Adhesions can be removed vaginally by abdominal hysterotomy or by blunt dissection or sharp severance at hysteroscopy. The operation selected varies with the severity and location of the adhesions. With therapeutic hysteroscopy, almost all intrauterine adhesions, and some dense marginal or multiple ones, have been bluntly removed vaginally under visual control. As a result of hysteroscopic synechiolysis, 246 of the 258 patients had the original form of their uterine cavity satisfactorily restored. To prevent recurrence, authors have reported various methods: endometrial transplant, transplantation of the fallopian tube, grafting of the fetal membrane, and insertion of an IUD. We used an IUD because the method was easy and useful for follow-up study by hysteroscopy. Most patients regained their original uterine contour, had increased menstrual flow, and regained their ability to conceive after hysteroscopic adhesiotomy. About one third of the patients were not cured of hypomenorrhea. Half the women who became pregnant had either an abortion or premature delivery. Eighteen percent of the women who delivered at term needed manual or instrumental removal of retained placenta.

The unsatisfactory prognosis after adhesiotomy in some patients may be due to insufficient recovery of endometrial function. Hysteroscopy often reveals a focal endometrial atrophy or scarring with little cyclic change. Pseudopregnancy was used for 3 to 4 mo immediately after synechiolysis in 51 patients; it did not ensure restored menstruation or fertility. Further studies are necessary to elucidate the causes and treatment of this endometrial dysfunction after lysis of intrauterine adhesions.

REFERENCES

1. Sugimoto O: Diagnostic and therapeutic hysteroscopy for traumatic intrauterine adhesions. Am J Obstet Gynecol 131:539, 1978
2. Sugimoto O: Diagnostic and Therapeutic Hysteroscopy. Tokyo, Igaku–Shoin, 1978

Hysteroscopic Treatment of Intrauterine Adhesions ■

42

Rafael F. Valle
John J. Sciarra

Since 1948, when Asherman described the syndrome that bears his name, the treatment of this condition did not change significantly until the advent of hysteroscopy.[1,2,4,5] Asherman had the foresight to recognize the potential value of hysteroscopy in the treatment of intrauterine adhesions. He wrote: "Hysteroscopy, which has so often been mentioned in the literature and just as often discarded, may be of use for this purpose. If it were possible to see the adhesions and to loosen them instrumentally, using the eye as a guide, the ideal method will have been found. We have the intention of trying out the practical application of this theoretical hypothesis."[2] Hysteroscopy is presently the accepted method for evaluating and treating intrauterine adhesions.[8,10,11] Previously an uncommon clinical diagnosis, Asherman's syndrome has become recognized as a frequent cause of repeated abortions and infertility in patients with postabortal or postpartum amenorrhea.[3,6,9] This article describes the use of hysteroscopy in the management of 61 patients with intrauterine adhesions.

MATERIALS AND METHODS

Between January 1975 and December 1980, hysteroscopy was used to treat 61 women with intrauterine adhesions. The patients' ages ranged from 20 to 37 yr, with a mean age of 22 yr. The preoperative obstetric histories included 59 miscarriages in 38 patients (45 in the first trimester and 14 in the second trimester) and 4 premature deliveries. All patients had a history of previous intrauterine trauma. Of the 59 who had had curettage after pregnancy, 14 were performed postpartum, 28 followed an incomplete abortion, 12 occurred during an elective abortion (5 in the first trimester and 7 in the second trimester), 2 had curettage for hydatidiform mole, and 3 had curettage for a missed abortion. One patient underwent myomectomy with entrance into the uterine cavity, and one had had a metroplasty for a septate uterus.

The main complaints were repeated abortion (38) and infertility (23); other symptoms included amenorrhea (14), hypomenorrhea (32), and dysmenorrhea (38). A hysterosalpingogram suggesting intrauterine adhesions had been performed on all patients before hysteroscopy. Ovulation was confirmed by biphasic basal body temperature studies, luteal phase serum progesterone, and a timed endometrial biopsy in those women who had cyclic menses. In the infertile patients, a standard infertility evaluation was performed, including semen analysis and postcoital test.

193

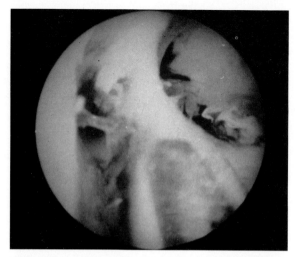

FIG. 42-1. Hysteroscopic view of an intrauterine adhesion in the right lateral upper portion of the uterus, partially occluding the uterotubal cone.

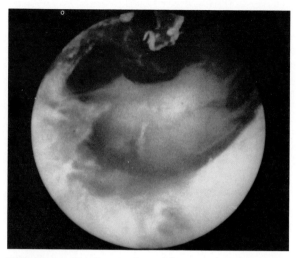

FIG. 42-3. Uterine cavity with normal architecture after lysis of adhesions.

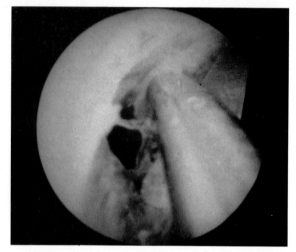

FIG. 42-2. Scissors guided through hysteroscopy to divide adhesions.

Hysteroscopy was performed in the early proliferative phase, but in 14 amenorrheic patients no special timing was attempted. Two types of hysteroscopes were used. The operating hysteroscope with a flexible scissors* (diameter, 7 French) was used in most patients. When thick adhesions were encountered, another operating hysteroscope,† one with a rigid

* Storz Instrument Company, Tuttlingen, West Germany.
† Eder Instrument Company

3-mm diameter scissors, was used (Figs. 42-1 to 42-3). Dextrose 5% in water and dextran 32% in dextrose 10% were used interchangeably for uterine distention. Dextran 70 (Hyskon) was used when observation was impaired by bleeding; otherwise, dextrose 5% in water was satisfactory. No electrocautery was necessary; division of adhesions did not produce major bleeding because most fibrotic bands were avascular.

Hysteroscopy was performed under general anesthesia in 59 instances, with simultaneous laparoscopy in 45 women who required extensive intrauterine dissections. In 14 others, filmy adhesions partially occluding the uterine cavity did not require laparoscopy. The use of laparoscopy was decided on at the time of dissection. Only two patients who had partial filmy adhesions underwent hysteroscopy under local anesthesia. Laparoscopy was added routinely when tubal blockage was seen on hysterosalpingography, regardless of the degree of intrauterine adhesion. After hysteroscopy, chromopertubation with indigocarmine was monitored during laparoscopy; suspected unilateral blockage was treated by selective chromopertubation. Following lysis of adhesions under hysteroscopic control, treatment included placing an intrauterine device (IUD) in 54 patients (Lippes loop in 49, Dalkon shield in

3, pleated membrane in 2) immediately post-operatively. In seven women no IUD was used because only filmy adhesions and partial uterine occlusion were present. A prophylactic antibiotic, 500 mg of ampicillin 4 times daily for 5 days, was given perioperatively. A regimen of estrogen (Premarin), 2.5 mg, twice a day for 26 days, with 10 mg of medroxy progesterone acetate (Provera) every day from days 22 through 26 of the cycle, was prescribed for 54 patients. The IUD remained in place for 2 mo, and the estrogen–progestogen therapy was continued for 3 cycles. Follow-up study did not include routine hysterosalpingography, except in 16 patients who preoperatively had thick adhesions completely or partially occluding the uterine cavity. Of these, 12 had recurrent but milder adhesions, but only 9 agreed to a second operation.

RESULTS

The classification of adhesions and their frequencies is set out in Table 42-1. The reproductive outcome of these 61 patients after hysteroscopic treatment included 23 term pregnancies, 5 patients pregnant but undelivered, 5 spontaneous abortions, and 1 ectopic pregnancy (Table 42-2). When 16 patients with mild intrauterine adhesions were treated, 10 (62.5%) achieved a term pregnancy. Most patients treated had moderate adhesions, that is, fibromuscular adhesions partially or totally occluding the uterine cavity. Of the 33 patients with moderate adhesions, 11 (33.3%) achieved a term pregnancy. Of 12 patients with severe intrauterine adhesions, only 2 term pregnan-cies occurred (16.6%), and there were 3 failures to restore the normal symmetry and architecture of the uterine cavity.

Of the 14 patients with a history of amenorrhea, 3 remained amenorrheic after hysteroscopy. Oligomenorrhea was corrected in all four women who had it before operation. Of the 32 patients with hypomenorrhea, 10 remained hypomenorrheic; of the 38 patients with dysmenorrhea preoperatively, 9 still complained of dysmenorrhea even after treatment and removal of their IUDs. Eleven patients had normal menses preoperatively, and 40 did after operation. There was a significant improvement in the obstetric performance postoperatively; 33 intrauterine pregnancies resulted, compared with none before therapy, but 5 women aborted. Fifty-nine spontaneous abortions had occurred in 38 patients preoperatively.

Table 42-1
HYSTEROSCOPIC CLASSIFICATION OF INTRAUTERINE ADHESIONS

TYPE OF ADHESIONS	OCCLUSION OF UTERINE CAVITY		TOTAL
	Partial	Complete	
Mild			
Thin, filmy (endometrial)	14	2	16
Moderate			
Thick, lined with endometrium (fibromuscular)	32	1	33
Severe			
Thick, solid, no endometrial lining (connective)	8	4	12

Table 42-2
REPRODUCTIVE OUTCOME AFTER HYSTEROSCOPIC TREATMENT OF INTRAUTERINE ADHESIONS IN 61 PATIENTS

TYPE OF ADHESIONS	PATIENTS	TERM PREGNANCY		MISCARRIAGE	ECTOPIC PREGNANCY	CHILD NOT YET BORN
		No.	%			
Mild	16	10	62.5	0	0	3
Moderate	33	11	33.3	3	1	2
Severe	12	2	16.6	2	0	0

In 8 of 33 patients with moderate adhesions, a recurrence was demonstrated, but only 6 accepted a second hysteroscopy; 5 patients had normal postoperative menstrual patterns, and 1 continued to have hypomenorrhea. Seven of 12 patients with severe adhesions developed recurrences, and 4 accepted a second treatment; 2 had normal postoperative menses, and 2 continued to exhibit hypomenorrhea. There were no recurrences in the 16 patients with mild intrauterine adhesions. There were two uterine perforations; one occurred during insertion of an IUD after lysis of intrauterine adhesions in a patient with severe Asherman's syndrome, and one occurred during uterine sounding in a patient with a completely occluded uterine cavity. The perforations were recognized at laparoscopy and did not require treatment. Hysteroscopic therapy could not be completed in three patients because of severe intrauterine adhesions.

DISCUSSION

For purposes of analysis, the 61 patients were grouped into three clinical categories depending on the severity of adhesions. Classification of adhesions was based on the degree of intrauterine involvement as shown by hysterosalpingography and the extent and type of adhesions found at hysteroscopy (see Table 42-1). Sugimoto's criteria were used to assess the components of adhesions during hysteroscopic diagnosis and therapy.[8] *Mild adhesions* are filmy but can produce partial or complete occlusion of the cavity. *Moderate adhesions* characteristically are thick fibromuscular bands covered with endometrium that bleed upon division and partially or totally occlude the uterine cavity. *Severe adhesions* are composed only of connective tissue, lack any endometrial lining, and do not bleed upon division; they may partially or totally occlude the uterine cavity. Although no attempt was made routinely to obtain tissue for analysis of the adhe-

sions, it was possible to perform a biopsy in 8 women with severe adhesions and in 15 others with fibromuscular adhesions. The histologic examination confirmed the visual appraisal of the adhesions from the 15 patients with fibromuscular adhesions and in 6 patients with connective tissue adhesions. Tissue from the remaining two patients with severe adhesions histologically was fibromuscular tissue.

CONCLUSION

The possibility of intrauterine adhesions after postpartum or postabortal curettage or any trauma to the uterine cavity suggests the need for early diagnosis. Best results are achieved with early therapy when adhesions are mild and filmy. Hysteroscopic lysis of intrauterine adhesions in this study proved superior to curettage. In patients with severe and extensive connective tissue adhesions, even division under hysteroscopic control was not satisfactory, and reproductive outcome remained poor.[7] To assist the clinician in predicting the outcome of therapy, a classification of the severity was based on the degree of intrauterine involvement on hysterosalpingography and the extent and type of adhesions found at hysteroscopy.

Concomitant laparoscopy is important, particularly in the treatment of patients with moderate and severe adhesions and when tubal occlusion is demonstrated by hysterosalpingography.

REFERENCES

1. Asherman JG: Amenorrhoea traumatica (atretica). J Obstet Gynaecol Br Emp 55:23, 1948
2. Asherman JG: Traumatic intra-uterine adhesions. J Obstet Gynaecol Br Emp 57:892, 1950
3. Klein SM, García CR: Asherman's syndrome: A critique and current review. Fertil Steril 24:722, 1973
4. Levine RU, Neuwirth RS: Simultaneous laparoscopy and hysteroscopy for intrauterine adhesions. Obstet Gynecol 42:441, 1973
5. March CM, Israel R, March AD: Hysteroscopic management of intrauterine adhesions. Am J Obstet Gynecol 130:653, 1978
6. Oelsner G, Amnon D, Insler V, et al: Outcome of pregnancy after treatment of intrauterine adhesions. Obstet Gynecol 44:341, 1974
7. Siegler AM, Kontopoulos VG: Lysis of intrauterine adhesions under hysteroscopic control. A report of 25 operations. J Reprod Med 26:372, 1981
8. Sugimoto O: Diagnostic and therapeutic hysteroscopy for traumatic intrauterine adhesions. Am J Obstet Gynecol 131:539, 1978
9. Toaff R, Ballas S: Traumatic hypomenorrhea–amenorrhea (Asherman's syndrome) Fertil Steril 30:379, 1978
10. Valle RF: Hysteroscopy in the evaluation of female infertility. Am J Obstet Gynecol 137:425, 1980
11. Valle RF, Sciarra JJ: Current status of hysteroscopy in gynecologic practice. Fertil Steril 32:619, 1979

Hysteroscopy in Asherman's Syndrome ■

43

Kees Wamsteker

Hysterography is not reliable in the diagnosis of intrauterine adhesions, whereas hysteroscopy enables the physician to see the extent of adhesions, select a therapeutic regimen, and offer a prognosis for fertility after treatment.[1,2] Treatment of patients with Asherman's syndrome to allow for subsequent pregnancy has been disappointing. Jewelewicz and colleagues reviewed the literature between 1948 and 1975 and found only 39% term deliveries in 351 pregnant women after they were treated for in-

trauterine adhesions. This chapter will report on a study from the Mariastichting, Haarlem, and the Women's Clinic of the University Hospital, Leiden, The Netherlands, of Asherman's syndrome detected by hysteroscopy in 36 patients with hypomenorrhea or amenorrhea (6), irregular menstrual pattern (2), infertility (21), or repeated abortion (7). Thirty-two patients already had hysterograms suggestive of intrauterine adhesions.

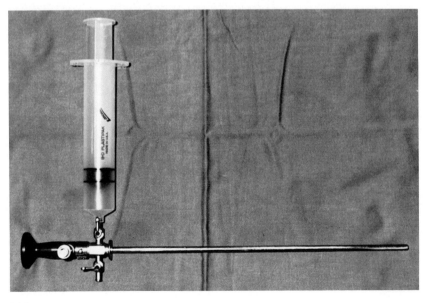

FIG. 43-1. A 5-mm Storz hysteroscope with syringe for injection of dextran 70 (Hyskon).

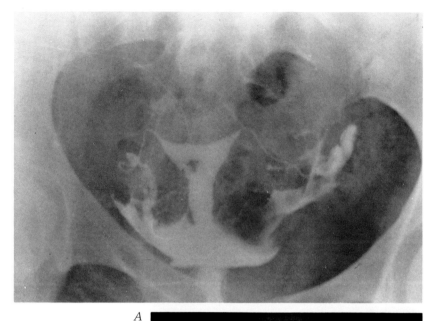

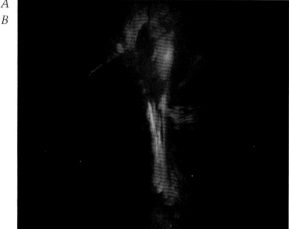

Fig. 43-2.   Hysterography showed a central defect; at hysteroscopy a definite bridge of tissue runs anterior –posterior.

A
B

MATERIALS AND METHODS

A special 5-mm hysteroscope* (Fig. 43-1) was used with 32% dextran 70 (Hyskon), which was injected manually to distend the uterine cavity. Intrauterine adhesions were lysed under vision with small scissors and biopsy forceps introduced into the cavity along the hysteroscope sheath. All hysteroscopic operations were performed under general anesthesia, and, in 15 patients with concomitant laparoscopy, this prevented inadvertent perforation of the myometrium. In 16 women, a Lippes Loop intrauterine device (IUD) was inserted immediately after the operation and left in place for 2 mo. Postoperative therapy consisted of antibiotics and hormones with a sequential contraceptive pill or conjugated estrogen tablets (Premarin), 2.5 mg/day, for 1 or 2 mo.

RESULTS

Classification of patients with Asherman's syndrome was based on hysteroscopic and hysterographic findings (Table 43-1). A grade I

* K.G. Storz, Tuttlingen, West Germany.

Asherman's syndrome consisted of minimal intrauterine adhesions that could be ruptured by the hysteroscope sheath alone. The significance of such intrauterine abnormalities is not clear. Patients with grades II, III, and IV all had firm adhesions that had to be cut by scissors or biopsy forceps. Marginal adhesions and endometrial scarring were also classified as Asherman's syndrome. When the lesions were extensive and associated with amenorrhea or hypomenorrhea (see Table 43-1), patients were considered grade IIIa. Examples of hystero-

Table 43-1

CLASSIFICATION OF ASHERMAN'S SYNDROME
IN 36 PATIENTS

GRADE	EXTENT OF INTRAUTERINE ADHESIONS	PATIENTS
I	Thin or filmy adhesions easily ruptured by hysteroscope sheath; uterotubal ostia normal	6
II	Single firm adhesion connecting two separate parts of the uterine cavity not lysed by hysteroscope sheath; occluding adhesions only at the internal cervical os; uterotubal ostia normal	11
III	Multiple firm adhesions connecting separate parts of the uterine cavity with unilateral obliteration of uterotubal ostium	11
IIIa	Extensive scarring of uterine cavity associated with amenorrhea or hypomenorrhea	2
IIIb	Combination of III and IIIa	
IV	Extensive firm adhesions agglutinating walls of the uterine cavity and obliterating uterotubal ostia bilaterally	6

graphic and hysteroscopic findings in women with different grades are shown in Figures 43-2 to 43-5. Of five patients with amenorrhea, three had a normal menstrual pattern after therapy. Two of the five had had grade II and one had had grade III adhesions; all later became pregnant. Of the two women with persistent amenorrhea, one had very extensive intrauterine adhesions with endometrial scarring and another had a very small uterine cavity after Beutner's operation for genital tuberculosis. Fertility after hysteroscopic lysis of adhesions could be studied in 27 women. One patient received no therapy, four did not wish to conceive, and four others were not followed.

Of 27 infertile patients, 17 conceived; other factors caused infertility in 6 of the remaining 10 patients. Of the three women with very low grade Asherman's syndrome, two did not conceive; no detectable reasons could be found for their infertility. Nine of 10 women with grade II Asherman's syndrome conceived; the tenth did not although she had a normal uterine cavity on hysteroscopy and on hysterography postoperatively. Five of eight women with grade III changes and two of six with grade IV changes later became pregnant. All other women had coexisting abnormalities that explained their persisting infertility. Of the 17 patients who conceived, 4 aborted and 1 had an ectopic pregnancy. The other 12 all had living children, with term deliveries in 11. One patient had a twin pregnancy and prematurely delivered two healthy children at 34 weeks' gestation. Two women who had cervical incompetency requiring cerclage had had this problem before hysteroscopy was performed. One of them had two abortions at 16 and 19 weeks and had had cerclage after a normal term delivery 5 yr before. After hysteroscopic lysis of adhesions she had an uneventful pregnancy with cerclage and term delivery. The other woman had had seven pregnancies without a living child and had a septate uterus with cervical incompetence. After a Tompkins operation, she developed Asherman's syndrome grade III, which was treated hysteroscopically. In her next pregnancy a cerclage was performed, and the patient delivered a living child at term. The remaining nine patients had uneventful pregnancies with term delivery of living children. A good correlation exists between the primary classification grade of Asherman's syndrome and fertility after therapy. Hysterograms of patients with extensive Asherman's syndrome before and after synechiectomy are shown in Figures 43-3 and 43-4.

COMMENT

Diagnosis and therapy of Asherman's syndrome have considerably changed since the introduction of new techniques for hysteroscopy. Hysterography is not reliable for diagnosis of intrauterine adhesions, and it is necessary to perform hysteroscopy in patients with abnormal hysterographic findings. A combination of hysteroscopic and hysterographic findings allows the intrauterine adhesions to be classified. An internationally accepted classification will be necessary to compare the results of therapy and to show a correlation between treatment and subsequent fertility.

The significance of thin filmy adhesions in the uterine cavity (grade I) is not known, although such adhesions seem to be a relatively frequent finding in eumenorrheic infertility patients.[3] For treatment of patients with Asherman's syndrome grades II, III, and IV, rigid, strong instruments and dextran 70 are required. A special 6-mm hysteroscope is being developed.

FIG. 43-3. (*A*) Before treatment, only a fingerlike projection of contrast material is seen. (*B*) After treatment, the normal shape of the cavity has been restored and both tubes are outlined.

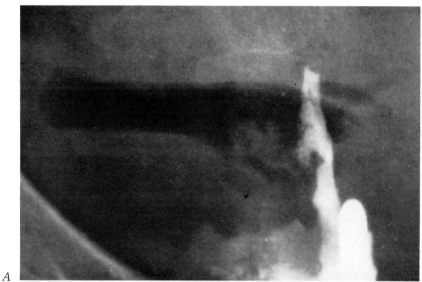

A

B

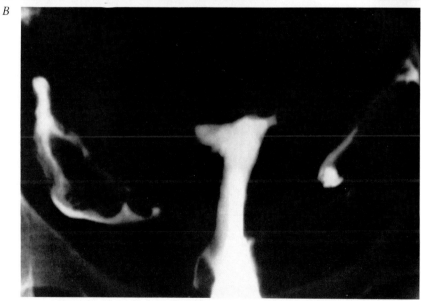

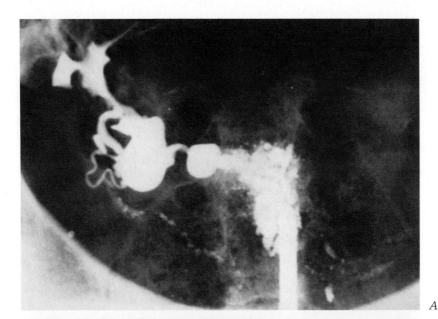

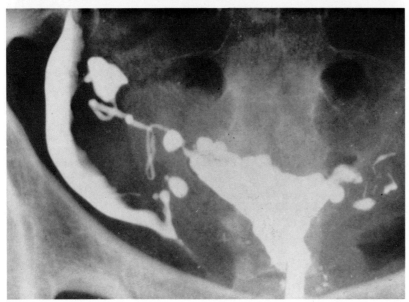

FIG. 43-4. (A) Hysterogram shows severely deformed corpus with myometrial intravasation (Asherman's syndrome grade IV). (B) After therapy, the cavity has a normal triangular appearance.

A

B

FIG. 43-5. (*A*) Hysterogram shows deformed uterine cavity and multiple irregular filling defects (Asherman's syndrome grade III). (*B*) Adhesions were confirmed by hysteroscopy.

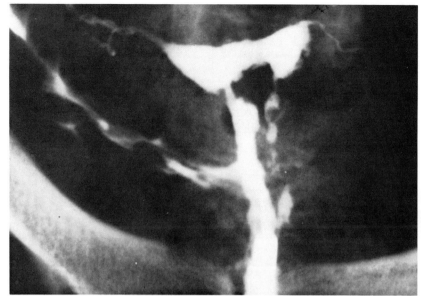

A

B

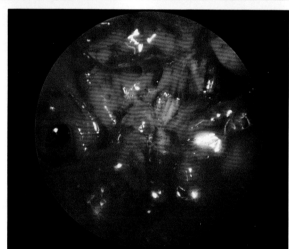

REFERENCES

1. Jewelewicz R, Khalaf S, Neuwirth RS, et al: Obstetric complications after treatment of intrauterine synechiae (Asherman's syndrome). Obstet Gynecol 47:701, 1976
2. March CM, Israel R, March AD: Hysteroscopic management of intrauterine adhesions. Am J Obstet Gynecol 130:653, 1978
3. Taylor PJ, Cumming DC, Hill PJ: Significance of intrauterine adhesions detected hysteroscopically in eumenorrheic infertile women and role of antecedent curettage in their formation. Am J Obstet Gynecol 139:239, 1981
4. Wamsteker K: Hysteroscopie. Thesis, University of Leiden, Holland, 1977

Hysteroscopic Management of Müllerian Fusion Defects ■

44

Alan H. DeCherney

Müllerian fusion defects are an important cause of abortion in the first trimester of pregnancy. These congenital abnormalities occur in approximately 5% of women, and 20% of these patients have reproductive problems. To date the accepted surgical treatment has been metroplasty, the Tompkins, Strassmann, or Jones type, with a reported 75% success rate. I have removed intrauterine septae responsible for habitual abortions transcervically, using the American cystoscopic resectoscope.*

MATERIALS AND METHODS

Fifteen patients who fulfilled the classic definition of habitual abortion were selected between July 1979 and July 1981. Their abortions occurred before 14 weeks of gestation. Preoperative evaluation included normal results from karyotypes on male and female partners, thyroid function studies, basal body temperature, endometrial biopsy specimens, and serum progesterone levels. Both partners were treated with broad-spectrum antibiotics. All patients had preoperative hysterosalpingograms that demonstrated either an arcuate or a septate uterus.

The procedure included resectoscopic removal of the uterine septum with concomitant laparoscopy under general anesthesia. The procedure was performed in the ambulatory surgical facility of the Yale–New Haven Hospital.

Dextran 70 (Hyskon) and a nonmodified fiberoptic, urologic, 8-mm (24 Fr) American cystoscopic resectoscope were used to examine the endometrial cavity. The septum was identified; if it was not too large, an attempt was made to excise it with electric cutting current from an Aspen Laboratory electrocautery unit.† The current flow was 30 watts/sec. In most instances the septum immediately became dessicated, reflecting its poor tissue integrity. Operability depended on a panoramic view and septum thickness.

During hysteroscopic examination, before resectoscopic dissection, a second operator performed a laparoscopy with carbon dioxide insufflation and a 5-mm standard laparoscope to view the uterine contour. The procedure was done during the follicular phase, and the tissue was sent to a pathologist. The septum was shaved to a level below the endometrium to permit endometrial regeneration in the area to fill the created gap.

No preoperative positive cultures for *Chlamydia* or *Mycoplasma* species were obtained. All patients had müllerian fusion defects on hysterosalpingogram. Two patients required an intrauterine Foley catheter postoperatively to

* American Cystoscope Makers Inc., Stamford, CT.

† Aspen Laboratories, Littleton, CO.

tamponade bleeding, but the catheter was removed 3 hr later without difficulty. All patients were given ampicillin, 500 mg 4 times daily, 1 day preoperatively and 5 days postoperatively and conjugated estrogen, 5 mg daily, for 30 days. No intrauterine device (IUD) was used to maintain separation of the uterine walls postoperatively.

RESULTS

Fifteen patients were selected for transcervical removal of the septum using the cystoscopic resectoscope. No serious intraoperative or postoperative complications occurred. All patients were followed. In four patients, the septum was too large for the procedure. Nine of the 11 remaining women conceived postoperatively and delivered at term—8 vaginally and 1 by cesarean section because of fetal distress. One patient had two subsequent first-trimester abortions, and one patient has been infertile during the 18 mo since the procedure. One patient had amenorrhea 8 wk after the resection but resumed menses spontaneously and has conceived. Five of the 11 women had postoperative hysterosalpingograms that demonstrated normal uterine cavities. An attempt to correlate the size of the fusion defect with feasibility of the operation from the preoperative hysterosalpingograms was not possible.

DISCUSSION

Habitual abortion means three consecutive abortions occurring at less than 20 weeks' gestation or at a fetal weight of less than 500 g. The incidence is approximately 1 : 200 women. Various causes include thyroid disease, inadequate luteal phase, chronic severe systemic disease, chromosomal abnormalities, chronic infections, and uterine anomalies. The 15 women discussed here had a uterine anomaly as the only cause of habitual abortion.

Hypothetically, abortion in patients with müllerian fusion defects is caused by a compromised blood supply in the septum. The fetus outgrows its nutritional supply if implantation occurs at that site. In the past, metroplasty was performed by removing the uterine septum (Jones and Strassmann) or by bisecting it, allowing it to retract laterally (Tompkins). Such patients can be successfully treated by a transcervical resectoscopic technique. Concomitant laparoscopy must be used because the external contour of the uterus cannot be seen on the hysterosalpingogram. A didelphic or bicornuate uterus cannot be operated on in this fashion. Perforation must be avoided to prevent thermal damage to intra-abdominal viscera. Gentile and Siegler have reported inadvertent bowel biopsy when they used the hysteroscope.[3]

Neuwirth in 1978 described hysteroscopic removal of submucous myomas by a similar technique, and Haning and co-workers have successfully removed a benign mesodermal tumor with the resectoscope.[4,5] Chervenak and Neuwirth in 1981 reported the successful removal of an intrauterine septum with this technique in two patients; they employed an IUD postoperatively, as did Edström and Fernström.[1,2] Haning and colleagues used glycine rather than dextran 70 because it mixes readily with blood and rinses bleeding rapidly out of view; it may also give a wider field of vision. Although no evidence exists to show that this operation causes Asherman's syndrome, we treated patients with conjugated estrogen to improve endometrial growth over the uterine defect.

The hysteroscopic procedure offers the patient a shorter hospitalization and a low complication rate. If successful, it obviates the necessity for later cesarean section and, possibly, postoperative intra-abdominal adhesions. Since the hysterogram cannot predict which patients will be amenable to this form of surgery, the final decision depends on the endoscopic findings.

Siegler and Kemmann in 1975 reported on removal of IUDs, treatment of Asherman's syndrome, and possibly transcervical hysteroscopic sterilization as possible uses of hysteroscopy.[6] Many reports describe removal of intrauterine lesions successfully, primarily pedunculated myomas and polyps.[1,2,5-7] To these can be added successful removal of intrauterine septae with a urologic resectoscope and electrocautery.

REFERENCES

1. Chervenak FA, Neuwirth RS: Hysteroscopic resection of the uterine septum. Am J Obstet Gynecol 141:351, 1981
2. Edström K, Fernström I: The diagnostic possibilities of a modified hysteroscopic technique. Acta Obstet Gynecol Scand 49:327, 1970
3. Gentile GP, Siegler AM: Inadvertent intestinal biopsy during laparoscopy and hysteroscopy. A report of two cases. Fertil Steril 36:402, 1981
4. Haning RV Jr, Harkins PG, Uehling DT: Preservation of fertility by transcervical resection of a benign mesodermal uterine tumor with a resectoscope and glycine distending medium. Fertil Steril 33:209, 1980
5. Neuwirth RS: A new technique for and additional experience with hysteroscopic resection of submucous fibroids. Am J Obstet Gynecol 131:91, 1978
6. Siegler AM, Kemmann E: Hysteroscopy. Obstet Gynecol Surv 30:567, 1975
7. Valle RF, Sciarra JJ: Current status of hysteroscopy in gynecologic practice. Fertil Steril 32:619, 1979

Combined Laparoscopy and Hysteroscopy in the Investigation of Infertility ■

45

Patrick J. Taylor
Arthur Leader
Ronald E. George

Many techniques have been used to assess the reproductive tract of the ovulatory infertile woman, among them laparoscopy, hysterosalpingography, endometrial biopsy, and, more recently in North America, hysteroscopy. The role of laparoscopy in ovulatory infertile patients is well established. Its superiority to hysterosalpingography in detecting peritoneal and peritubal causes of infertility has been demonstrated in several studies.[2,6,7,10,11] Hysterosalpingography can provide useful information on the uterine cavity not available from laparoscopy and is used by many gynecologists in the preliminary investigation of the nonovulatory causes of infertility in women. In some instances, the hysterosalpingogram may be ambiguous or the findings may be difficult to interpret. Hysteroscopy provides a safe method for both the rapid and accurate diagnosis and the treatment of many abnormalities of the uterine cavity.[3–6] Recent studies have demonstrated the increased accuracy of hysteroscopy over hysterosalpingography in the diagnosis of uterine lesions that may contribute to and perhaps cause female infertility.[8,10,12]

We have reported on combined laparoscopy and hysteroscopy in 169 women.[1] These 169 patients were included in the present prospective study of 602 women who underwent combined laparoscopy and hysteroscopy as part of the assessment of primary or secondary infertility or previous sterilization.

MATERIALS AND METHODS

We studied 602 patients ranging in age from 18 to 38 yr; 300 complained of primary infertility and 221 of secondary infertility, and 81 requested a reversal of a previous tubal ligation. The duration of infertility ranged from 7 to 144 mo.

All the patients attended the University of Calgary Endocrine/Infertility Clinic. A routine full assessment was made of all patients and included a history and physical examination, the detection of presumptive evidence of ovulation by basal body temperature graphing, serum progesterone assays, and, when indicated, a timed endometrial biopsy. Two semen analyses were performed on each male partner after a complete history and physical examination had been recorded. A postcoital test was carried out at the appropriate time in the second, apparently normal ovulatory cycle.

Patients with evidence of anovulation were excluded from the study. No couples with a male causative factor were included. Also excluded from the study were those patients who either conceived while under investigation or who voluntarily withdrew from the program.

The remaining patients were examined endoscopically within 3 mo of the initial visit. The procedures were carried out under general anesthesia on a day-care basis as previously described.[9] The surgeons worked as a team: cervical dilatation and pneumoperitoneum introduction were simultaneous; the laparoscope and hysteroscope were introduced simultaneously as well, allowing for intra-abdominal monitoring of the hysteroscopic maneuvers. Dextran 70 (Hyskon) was used routinely to distend the uterus. Chrompertubation was performed with the Valtchev mobilizer.* In no instance was dye leakage a problem, despite previous cervical dilatation. The findings were recorded on a standard coding sheet. The data were processed by the Academic Computing Services of the University of Calgary, which also assisted with data analysis.

RESULTS

Laparoscopy was performed successfully in 598 patients. One failure occurred in a patient in whom the diagnosis of early pregnancy was made at the time of hysteroscopy.[1] Under these circumstances, no attempt was made at laparoscopy. In two patients, obesity prevented successful introduction of the laparoscope, and in one patient preperitoneal emphysema prevented successful laparoscopy. The failure rate for laparoscopy was 0.67%.

In the infertile group of 521 patients, laparoscopy was performed successfully in 518. Of these examinations, 333 (64.3%) were judged to reveal lesions sufficiently severe to be considered to have caused infertility (Table 45-1). We found that 188 of the 300 patients (62.7%) with primary infertility and 145 of the 221 patients (65.6%) with secondary infertility had a tubal or peritoneal factor. In addition, two women with secondary and one with primary infertility had abnormalities of müllerian development. The specific lesions detected laparoscopically are shown in Table 45-2.

Hysteroscopy was performed successfully in 587 patients. In the patient with an early pregnancy, hysteroscopy was considered a failure. Failure in the other 14 patients occurred for the following reasons: air bubbles in the medium (3), failure of cervical dilatation (9), and blood obscuring the field of view (2). The

* Conkin Surgical Instruments, Toronto, Canada.

Table 45-1

LAPAROSCOPIC FINDINGS IN 602 WOMEN

INFERTILITY	NORMAL	ABNORMAL	FAILED	TOTAL
Primary	112	188	0	300
Secondary	73	145	3	221
Previous sterilization		80	1	81

Table 45-2

LAPAROSCOPIC ABNORMALITIES IN 518 INFERTILE WOMEN

ABNORMALITY	PRIMARY INFERTILITY (N = 300)	SECONDARY INFERTILITY (N = 218)
Adhesions		
Unilateral	26	28
Bilateral	94	81
Phimosis		
Unilateral	18	21
Bilateral	24	14
Hydrosalpinx		
Unilateral	29	20
Bilateral	27	39
Cornual occlusion		
Unilateral	18	8
Bilateral	2	9
Endometriosis		
Unilateral	37	15
Bilateral	37	15
Fibroids	15	10
Müllerian abnormality	1	2

failure rate was 2.5%. There was one uterine perforation that was seen laparoscopically and treated successfully by observation. Suture repair of a cervical laceration was required in 2 patients for a 0.67% complication rate, when the detection of pregnancy is also considered to be a complication.

Intrauterine abnormalities were detected in 203 of 506 successfully completed hysteroscopies in the infertile group (40%) and in 27 of the 81 patients requesting reversal of a previous sterilization (33.3%). Ninety-nine of 291 patients (34.0%) with primary infertility and 104 of 215 patients with secondary infertility (48.4%) had hysteroscopically recognizable lesions (Table 45-3).

The specific nature of the lesions detected hysteroscopically is shown in Table 45-4. Because multiple lesions were detected in several patients, these are expressed individually; hence the total number of detected abnormalities exceeds 333. Table 45-5 shows that 62 of 505 women (12.3%) who would have been assessed as laparoscopically normal with primary or secondary infertility were found to have uterine lesions. In addition, 167 of 403 women (41.4%) with pelvic abnormalities had hysteroscopically identifiable lesions.

DISCUSSION

Laparoscopy and hysteroscopy have been shown to play an important role in the investigation of ovulatory infertile women in several studies. The combined endoscopic procedures provide complete information on the status of these patients' reproductive tracts while adding little operating time to the laparoscopy.

Although laparoscopy in conjunction with hysterosalpingography is still the most common investigative combination in such patients, consideration should be given to hysteroscopy at the time of laparoscopy. Hysteroscopy is a safe method for the direct, rapid, and accurate diagnosis of intrauterine lesions and has low failure (2.5%) and complication (0.67%) rates. Hysteroscopy may allow the physician to diagnose small and possibly insignificant abnormalities not evident on hysterosalpingography, but it has also shown that the artifacts of hysterosalpingography are not evident on hysteroscopy.[3,9] When others have compared hysteroscopy to hysterosalpingography, an accuracy rate of 50% to 62% has been noted for the latter.[12] Hysteroscopy provides the gynecologist with the opportunity not only to visualize the abnormality but also to correct it in many cases.[6]

To what extent intrauterine filmy adhesions and polyps contribute to a patient's infer-

Table 45-3
HYSTEROSCOPIC FINDINGS IN 602 WOMEN

INFERTILITY	NORMAL	ABNORMAL	FAILED	TOTAL
Primary	192	99	9	300
Secondary	111	104	6	221
Previous sterilization	54	27	0	81

Table 45-4
HYSTEROSCOPIC ABNORMALITIES IN 587 WOMEN

ABNORMALITY	PRIMARY INFERTILITY (N = 291)	SECONDARY INFERTILITY (N = 215)	PREVIOUS STERILIZATION (N = 81)
Adhesions			
Cervix	1	2	0
Uterus	44	68	12
Polyps			
Cervix	2	2	0
Uterus	45	28	15
Fibroids (uterus)	5	6	2
Septa			
Cervix	0	1	0
Uterus	1	3	0
Total	98 (33.7%)	110 (51.2%)	29 (35.8%)

Table 45-5
COMBINED LAPAROSCOPIC AND HYSTEROSCOPIC FINDINGS IN 585 WOMEN

INFERTILITY	BOTH NORMAL	LAPAROSCOPY NORMAL, HYSTEROSCOPY ABNORMAL	LAPAROSCOPY ABNORMAL		TOTAL
			Hysteroscopy normal	Hysteroscopy abnormal	
Primary	80	30	112	69	291
Secondary	40	32	70	72	214
Tubal			54	26	80

tility is not known.[4,5] It has been suggested but not proved that these lesions are significant, and we are presently assessing that in our patients. In our study a significant number of women with secondary infertility (P < 0.01; χ^2 test) had abnormal hysteroscopic findings when compared to either women with primary infertility or a previous sterilization.

The nature of these lesions did not show the statistical significance between primary and secondary infertility that was evident when each of both groups was compared with previously sterilized women. If hysteroscopic lesions contribute to or perhaps cause a woman's infertility, then the overall detection rate of 78% for either uterine or peritubal lesions or both makes a strong argument for the combined approach. For women considered suitable for reversal of a previous sterilization by tubal surgery, awareness and treatment of hysteroscopic lesions may have a role in altering the outcome.

REFERENCES

1. Cumming DC, Taylor PJ: Combined laparoscopy and hysteroscopy in the investigation of the ovulatory infertile female. Fertil Steril 33:475, 1980
2. Maathuis JB, Horbach JGM, van Hall EV: A comparison of the results of hysterosalpingography and laparoscopy in the diagnosis of fallopian tube dysfunction. Fertil Steril 23:428, 1972
3. Rosenfeld DL: A study of hysteroscopy as an adjunct to laparoscopy in the evaluation of the infertile woman. In Phillips JM (ed): Endoscopy in Gynecology, pp 337–340. Downey, CA, American Association of Gynecologic Laparoscopists, 1978
4. Sugimoto O: Hysteroscopy. V. Endometrial polyps. Obstet Gynecol Ther 24:217, 1972
5. Sugimoto O: Diagnostic and therapeutic hysteroscopy for traumatic intrauterine adhesions. Am J Obstet Gynecol 131:539, 1978
6. Sugimoto O: Diagnostic and Therapeutic Hysteroscopy. Tokyo, Igaku–Shoin, 1978
7. Swolin K, Rosencrantz M: Laparoscopy vs hysterosalpingography in sterility investigation: A comparative study. Fertil Steril 23:270, 1972
8. Taylor PJ: Correlations in infertility: Symptomatology, hysterosalpingography, laparoscopy and hysteroscopy. J Reprod Med 8:339, 1977
9. Taylor PJ, Cumming DC: Hysteroscopy in 100 patients. Fertil Steril 31:301, 1979
10. Taylor PJ, Cumming DC: Laparoscopy in the infertile female. Curr Probl Obstet Gynecol 2:3, 1979
11. Templeton AA, Kerr MG: An assessment of laparoscopy as the primary investigation in the subfertile female. Br J Obstet Gynaecol 84:760, 1977
12. Valle RF: Hysteroscopy in the evaluation of female infertility. Am J Obstet Gynecol 137:425, 1980

Carbon Dioxide Hysteroscopy Before Tubal Microsurgery ■

46

Michael Dolff

MATERIALS AND METHODS

Between January 1980 and August 1981 I performed carbon dioxide hysteroscopic investigations, in addition to hysterosalpingography and laparoscopy, on 98 patients at the UFK-Düsseldorf to evaluate tubal causes of sterility. Morphologic findings such as intramural polyps or functional blockage of the tubocornual junction can be seen by direct observation of the tubal angle. Carbon dioxide hysteroscopy was performed in the technique introduced by Lindemann.[1]

To clarify the tubal cause of sterility the following factors are important during hysteroscopy:

Intracavitary pressure
Carbon dioxide flow rate
Leakage of mucus and bubbles through the tubal ostia
Salpingocatheterization
Motility of the tubal angle

Intracavitary pressure and carbon dioxide flow are physically interdependent variables. In patients whose tubes are obstructed, the pressure increases to 150 mm Hg to 200 mm Hg with an automatic fall in the carbon dioxide flow rate.

The static behavior of bubbles in front of the tubal ostia is demonstrable. Leakage of mucus and bubbles can be spontaneous or delayed. Delayed leakage is seen mainly in patients with sactosalpinx or hypoplastic, phimotic, or adherent tubes; I encountered it in one patient with salpingitis isthmica nodosa. The differential diagnosis is clarified only by laparoscopy or laparotomy. Salpingocatheterization of the tubal angle and the tubocornual

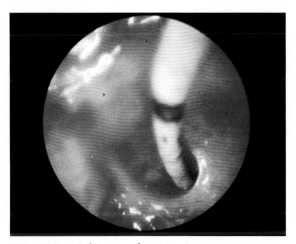

FIG. 46-1. Salpingocatheterization.

junction with a no. 3 Charrière ureteral catheter indicates that the tubes may be blocked close to the uterus.

Spontaneous contractions of the tubal angle were observed in several patients during hysteroscopy. Induced contractions during salpingocatheterization might be correlated with intensified motility of the tubal angle and the tubocornual junction. Intramural spasm during hysteroscopy can be differentiated from organic cornual blockages. The inability to induce contractions of the tubal angle by its catheterization is presumptive evidence of a postinflammatory fibrosis.

RESULTS

Laparotomies were performed in 401 women thought to have tubal blockage because of findings at hysterosalpingography or laparoscopy or both. Fifteen patients (3.7%) had patent tubes at laparotomy. The erroneous diagnosis had been made from both hysterosalpingographic and laparosopic findings in 11 patients and in 2 by one or the other procedure. Seven of the 15 patients had had hysteroscopy before operation, and no evidence of anatomic tubal obstruction was detected in 6 (86%). In one instance a fundal myoma had misled the hysteroscopist because the tube proved patent.

Functional blockage (spasm) was the cause of erroneous findings in hysterosalpingograms and at laparoscopy in ten patients. In three instances the tubes were hypoplastic; twice a "valve" mechanism caused functional blockage, and in one patient both tubocornual junctions were distorted by a fundal myoma.

Three case reports follow.

CASE 1

A patient complained of infertility for 1½ yr. The diagnosis of cornual blockage was made from laparoscopic and hysterosalpingographic findings. Carbon dioxide hysteroscopy with salpingocatheterization showed a cornual blockage caused by spasm that was confirmed on minilaparotomy.

CASE 2

A patient complained of infertility for 4 yr. The diagnosis of cornual blockage was made at laparoscopy and from repeated hysterosalpingograms. Carbon dioxide hysteroscopy with tubal catheterization showed right cornual spasm and a cornual polyp that prolapsed while the tip of the catheter was introduced into the left horn. The polyp was removed at hysteroscopy, and the patient subsequently underwent lysis of pelvic adhesions.

CASE 3

A patient underwent salpingo-oophorectomy because of tubal pregnancy and tubal implantation on the opposite side because of cornual blockage. Carbon dioxide hysteroscopy showed a normal uterine cavity and a normal tubal angle on the side of implantation. The tip of the catheter was inserted 2 cm into the implant (Fig. 46-1). No sutures from the tubal implantation were observed. An isthmic—isthmic anastomosis was performed. The microscopic findings of the resected tube showed no inflammation.

REFERENCE

1. Lindemann HJ: Pneumometra für die Hysteroskopie. Geburtshilfe Frauenheilkd 33:18, 1973

HYSTEROSCOPY AND PREGNANCY

V

Although pregnancy is a relative contraindication to hysteroscopy, Gallinat, and Wagner and Schweppe, show the successful application of the technique to resolve difficult clinical problems. Women who conceive while wearing an intrauterine device (IUD) are examined before their pregnancies are terminated. These authors are able to locate the position of an IUD and remove it in selected instances without disturbing the pregnancy. Most of the gestations continue to term without any untoward effects. The application of embryoscopy enables the study of early intrauterine fetal development and implantation sites and has potential clinical value. The technique is not simple nor without hazard; it should be considered experimental and limited at present to patients whose pregnancies are scheduled for termination by abortion.

The other contributions in this section are by Lueken and by Salat-Baroux and coworkers. They report on the results of postabortal hysteroscopy in an effort to study whether suction and sharp curettage allow for complete uterine evacuation in elective abortion and to detect intrauterine changes after spontaneous abortion. Although complete evacuation occurs most often after suction curettage, mild intrauterine adhesions are detected in many instances.

These investigators do not suggest hysteroscopic examination as a routine method to study the uterine cavity after abortion, but new information is contained in both these presentations. It is fascinating to realize the ability of the hysteroscopist to see the uterine cavity so clearly immediately after curettage for abortion.

Hysteroscopy in Early Pregnancy ■

47

Adolf Gallinat

There are three groups of indications for hysteroscopy during early pregnancy: to study an intrauterine device (IUD) in relation to the early implantation, to perform embryoscopy, and to evaluate the "disturbed" pregnancy.

PREGNANCY AND AN INTRAUTERINE DEVICE

An intrauterine pregnancy can occur despite the presence of an IUD in between 1% and 4% of patients. The IUD should be removed because of the possible complication of a septic abortion or a possible teratogenic effect from copper-bearing devices.[1,12,14] Secondary dislocation and tail retraction are caused by the growth of the uterus (Fig. 47-1) if the IUD is not extracted promptly.[7] The presence of the IUD is recognizable by ultrasound in 96% of women; at hysteroscopy the device should be removed. If abortion is indicated, evacuation is accomplished by suction. An attempt to extract the IUD by suction can fail and cause complications; the device can be pushed into the soft uterine wall.[2] The pregnancy can proceed even after removal of the IUD, and term pregnancies and deliveries without complications have been reported.[11,13] After carbon dioxide hysteroscopy, bleeding can be provoked through the tearing of the placenta by pneumometra.[2]

INTRAUTERINE DEVELOPMENT OF THE AMNIOTIC SAC AND EMBRYOSCOPY

Carbon dioxide hysteroscopy was done before elective abortion between the 5th and 12th wk of gestation to study the blastocyst (its growth, site of implantation, junction of the decidua parietalis with capsularis) and the optical changes of the amniotic sac. Only dilatation up to Hegar no. 5 and to the level of the internal os was carried out. A 4-mm Hopkins integrated optic in a 5-mm shaft was used. For photographic documentation, a xenon light source and integrated optics were necessary. After the tenth week of pregnancy an 11-mm foroblique optic was used. Because this endoscope has a comparatively small opening angle, the three-dimensional effect was reduced to a minimum and the smallest details were clearly visible. When hysteroscopy was begun, ergotamine was injected to prohibit extreme uterine expansion. With a contraction, the intrauterine pressure increased simultaneously, enabling better visibility. Immediately after hysteroscopy abortion was performed by suction.

Carbon dioxide hysteroscopy gives the same excellent view in pregnant and nonpregnant patients, although different physical principles exist. The cavity is slit- rather than pear-shaped in the nonpregnant uterus. An obvious increase in size occurs in pregnancy, the gas flow is higher, and the intrauterine pressure is lower (between 5 mm Hg and 10 mm Hg); shortly after mucus settles on the walls, gas bubbles are no longer a problem. The implantation locations are on the front and rear walls, the fundal area, and, sometimes, on the side wall. I have performed hysteroscopy on only a few patients during the fifth and sixth weeks of gestation.

The site of the blastocystic implantation is seen as a small knoll. The anatomic transition from parietal to capsular decidua known in embryology is not visible. Likewise, no other signs (e.g., color differences in the endometrium) are evident. In the case of lateral implantation, the knoll is hardly visible because of the smaller radius of curvature. The best panoramic view occurs in the seventh week of gestation, when the cavity is slightly enlarged and the blastocyst is clearly evident (Fig. 47-2). The shape is that of an igloo. The transitional angle at the adhesion point is almost 90 degrees. The covering decidua shows a different color—it gleams dark with a greenish tinge.

The amniotic sac grows wider in the eighth or ninth week and no longer protrudes like a knoll into the cavity. The surface of the amnion becomes more freckled, lighter, and more transparent. With implantation of the blastocyst on the anterior lateral wall, the gestational sac hangs in a drop shape down to the posterior wall (Fig. 47-3). If implantation is located on the posterior wall, the blastocyst fills the troughlike base of the cavity.

It is no longer possible to view the total blastocyst in the 10th to 11th wk of gestation. There is now considerably less empty space in the cavity. The endoscope slips past the amniotic sac, which protudes tensely. The fundus and posterior wall are hardly depictable. In posterior implantation, the blastocyst fills out half the cavity from wall to wall. Its surface resembles compact clouds, such as those seen from an aircraft (Fig. 47-4).

The panoramic view deteriorates and the amniotic sac and cavity only grow proportionally in the 12th wk.[4] No further changes in shape occur. The top surface of the amnion is gray to white, and its translucency permits a view of the amniotic cavity, provided that the surface reflection can be eliminated. For this, a direct contact of endoscopic lens on the membrane is necessary. Transcervical extra-amniotic embryoscopy has been made possible with this technique.

For embryoscopy, the shaft was altered by installing a glass ball over the lens to avoid traumatic effects and ensure full contact with the surface of the amniotic sac.[3] The convex glass top prevents the collection of mucus and bubbles. Embryoscopy is performed without carbon dioxide insufflation. After inserting the endoscope it is easy to identify the amniotic sac from its typical surface structure of decidua capsularis. With the help of the endoscope, a translucent spot can be located. Depending on lens width and size of amniotic cavity, the embryo can be observed totally or in part (Figs. 47-5 and 47-6). Its movements up to the tenth week are slow and involve only the upper limbs. The legs at this time are like folded paddles. The inspection of the entire embryo is simplified through its lack of movement (Fig. 47-7). From the 11th wk on its movements increase considerably, the overall view improves, and the amniotic sac becomes more transparent.[9] The amniotic fluid is always clear and rarely yellowish (Fig. 47-8).[5,8,10] Transcervical extra-amniotic embryoscopy is used exclusively for scientific research because only large superficial malformations can be detected and the strong, cold light can damage the fetal eye. Practical application remains minimal.

THE DISTURBED PREGNANCY

Pregnant women scheduled for first-trimester abortion who complained of bleeding were examined by carbon dioxide hysteroscopy to locate the origin and cause. Depending on the site of bleeding, four different types of disturbed pregnancy were distinguished (Table 47-1).

Table 47-1
TYPES OF BLEEDING BASED ON LOCATION
IN 16 PATIENTS

TYPE	DEFINITION	NO. OF PATIENTS
A	Bleeding from decidua parietalis without organic alteration	6
B	Endometrial disturbances	3
C	Bleeding inside amniotic sac without decidua parietalis involvement	4
D	Decidua capsularis bleeding	3

TYPE A

Bleeding from the decidua parietalis without obvious organic alterations was termed a type A disturbance. Four patients in the seventh to ninth weeks of gestation in whom bleeding began 2 or 3 days before hysteroscopy were examined and showed a diapedesis from the decidua parietalis (Fig. 47-9). The amniotic sac was normally developed and apart from the bleeding area. There was no pathologic finding in the cavity. In two patients an IUD was in place, the amniotic sac was normally developed, and the bleeding was caused by friction between the device and the decidua parietalis.

TYPE B

Local disturbances comprised a type B disturbance. In three patients, bleeding came from a submucous fibroid. The blastocyst was away from the bleeding and normally developed. Slight bleeding was found in two of these patients at the time of expected menstruation.

TYPE C

Bleeding inside the amniotic sac without involvement of decidua parietalis was termed a type C disturbance. Two patients at 8 and 9 wk of gestation had hematomas partially filling the amniotic cavity. The blood had dropped into the cavity, passing through the amniotic wall (Fig. 47-10). It was not clear whether membranes ruptured. The decidua parietalis was completely normal. In two other women in their seventh and ninth weeks, the bleeding started out of the amniotic sac and the surrounding decidua parietalis. No abnormality was seen in the cavity.

TYPE D

Decidua capsularis bleeding was considered a type D disturbance. Three patients in their eighth and tenth weeks showed bleeding from the degenerating decidua capsularis. In places, a chorion laeve could be seen clearly (Fig. 47-11). Embryoscopy was possible. The amniotic cavity was not affected, and the decidua parietalis was smooth.

If there is bleeding out of the decidua parietalis and the endometrium appears normal, a hormonal cause must be assumed. A psychologic influence before a planned abortion may be a possible reason. Slight temporary changes in hormonal pattern can also affect bleeding in specific areas. This type of bleeding sometimes is noted during pregnancy at the time menstruation could have been expected and is similar to the spotting around ovulation. During hysteroscopy there is slight bleeding from the endometrial surface. Hormonal therapy is successful. When the amniotic sac and decidua are normal and a fibroid is seen, the covering endometrium becomes thinly stretched. Larger blood vessels can rupture and cause bleeding. In these patients early pregnancy is not involved. The indication for antifibrinolytic agents should be considered. When the blood reaches the amniotic cavity, retention of the pregnancy is unlikely. Endocrinologic abnormalities can disturb the surrounding area. If the blastocyst is implanted on or near a submucous myoma, polyp, or synechia, the placenta cannot develop normally and bleeding into the amniotic sac ensues.

Besides these four types of threatened abortion, the most frequent finding in a "disturbed" early pregnancy is the failure in the initial stage of development in which an amniotic sac is not seen or is empty and the only therapy is dilatation and curettage (Fig. 47-12).

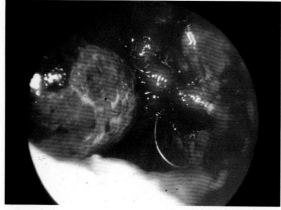

FIG. 47-1. Secondary dislocation and tail retraction are caused by uterine growth.

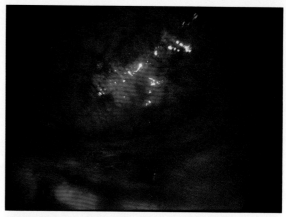

FIG. 47-4. Another illustration of posterior implantation of blastocyst.

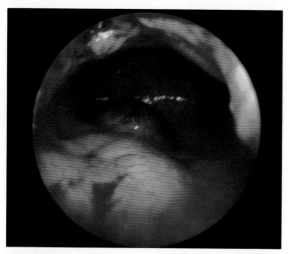

FIG. 47-2. Cavity is slightly enlarged, and blastocyst is clearly evident.

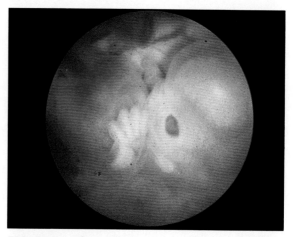

FIG. 47-5. The embryo is observed.

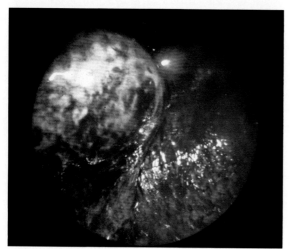

FIG. 47-3. Posterior implantation of blastocyst. Surface resembles compact clouds.

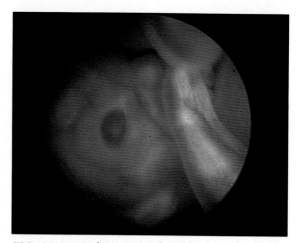

FIG. 47-6. Embryo, 8 weeks old.

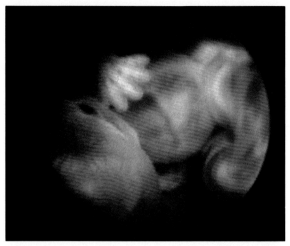

FIG. 47-7. Inspection of the entire embryo is simplified by lack of movement.

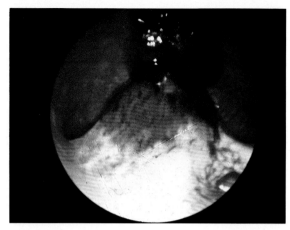

FIG. 47-10. Blood dropped into the cavity, passing through the amniotic wall.

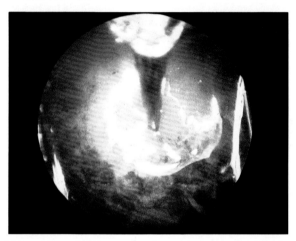

FIG. 47-8. Puncture of the amniotic sac (ninth week of gestation).

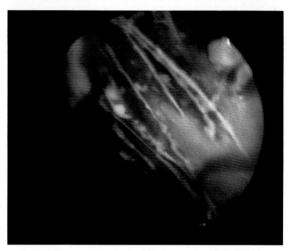

FIG. 47-11. A chorionic laeve is clearly seen.

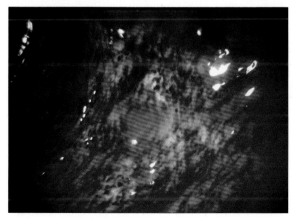

FIG. 47-9. Examination showed diapedesis from the decidua parietalis.

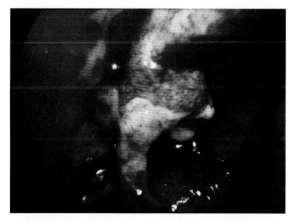

FIG. 47-12. Abnormal early gestational sac is no longer oval.

COMMENT

It is clear that bleeding in the early stages of pregnancy stems from various causes. Some are comparatively harmless and can be treated without risk. Others, such as local vascular diseases with resulting coagulation disorders, require treatment with antifibrinolytic drugs. Finally, bleeding caused by organic intrauterine abnormality does not allow the normal progress of pregnancy. Since the precise cause of bleeding associated with a pregnancy cannot always be discovered, the presence of an amniotic sac on ultrasound indicates therapy. The medications of choice are hormonal and antifibrinolytic agents.

REFERENCES

1. Cates W, Ory HW, Rochat RW, et al: The intrauterine device and deaths from spontaneous abortion. N Engl J Med 295:1155, 1976
2. Gallinat A, Lueken RP, Lindemann HJ: Komplikationen mit Intrauterinpessaren. Sexualmedizin 7:215, 1978
3. Gallinat A, Lueken RP, Lindemann HJ: A preliminary report about transcervical embryoscopy. Endoscopy 10:47, 1978
4. Lindemann HJ, Lueken RP: Development of the blastocyst as seen by hysteroscopy and the transcervical extraamniotic embryoscopy. Presented at the Ninth World Congress of Gynecologists and Obstetricians, Tokyo, 1979
5. Lindemann HJ, Lueken RP: Transcervical amniocentesis via hysteroscopy within the first three months of pregnancy. In Phillips JM (ed): Endoscopy in Gynecology, p 341. Downey, CA, American Association of Gynecologic Laparoscopists, 1978
6. Lindemann HJ: Atlas der Hysteroskopie. Stuttgart, Gustav Fischer, 1980
7. Lueken RP, Lindemann HJ: Diagnosis and treatment of lost IUDs using CO_2 hysteroscopy. Endoscopy 9:119, 1977
8. Lueken RP, Krieg M: Transcervical amniocentesis for quantitative determination of alphafetoprotein in the first trimester of pregnancy. In Weitzel HK, Schneider J (eds): Alpha-Fetoprotein. Stuttgart, Georg Thieme Verlag, 1979
9. Mohri TC, Mohri C, Yamadori F: The original production of the glassfibre hysteroscope and a study on the intrauterine observation of the human fetus, things attached to the fetus and the inner side of the uterus wall in late pregnancy and the beginning of delivery by means of hysteroscopy and its recording on the film. J Jpn Obstet Gynecol Soc 15:87, 1968
10. Mohri T: Our 25 years experiences with endoscopes. Tokyo, Jinmu Shobo, 1975
11. Tatum HJ, Schmidt FH, Jain AK: Management and outcome of pregnancies associated with the copper intrauterine device. Am J Obstet Gynecol 126:869, 1976
12. Van der Pas H: Die ambulante Hysteroskopie als Untersuchungsmethode in der Gynäkologie. Keitum/Sylt, Keitumer Kreis, 1980
13. Wagner H: Lost IUD. Keitum/Sylt, Keitumer Kreis, 1980
14. Zielske F, Becker K, Knauf P: Schwangerschaften bei intrauterinpessaren. Geburtshilfe Frauenkeilkd 37:473, 1977

The Influence of Intrauterine Device Displacement on the Pregnancy Rate ■ 48

Horst Wagner
Karl W. Schweppe

The contraceptive effect of intrauterine devices (IUDs) can be attributed to several factors. One important factor is the inflammatory, foreign-body reaction on the surface of the endometrium. The contraceptive safety is proportional to the extent of the endometrial reaction. This in turn depends, with nonmedicated IUDs, on the surface area of the IUD and, in copper-bearing IUDs, on the release rate of copper.[2] The effectiveness of an IUD is reduced by displacement, and its early detection and correction can reduce the rate of unplanned intrauterine pregnancy considerably. A Pearl index of less than 1 was found in patients monitored by ultrasound, and ultrasound is the most suitable method to see the intracavitary position of an IUD because it allows for safe, rapid, and noninvasive detection of its position (Fig. 48-1).[1]

Intrauterine displacement has been observed in some pregnant women, the rate being highest in the first 4 mo of use and thereafter showing a rather constant level (Fig. 48-2). Three factors are mainly responsible for pregnancies occurring in women wearing IUDs: intrauterine displacement or expulsion, insertion of the IUD at an early stage of an existing pregnancy, and a too-slow release rate of copper.

MATERIALS AND METHODS

Women who conceived an intrauterine pregnancy while wearing an IUD were examined before the pregnancy was terminated. The length of gestation ranged from 4 to 12 wk. The methods used were ultrasound and hysteroscopy; hysterography was not used because it was considered too invasive. Each patient was initially examined by sonogram. If the IUD was shown clearly outside the gestational sac or in the upper part of the cervix, displacement had occurred (Fig. 48-3). If the IUD echo was close to the gestational sac or between the sac and uterine wall, pregnancy was considered caused by IUD failure (Fig. 48-4). False-positive echoes caused by decidual or amniotic reflections were higher from the ninth week of pregnancy on (Fig. 48-5), and the intrauterine position of the IUD was misinterpreted in three such patients. Hysteroscopy proved more reliable in this situation. The uterine probe was introduced into the cervical canal if the IUD was lying intracervically, preventing its further displacement. After dilatation of the cervical canal and introduction of the hysteroscope, the uterine cavity was slowly inflated by carbon dioxide; a pressure of 100 mm Hg was suffi-

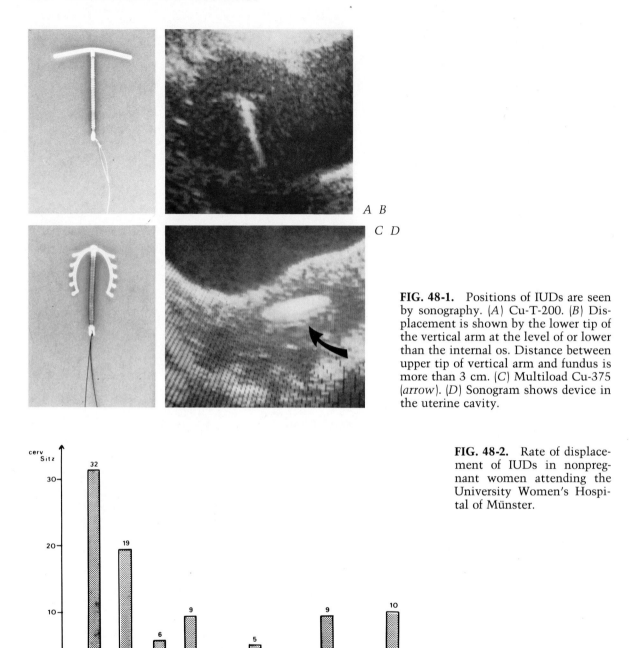

A B
C D

FIG. 48-1. Positions of IUDs are seen by sonography. (*A*) Cu-T-200. (*B*) Displacement is shown by the lower tip of the vertical arm at the level of or lower than the internal os. Distance between upper tip of vertical arm and fundus is more than 3 cm. (*C*) Multiload Cu-375 (*arrow*). (*D*) Sonogram shows device in the uterine cavity.

FIG. 48-2. Rate of displacement of IUDs in nonpregnant women attending the University Women's Hospital of Münster.

cient. If the IUD was distant from the gestational sac, the pregnancy was the result of IUD displacement (Fig. 48-6). If the IUD lay partially or completely between the placenta and the uterine wall, or above the sac in the fundus, pregnancy resulted from IUD failure. It was often possible to see only part of the vertical or horizontal arms and occasionally only the threads (Figs. 48-7 and 48-8). The IUD could not be located if it was above the sac in the

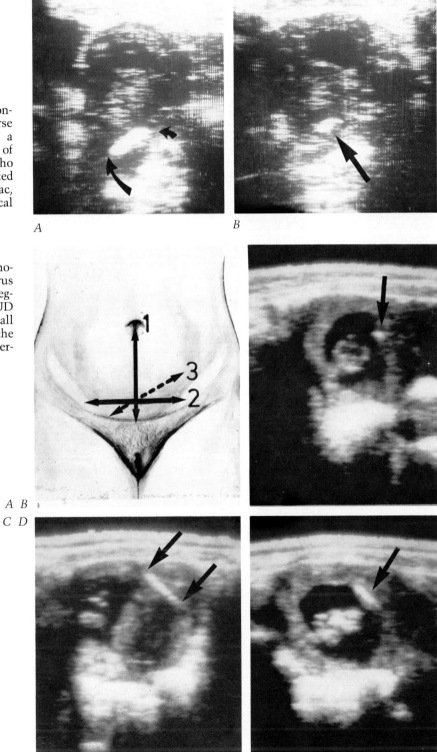

FIG. 48-3. Sonographic longitudinal (A) and transverse section (B) appearance of a uterus in the eighth week of pregnancy. The IUD echo (arrows) is clearly separated from the gestational sac, lying almost in the cervical canal.

FIG. 48-4. (A) Three sonographic sections of a uterus in the eighth week of pregnancy. (B), (C), (D) The IUD echo (arrows) is present in all three sections between the gestational sac and intrauterine wall.

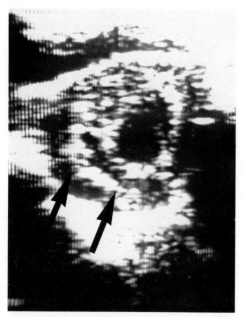

FIG. 48-5. Longitudinal section of a uterus in the ninth week of pregnancy. Echo (*arrows*) beneath the sac could have been caused by an IUD but is a reflection of the decidual surface.

fundus. In one patient an intracervical Cu-T-200 had disappeared below the decidual surface and could not be identified by hysteroscopy (Fig. 48-9). Displaced IUDs were found in 32 of 50 patients, but in 4 the IUDs had been expelled without the patients' knowledge. They had used tampons. In 13 instances the IUD showed partial association with the gestational sac, and in 5 others the device could not be seen on hysteroscopy because it was positioned either above the gestational sac or between the placenta and the uterine wall. In three instances the IUD had been inadvertently inserted in pregnant patients.

Intrauterine displacement and partial or complete IUD expulsion permitted pregnancy in 29 of the 50 patients. Until recently in Germany, pregnancy in women with an IUD was interrupted. Currently it is considered sufficient to remove the IUD to reduce the risk of infection and abortion and to culture the IUD for bacteria. If cultures are negative and no abortion occurs, the pregnancy is allowed to

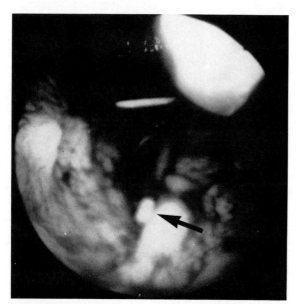

FIG. 48-6. Hysteroscopic view of a Cu-T-200 lying free (*arrow*) in the uterine cavity above the internal os with threads folded back into the cavity.

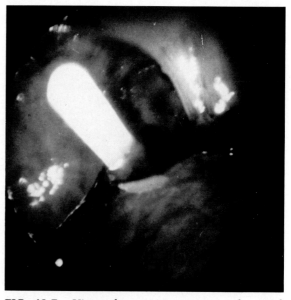

FIG. 48-7. View of a uterine cavity in the ninth week of pregnancy with a Cu-T-200 *in situ*; part of the horizontal arm can be identified.

continue, with no increased risk to mother or fetus.

If the thread is visible in the cervical canal, removing the device presents no problem. The thread usually retracts into the cavity after 6 to 7 wk of gestation, and the device must be located and removed. Other methods used to locate and extract an IUD and their results are summarized in Table 48-1.

COMMENT

Hysteroscopy is the safest and least traumatic method for locating and extracting IUDs in pregnant women. When the IUD is separate from nidation, it was always possible to remove it without damaging the fetus.[3] Hysteroscopy is particularly suitable for those women who wish to continue pregnancy. Intravenous (IV) antibiotics are given to patients who are

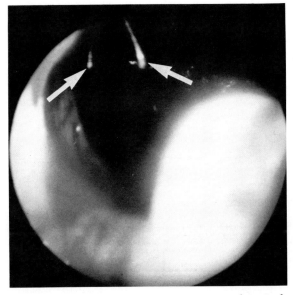

FIG. 48-8. View of a uterine cavity in the ninth week of pregnancy. Only ends of threads (*arrows*) of the IUD are visible.

Table 48-1
METHODS FOR DETECTING AND REMOVING IUDs IN PREGNANT WOMEN

METHODS	NO. OF PATIENTS	GESTATIONAL WK (RANGE)	EXTRACTION SUCCESSFUL		PREGNANCY UNDISTURBED		REMARKS
			Yes	No	Yes	No	
Localization by palpation with a probe; extraction by special forceps	16	5.6–10.5	9	7	8	8	Trauma to pregnancy in successful or failed extractions
Localization by sonography; extraction by special forceps	12	7.2–9.6	8	4	5	7	Trauma to pregnancy possible when extraction successful; trauma to pregnancy when extraction failed
Localization by x-ray film; extraction by special forceps	8	8.2–10.3	7	1	7	1	Trauma to pregnancy when extraction failed
Localization and extraction by hysteroscopy	18	7.1–11.3	18	0	14	4	Trauma to pregnancy when IUD located in area of nidation or high in the fundus and covered by decidua or gestational sac
Total	54	5.6–11.3	42	12	34	20	

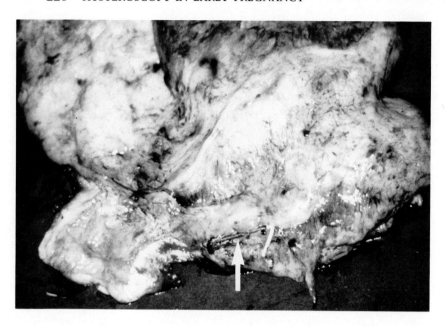

FIG. 48-9. Section of pregnant uterus removed by vaginal hysterectomy. In lower segment, the Cu-T-200 (*arrow*) is completely covered by decidua. Area of nidation and sac are separated from the IUD.

informed of possible risks from the operative procedure. Dilatation of the cervical canal and expansion of the uterine cavity with carbon dioxide have not been associated with an increased risk of abortion or malformation. If the intrauterine carbon dioxide pressure is too high, it could cause placental disruption. At hysteroscopy the light could have an adverse effect on the fetal eye, although no harm has been reported after a delivery following fetoscopy; three healthy children have been born in our clinic after hysteroscopy.

REFERENCES

1. Schmidt EH, Wagner H, Quakernack K: Ergebnisse der Lageüberwachung von Intrauterinpessaren durch Ultraschall. Geburtshilfe Frauenheilkd 39:134, 1979
2. Wagner H: Derzeitiger Stand der Intrauterinpessaranwendung. In Beller FK (ed): Fortschritte in der Geburtshilfe und Gynäkologie. Karlsruhe, G Braun, 1979
3. Wagner H, Schweppe KW, Kronholz HL, et al: Möglichkeiten der Extraktion von Intrauterinpessaren bei eingetretener Schwangerschaft. Med Welt 31:1317, 1980

Management of the Lost Intrauterine Device with Hysteroscopy ■

49

Rolf Peter Lueken

The use of intrauterine devices (IUDs) as contraceptives is important in family planning.[2,4] The efficacy of the IUD depends on patient acceptance and IUD shape and position.[5,6] The size of the IUD must correspond with the size of the uterine cavity. Only in a normal uterus can a correctly placed IUD revert to its original shape and find its proper position. When the uterine cavity and the IUD do not accommodate each other, the device may assume an abnormal position.[8,9] Such a position may be oblique, transverse, upside down, intracervical, or intramural. These displacements can cause side-effects, such as uterine cramps and spotting. Intrauterine abnormalities such as synechiae, polyps, and fibroids predispose to misplacements and side-effects.[16,17]

A thread or tail is generally attached to the IUD to make checking its presence and its removal easier. Some authors prefer threadless IUDs because of their concern about ascending intrauterine infection.[7,12] When threads are not visible or palpable, a search is made to locate the device. It may have fractured, penetrated, or perforated the uterine wall or have been expelled. The tail can retract or tear off. This uncertainty causes stress and concern for the patient and her physician.[3]

Ultrasound is usually the first step in locating an IUD unless the thread was torn off or the device fractured during attempted extraction. Then a carbon dioxide hysteroscopy is performed without prior ultrasound; in 96% of such patients in one series the precise position of the IUD could be seen.[13] As long as the IUD is in the correct position and its effectiveness has not been lost, it can be left *in situ*. When the device cannot be seen, carbon dioxide hysteroscopy should be performed. The threads are either pulled into the cervical canal or the device is extracted under hysteroscopic control. If the IUD cannot be detected by ultrasound or hysteroscopy, an x-ray film of the abdomen and a hysterosalpingogram should be taken.

Tail retraction can be caused by pregnancy. To avoid a potential septic abortion, IUD extraction is indicated and is performed during hysteroscopy.[1] The pregnancy may then safely continue. Wagner reported 14 undisturbed pregnancies after performing hysteroscopy to remove IUDs.[21] When an induced abortion is scheduled, IUD extraction is recommended hysteroscopically before evacuation by suction.[10]

Since 1975, I have seen 310 patients with IUD problems, 115 of them with tail retractions. In 52 of those 115, the missing tails were eased out through the cervix and the IUDs left in place. In the other 63 patients, discrepancies between the size and shape of the uterus and the IUD were observed. Only rarely was the displacement caused by a pathologic condition or malformation. In 96 patients, the tails were torn off during attempted extraction. In 26 women remnants of IUDs, such as the T-bar of the Cu-T device, were found. In 44 pregnant women with "lost" IUDs, the device was removed hysteroscopically after previous ultrasound followed by suction curettage. An IUD *in situ* associated with a pregnancy not seen within the uterine cavity suggests an ectopic pregnancy.

Thirty-seven patients underwent hysteroscopy because of severe side-effects from the IUD. Even a proper device, correctly inserted, will cause symptoms when pathologic conditions exist in the uterine cavity. Myomas, polyps, and synechiae cause some of these side-effects.

Thirteen patients had stringless uterine devices that could not be removed in the physician's office even with the aid of hooks and other forceps. Self-made plastic rings and Ota and Grafenberg rings were removed hysteroscopically. In five patients the IUD was found in the abdomen. Three of these IUDs could be removed at laparoscopy, but in the other two patients a laparotomy was indicated because of serious bowel injury.

COMMENT

Hysteroscopy is a safe, simple operation performed to solve problems associated with intrauterine devices.[10,14,15,18–20] The investigation should generally commence with ultrasound, less frequently with hysteroscopy, and rarely with x-ray study of the lower abdomen. The ideal way to prevent complications from an IUD is to perform hysteroscopy before insertion to see the size, shape, and condition of the uterine cavity and thus decide on the type of device most suitable for the patient.[11]

REFERENCES

1. American College of Obstetricians and Gynecologists: Technical Bulletin, August 1974
2. Gallinat A, Lueken RP, Lindemann HJ: Komplikationen mit Intrauterinpessaren. Sexualmedizin 7:215, 1978
3. Hepp H: Zum Problem des "verlorenen" Intrauterinpessars. Geburtshilfe Frauenheilkd 37:653, 1977
4. Huber SC, Piotow P, Orlans B, et al: IUDs reassessed— a decade of experience. Popul Rep B/2:21, 1975
5. Lindemann HJ, Gallinat A, Lueken RP: Intrauterinpessare in Situ. Coloratlas. Oberschleissheim, Germany, Nourypharma, 1980
6. Lindemann HJ: Atlas der Hysteroskopie. Stuttgart Gustav Fischer, 1980
7. Lindemann HJ: Das fadenlose IUD. Helsinki–Kiel–Grafenberg Symp 19:26, 1980
8. Lueken RP: Position und Kinetik von Intrauterinpessaren. Keitumer Kreis 2:4, 1980
9. Lueken RP, Lindemann HJ: Diagnosis and treatment of lost IUDs using CO_2-hysteroscopy. Endoscopy 9:119, 1977
10. Lueken RP, Lindemann HJ: Problems with IUDs: Use of hysteroscopy. Proceedings of the First National Congress on Gynaecological Endoscopy, Vol 14, p 16. Bombay, 1979
11. Lueken RP: Hysteroskopische Operationen. III. Europäischen Kongress für Endoscopie, West Berlin, 14:17, 1981
12. Mohr J: Idealform des Intrauterinpessars. Keitumer Kreis 2:4, 1980
13. Quakernack K, Schmidt EH, Lieder B, et al: The identification of IUDs by ultrasound in the uterine cavity. Europ J Obstet Gynecol Reprod Biol 4:203, 1975
14. Siegler AM, Kemmann EK: Hysteroscopic removal of occult intrauterine contraceptive devices. Obstet Gynecol 46:604, 1975
15. Siegler AM, Kemmann EK: Location and removal of misplaced or embedded intrauterine devices by hysteroscopy. J Reprod Med 16:139, 1976
16. Taylor PJ, Cumming DC, Hill PJ: Significance of intrauterine adhesions detected hysteroscopically in eumenorrheic infertile women and the role of antecedent curettage in their formation. Am J Obstet Gynecol 139:239, 1981
17. Valle RF, Sciarra JJ: Hysteroscopy: A useful diagnostic adjunct in gynecology. Am J Obstet Gynecol 122:230, 1975
18. Valle RF, Freeman DW: Hysteroscopy in the localization and removal of intrauterine devices with "missing strings." Contraception 11:161, 1975
19. Valle RF, Freeman DW: Hysteroscopy in the management of the "lost" intrauterine device. Adv Plan Parent 10:164, 1975
20. Valle RF, Sciarra JJ, Freeman DW: Hysteroscopic removal of intrauterine devices with missing filaments. Obstet Gynecol 49:55, 1977
21. Wagner H: Lost IUD. Keitumer Kreis 2:4, 1980

Hysteroscopy after Abortion by Suction and Conventional Curettage ■

50

Rolf Peter Lueken

MATERIALS AND METHODS

The advantages of abortion by suction curettage are simplicity, minimal blood loss, and speed. In the United States termination of pregnancy is performed by suction evacuation in 95% of all elective abortions.[4] In the Federal Republic of Germany in 1977, suction and conventional curettage were used equally. To compare the methods for thoroughness in clearing the uterine cavity, hysteroscopy was performed immediately after each of these procedures. In 130 patients termination of pregnancy was performed between the 7th and 12th wk of gestation. No selections were made by parity. The uterus was evacuated by suction in 74 patients and by conventional methods in 56 others. A no. 8 Karman catheter was used up to the 8th wk, and a no. 10 was used from the 8th to 12th wk of gestation. The cervix was dilated one size larger than the catheter. Maximal Hegar no. 11 enabled smooth passage of the catheter. The negative aspiration pressure was 0.6 kg/cm to 0.8 kg/cm.[2] Before aspiration, 6 IU of oxytocin was given intravenously (IV).

Hysteroscopy with a modified Lindemann technique was performed immediately after the evacuation with an additional 6 IU of oxytocin.[1] Producing a pneumometra in a pregnant uterus presents various physiologic and technical problems. In a nonpregnant uterus the slit-shaped cavity is distended with carbon dioxide gas up to pear size without any increase in the volume of the uterus; only its shape is altered. In a pregnant uterus the soft myometrium gives little resistance to increasing pressure. The resulting intrauterine pressure varies between 5 mm Hg and 10 mm Hg, whereas in a nonpregnant uterus the pressure reaches 40 mm Hg to 60 mm Hg. Less resistance requires gas flow to be increased up to 70 ml/min because a larger surface for gas absorption exists, open vessels are present, and myometrium has a special softness. After suction and conventional curettage, more blood is present than in the usual hysteroscopic examination. Generally blood and gas bubbles disappear immediately, but in the recently pregnant uterus they linger for a rather long time because of low uterine pressure. Additionally, the higher gas flow predisposes to bubbles. Within 3 min, residual blood collects in the lowest part of the cavity, generally on the posterior wall. The contracting myometrium compresses the blood vessels, and the uterine pressure prevents oozing from the capillaries. Remnants of tissue were sent for histologic examination.[2] Visibility was sufficient to ascertain exact information about the completeness of the evacuation.

RESULTS

In 67 of 74 suction evacuations, the cavity was completely empty, the endometrial surface was smooth, and the structure of myometrium could easily be identified. In the other seven patients small remnants were seen. Histologic diagnosis of these samples revealed decidual tissue and, in two instances, products of conception. Hysteroscopy after the 56 conventional curettages showed only 8 clean cavities. All other patients showed remnants and furrowed and rough uterine walls. In 26 instances curettage was repeated. Histologic diagnosis of these remnants showed mainly decidual tissue with occasional products of conception. No complications were observed during curettage, follow-up hysteroscopy, or postoperatively. Histologic examination of extirpated uteri immediately after suction proved that a complete evacuation is achieved only by suction and not by conventional curettage.[3]

COMMENT

The quality of hysteroscopic documentation in a pregnant uterus clearly differs from that in the nonpregnant one. The increased size of the cavity and vascularity absorb light, so that photographic documentation is not possible with the usual light. Special optics and light sources are therefore required.

REFERENCES

1. Lindemann HJ, Gallinat A: Physikalische und physiologische Grundlagen der CO_2-Hysteroskopie. Geburtshilfe Frauenheilkd 36:729, 1976
2. Lueken RP, Gallinat A, Lindemann HJ: Hysteroskopishe Untersuchungen nach Aspirations und instrumenteller Kürettage für den Schwangerschaftsabbruch. Geburtshilfe Frauenheilkd 37:776, 1977
3. Schweppe KW, Wagner H, Beller FK: Schwangerschaftsunterbrechung durch Saugkürettage im Vergleich zur konventionellen Metallkürette. Med Welt 31:479, 1980
4. Tietze C: Therapeutic abortions in the United States. Am J Obstet Gynecol 101:784, 1968

Postabortal Hysteroscopy ■ 51

Jacques Salat-Baroux
Jacques E. Hamou
Serge Uzan
Jean M. Antoine

The aim of this hysteroscopic study was two-fold: to check local sequelae of uncomplicated cases of elective abortions and to detect early complications of spontaneous or induced abortions with sequelae. Correlations between hysteroscopic, hysterographic, and sonographic data were sought. The main interest of this study was to establish a therapeutic approach when complications occurred and consequently to reduce sequelae, especially synechiae.

Two studies were performed between April 1978 and September 1979. The first included 118 patients who had had elective abortions before 10 wk of gestation.[3] Table 51-1 summarizes the techniques used, duration of pregnancy, and previous pregnancies. The second study included 33 women; 13 had had complications after spontaneous abortion and 20 had had complications after elective abortion.

MATERIALS AND METHODS

A 4-mm Storz microhysteroscope designed by Hamou was used. Carbon dioxide was instilled with a constant gas flow at 30 ml/min at variable gas pressures, not over 100 mm Hg.[1,3] The initial hysteroscopy was performed 15 days after the abortion. Patients had sequential hysteroscopy weekly until a normal uterine cavity was seen. All patients received norethindrone (Nor-Q.D.) for two menstrual cycles. If residual products of conception were found, sonography was performed. In the absence of endometritis, hysterograms were done and a biopsy was taken.

RESULTS

Residual adhesions were found in the uteri of 25 of 118 women who had had uncomplicated abortions. In 13 uteri only one wall was involved, but in 12 others bridgelike formations were seen (Table 51-2). The types encountered are shown in Figure 51-1. After 4 wk, no intrauterine residues were seen. All uterine cavities appeared normal after the first menses. In 22 instances hysterograms were done; 13 of them agreed with hysteroscopic findings. On seven hysterograms no abnormalities were seen, but residual tissue was detected in the cavity endoscopically; in two other instances false-positive hysterograms were noted (Table 51-3). The agreement was graded between the sonograms and hysteroscopy in that 30 of 38 patients showed similar results; 7 had false-negative sonograms and 1 had a false-positive test (Table 51-4). The vacuity line is a very reliable sonographic finding (Fig. 51-2).

Comparisons made between hysteroscopy and biopsy in 18 patients showed trophoblastic tissue only once (Table 51-5). Most of the intra-

Table 51-1

TECHNIQUES OF ABORTION, DURATION OF
PREGNANCY, AND PARITY IN 118 WOMEN WHO
HAD ELECTIVE ABORTIONS

Method of Abortion
Aspiration: 55 patients
Aspiration & curettage: 61
Curettage: 2

Duration of Pregnancy
6 wk: 2 patients
6–8 wk: 95
9–10 wk: 21

Previous Pregnancies
0: 24 patients
1–2: 77
3 or more: 17

Table 51-2

FINDINGS IN 118 PATIENTS WITH ELECTIVE ABORTIONS

RESULTS	SEQUENTIAL HYSTEROSCOPIES (WEEKLY)			
	First	Second	Third	Fourth
No. of patients	118	33	17	7
Uterus empty	19	6	8	7
Blood clots	6	0	0	0
Minimal residual tissue	42	18	5	0
Minimal residual adhesions	25	9	4	0

Table 51-3

HYSTEROSCOPIC AND HYSTEROGRAPHIC FINDINGS IN 22 PATIENTS

HYSTEROGRAPHY	HYSTEROSCOPY			
	Minimal Residual Tissue	Moderate Residual Tissue	Small Synechiae	Moderate Synechiae
Normal	2	4	1	0
Minimal residual tissue	3	1	0	0
Moderate residual tissue	3	4	0	0
Synechiae, small	0	0	2	0
Lacunae (moderate synechiae)	2	0	0	0

Table 51-4

SONOGRAPHIC AND HYSTEROSCOPIC FINDINGS IN 38 PATIENTS

SONOGRAPHY	HYSTEROSCOPY		
	Blood Clots	Minimal Residual Tissue	Moderate Residual Tissue
Vacuity line (20)	0	17	3
Normal cavity (8)	0	4	4
Residual tissue (10)	1	6	3

Table 51-5
HISTOLOGIC AND HYSTEROSCOPIC FINDINGS IN 18 PATIENTS

HISTOLOGY	HYSTEROSCOPY	
	Minimal Residual Tissue	Moderate Residual Tissue
Endometrium only (10)	9	1
Decidua (7)	5	2
Products of conception (1)	0	1

Table 51-8
HISTOLOGIC AND HYSTEROSCOPIC DIAGNOSES

HISTOLOGY	HYSTEROSCOPY	
	Minimal Placental Tissue	Moderate Placental Tissue
Decidua (4)	1	3
Products of conception (4)	0	4

Table 51-6
HYSTEROSCOPIC FINDINGS IN 33 WOMEN WITH COMPLICATIONS AFTER ABORTION

SIGNS	HYSTEROSCOPIC FINDINGS							
	Normal	Clots	Minimal Residual Tissue	Moderate Residual Tissue	Endo-metritis	Adhe-sions	Atrophy	Hyper-plasia
Bleeding only (11)	0	0	2	4	1	0	1	3
Bleeding and other signs (6)	1	0	0	3	1	0	0	1
Fever, pain without bleeding (1)	0	0	1	0	0	0	0	0
Amenorrhea (15)	1	0	0	1	0	11	2	0

Table 51-7
SONOGRAPHIC AND HYSTEROSCOPIC FINDINGS IN 10 COMPLICATED CASES

SONOGRAPHY	HYSTEROSCOPY					
	Normal	Clots	Minimal Residual Tissue	Moderate Residual Tissue	Endometritis	Adhesion
Vacuity line (4)	1	0	2	0	0	1
Minimal residual tissue (2)	1	0	0	1	0	0
Moderate residual tissue (4)	0	0	0	4	0	0

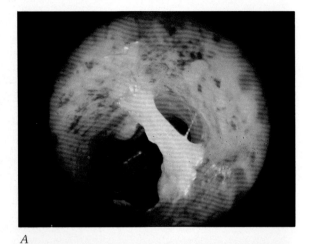

A

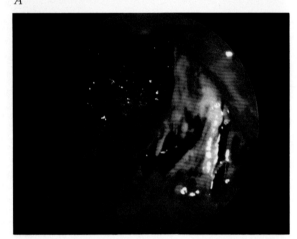

B

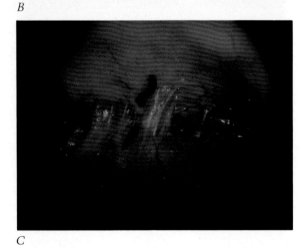

C

FIG. 51-1. Intrauterine adhesions are seen during endoscopy of postabortal patients. (*A*) Mild. (*B*) Moderate. (*C*) Severe.

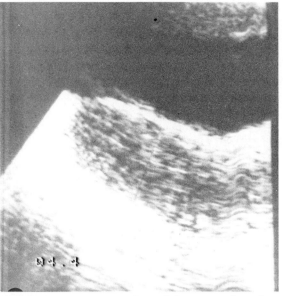

FIG. 51-2. Continuous line of the uterus (less than 1.5 mm thick).

uterine formations seen on hysteroscopy proved to be endometrial tissue. Hysteroscopy was performed after curettage for abortion in 33 patients because of bleeding in 18 instances. Mainly isthmic synechiae were found associated with amenorrhea (Table 51-6). Comparisons were made between the findings on ultrasound and hysteroscopy (Table 51-7); sonography seems reliable when the uterine cavity is empty. Residual products of conception were found in four patients (Table 51-8).

COMMENTS

In 118 patients who had undergone elective, uncomplicated abortions, most residual intrauterine strands or adhesions disappeared spontaneously within 1 mo. In cases of slight postabortal bleeding, repeated curettage is unnecessary. Hysterography is not reliable or indicated in such patients, but sonograms can help confirm an empty cavity. The postoperative hysteroscopic appearance of the uterus was virtually the same no matter which of the three techniques was used to evacuate the uterus. When postabortal bleeding is associated with fever and pain, retention of products of conception should be suspected. In such patients, hysteroscopy is a simple, inexpensive, and autraumatic procedure, enabling an immediate diagnosis. Treatment under hysteroscopic control may prevent the formation of synechiae by removal of residual fibrononecrotic tissue. When postabortal amenorrhea occurs, hysteroscopy can disclose the existence of synechiae and correct the condition at an early stage.[2,4]

REFERENCES

1. Lindemann HJ: CO_2 hysteroscopy today. Endoscopy 11:94, 1979
2. March CM, Israel R, March AD: Hysteroscopic management of intrauterine adhesions. Am J Obstet Gynecol 130:653, 1978
3. Siegler AM, Kemmann EK, Gentile GP: Hysteroscopic procedures in 257 patients. Fertil Steril 27:1267, 1976
4. Sugimoto O: Diagnostic and therapeutic hysteroscopy for traumatic intrauterine adhesions. Am J Obstet Gynecol 131:539, 1978

HYSTEROSCOPY AND STERILIZATION

VI

In six chapters describing hysteroscopic sterilization with the silicone plug, the authors share their experiences with over 800 operations. The standard technique involves uterine distention with high-molecular-weight dextran, local anesthesia with a paracervical nerve block, and various ancillary medications depending on the patient. Limited success was achieved in overcoming tubal spasm using glucagon and naproxen. These operations, although readily performed in an outpatient facility or an office, require about 45 min to 1 hr and expert assistance to mix the silicone precisely and measure its consistency. The proponents of this experimental method of sterilization cite the use of local rather than general anesthesia, minimal pain or sequelae, and successful bilateral plugs on first attempts in over 80% of operations. Thus far few tubal pregnancies have been reported, and intrauterine pregnancies seem rare if normal implants are *in situ.* An inadequate plug can be replaced, and the procedure seems repeatable with no increased risk to the patient.

However, an expert hysteroscopist is needed so that both tubal orifices can be located consistently, and the assistant must be careful with the timing of the mix. Obviously, these technical problems can be solved with experience and a ready-made recipe. Women must be informed that the procedure is still experimental and that repeated applications may be required; many women may not be suitable candidates. Expulsions are prevented because of the dumbbell configuration of the formed silicone. Although some authors speculate about reversibility, it is important to emphasize that no evidence shows, as yet, that the method is reversible. Potentially the uterine bulbous end is removable and then the distal part can be flushed into the peritoneal cavity or moved along by tubal contractions.

Brundin describes a carbon dioxide hysteroscopic method of sterilization in 22 women using a hydrogelic winged device to prevent expulsion of the plug. The method causes no untoward effects, and insertions fail only in patients with very narrow tubal ostia.

The Quest for a Hysteroscopic Method of Sterilization ■

52

Alvin M. Siegler

For more than a century, physicians have searched for a way to occlude the fallopian tubes at their uterotubal junction. The width of the ostia in the intramural segment is less than 0.5 mm; the lumen is lined with a simple endosalpinx of low-columnar cells. The three-layered surrounding muscular wall is the thickest area of the fallopian tube; it is about 2 cm long. Although no anatomic sphincter has ever been identified, hysterosalpingograms often show a small triangle whose base is toward the uterus and apex toward the tubal isthmus, with straight or convex side walls. An interruption in the tubal continuity is sometimes referred to as a sphincter. It usually occurs at the base of the triangle and separates it from the intramural segment. An anatomic basis for this radiologic finding seems to be a fold at the transition between the endometrium and endosalpinx.[25]

Access to the tubal ostia for sterilization has been by indirect transuterine techniques and through direct observation. As early as 1849, Froriep infused a solution of silver nitrate into the uterine cavity to occlude the ostia.[7] Subsequently, Kocks in 1878 reported his early attempts at transuterine sterilization by cauterizing the tubal ostia at the cornua.[10] Similar reports of selectively treating each tubal opening with specially designed probes and balloons without benefit of direct observation have appeared.[2,5,9,20,24] Since permanent tubal occlusion and sterilization occurred in only about 80% of these patients, the results were considered unacceptable. Various chemical substances, adhesives, sclerosing agents, and silicone rubber plugs have been used.[1,4,7,17–19,28] The endosalpinx has a remarkable ability to regenerate, and these materials could not produce permanent blockage. In addition, some of these procedures required multiple applications, sometimes weekly, and a follow-up hysterosalpingogram to observe their occlusive effect.[28] Occasionally, despite radiographic evidence of proximal tubal obstruction, subsequent recanalization occurs and pregnancy becomes possible. Other indirect methods include endometrial ablation by cryosurgery with probes, injection of supercooled liquids, and application of solid carbon dioxide.[6] These techniques have been mostly abandoned because of difficulty in achieving effective endometrial destruction and tubal obliteration and the consequent development of intrauterine synechiae. Although transcervical indirect methods have intrigued investigators for many years, the few clinical studies with chemical agents such as quinacrine, methylcyanoacrylate, paraformaldehyde, plugs of various types, thermal energy, and freezing have not shown impressive results.[5,6,9,10,17,18,24,27,28] Complications from these procedures included hemorrhage, salpingitis, peritonitis, and intestinal injury, and even death has occurred.[8]

The endoscopic or direct visual approach to the tubal ostia for sterilization was initially suggested by von Mikulicz-Radecki and Freund in 1927, who cited the need to destroy the endosalpinx plus part of the myometrium to prevent regeneration and recanalization after cauterization of the intramural tubal segments in experimental animals. They did a few of these operations and followed them soon afterward with a hysterectomy to study the effect of coagulation on the tissue.

Schroeder in 1934 was the first physician to report the results of hysteroscopic tubal sterilization by electrocoagulation as defined by a follow-up hysterosalpingogram 2 wk postoperatively.[22] Since both women he operated on showed tubal patency, this procedure was considered a failure and the patients were subsequently sterilized at laparotomy. Norment described attempts at tubal sterilization by fulguration of the cornual ostia under hysteroscopic control, but he never disclosed the number of patients treated or the results.[15]

The potential advantages of tubal sterilization by hysteroscopy are the avoidance of hospitalization, of general anesthesia, of entering the peritoneal cavity, and of an abdominal scar.

In 1973 a workshop on hysteroscopic sterilization was convened in Minneapolis, where 17 world experts discussed their hopes for this new technique.[23] It was hoped that the method would become available for mass outpatient application as an economically sound investment—safe, effective, and easily learned. However, the preliminary findings revealed that patients had to be treated in the immediate postmenstrual phase, days 5 to 9 of the cycle, because all investigators noted difficulty in routinely finding the tubal opening during the secretory phase. Furthermore, locating the tubal ostium was crucial. When it is clearly seen, it is easy to insert the probe and perform electrocoagulation. Results were excellent with experience, but probably 75 to 100 operations were advised before ostial identification became consistent. A slow interstitial electrosurgical destruction was the method of choice, with the active end of the probe being 5 mm to 8 mm long and 1 to 2 mm in diameter. No uniformity of opinion or findings on factors of time and wattage emerged at this symposium.

The number of treated patients and the duration of follow-up study were insufficient to permit any conclusions on the efficacy of the method for permanent sterilization. Was the medium the key element? Carbon dioxide, dextran, polyvinylpyrrolidone, dextrose 5%, and physiologic saline had all been used to distend the uterine cavity for ostial identification.

The number of operations performed grew slowly, and cautious optimism continued to be expressed. Sugimoto performed 38 of these operations, but no follow-up results were noted.[26] Despite some of the aforementioned shortcomings, Neuwirth believed the effectiveness of the procedure could be improved, enabling it to compete with some established sterilization techniques.[14] In a report of initial studies in 93 patients who underwent electrosurgical sterilization under hysteroscopic control with dextran 32% as the distending medium, Neuwirth noted that the procedure proved safe and simple. Effectiveness was limited because postoperatively three patients were found to have both tubes patent and 16 others had at least one open tube, making the failure rate 20%.

Perhaps the most impressive contribution to the subject of hysteroscopic tubal sterilization appeared in 1976 by Quiñones and co-workers.[16] These authors reported on 930 hysteroscopic tubal sterilizations in which they used electrosurgical energy. The prerequisites for this operation were that the patient be in the follicular phase of the cycle, that adequate uterine distention (intrauterine pressure of 100 mm Hg be achieved, and that electrocoagulation be precise (25 watts at the end of the probe for 8 to 10 sec). The Silastic-tip electrode was inserted 6 mm into the intramural portion of the tube. Vaginitis, cervicitis, myomas, or uterine abnormalities that distorted the cavity were contraindications to the procedure. The operation was done under local paracervical block. Patients were discharged 20 min postoperatively and could resume usual activities the following day. Only one minor complication was reported. Temporary contraception with either intrauterine devices (IUDs) or oral contraceptives was advised until a hysterosalpingogram, taken 12 to 14 wk postoperatively, confirmed occlusion. Hysterosalpingograms were performed on 552 women; 115 (17.3%) showed unilateral or bilateral patency. These women were resterilized by the same technique, and 112 (98%) of them subsequently had bilateral tubal occlusion. No pregnancies occurred in 513 patients who had bilateral occlusion and who were followed for 1 yr. Of six pregnancies reported from the entire group, three occurred in the interstitial segment.

Lindemann and Mohr observed at least 1 patent tube in 33 of 124 women on hysterosalpingography 12 wk postoperatively.[11] Since pregnancy was rare, they initially hypothesized a functional sterility caused by destruction of the tubal sphincter. Presumably the fertilized ovum could not remain in the tube for the 4 days required for maturation before implantation. Histologic studies of some cauterized segments showed significant endosalpingeal destruction. These authors stated that a postoperative pregnancy might represent a failure to detect patency by hysterosalpingography because recanalization was doubtful.

In a subsequent report on 580 patients studied postoperatively with hysterosalpingography, Lindemann noted that 14% of them had at least one patent tube.[12] Rimkus and Semm reported results from 50 operations, with 49 of their patients having follow-up hysterosalpingograms.[21] At least 1 patent tube was seen in 61%; in 2 instances the thermal probe perforated the uterus; and 5 intrauterine pregnancies occurred. The hysterosalpingograms in these women did not show any intramural segment, in contrast to the type of x-ray films seen after tubal sterilization by either laparoscopy or laparotomy. Theoretically, a pregnancy occurring after such a picture indicates that the blocked tubes became recanalized or that the hysterosalpingogram was inadequately done or, in fact, caused tubal patency.

Tubal sterilization by hysteroscopy using thermal energy fell into disfavor after publication of the results of a collaborative study.[3] The authors noted a high patency rate when cautery was used; more important, serious complications were noted. Ten collaborators reported between 6 and 298 cases (a total of 773 operations), with an overall failure rate of 33%. Even in 349 women whose hysterosalpingograms showed closed fallopian tubes bilaterally, 11 pregnancies were reported. Second sterilizations were done in 27% of the patients; a persistent patency was noted in 18% of these women. Sixteen patients had a third sterilization by hysteroscopy with electrosurgical energy, and 3% of them continued to show some patency. The major complications included seven uterine perforations, six ectopic pregnancies, seven bowel damages and peritonitis; one mortality was caused by an unrecognized bowel perforation. Only 25% of the patients were followed for more than 6 mo. These authors concluded that hysteroscopic tubal sterilization with electrosurgery is neither simple nor an outpatient procedure. Instead, it requires a highly skilled gynecologist, and the patient must be in the follicular phase of the menstrual cycle for proper ostial identification. Problems with electrocautery for tubal sterilization also include the lack of an objective endpoint, variability in electrodes and generators, and the unknown influence of the medium surrounding the electrode.

REFERENCES

1. Corfman PA, Richart RM, Taylor HC Jr: Response of the rabbit oviduct to a tissue adhesive. Science 148:1348, 1965
2. Corfman PA, Taylor HC Jr: An instrument for transcervical treatment of the oviducts and uterine cornua. Obstet Gynecol 27:880, 1966
3. Darabi KF, Richart RM: Collaborative study on hysteroscopic sterilization procedures. Obstet Gynecol 49:48, 1977

4. Davis RH, Platt HA, Moonka DK, et al: Chronic occlusion of the monkey fallopian tube with silicone polymer. Obstet Gynecol 53:527, 1979

5. Dickinson RL: Simple sterilization of women by cautery stricture at the intrauterine tubal openings, compared with other methods. Surg Gynecol Obstet 23:203, 1916

6. Droegemueller W, Green BE, Davis JR, et al: Cryocoagulation of the endometrium at the uterine cornua. Am J Obstet Gynecol 131:1, 1978

7. Froriep R: Zur Vorbeugung der Notwendigkeit des Kaiserschnitts und der Perforation. Notiz Geb Natur Heilk 11:9, 1849

8. Hulka JF, Omran KF: Cauterization for tubal sterilization. In Richart RM, Prager DJ (eds): Human Sterilization, p 313. Springfield, IL, Charles C Thomas, 1972

9. Hyams MN: Sterilization of the female by coagulation of the uterine cornu. Am J Obstet Gynecol 28:96, 1934

10. Kocks J: Eine neue Methode der Sterilisation der Frauen. Zentralbl Gynaekol 2:617, 1878

11. Lindemann HJ, Mohr J: Tubensterilisation per Hysteroskop. Sexualmedizin 3:122, 1974

12. Lindemann HJ: Hysteroskopie. In Frangeheim H (ed): Die Laparoskopie in der Gynäkologie, Chiurgie und Pädiatrie. Stuttgart, Georg Thieme Verlag, 1977

13. Mikulicz-Radecki F von, Freund A: Ein neues Hysteroskop und seine praktische Anwendung in der Gynäkologie. Geburtshilfe Gynaekol 92:13, 1927

14. Neuwirth RS: Hysteroscopy, pp 64–69. Philadelphia, WB Saunders, 1975

15. Norment WB: The hysteroscope. Am J Obstet Gynecol 71:426, 1956

16. Quiñones RG, Alvarado DA, Ley E: Hysteroscopic sterilization. Int J Gynaecol Obstet 14:27, 1976

17. Rashkit B: The scope of liquid plastics and other chemicals for blocking the fallopian tubes. In Richart RM, Prager DJ (eds): Human Sterilization. Springfield, IL, Charles C Thomas, 1972

18. Reed TP, Erb RA: Hysteroscopic oviductal blocking with formed-in-place silicone rubber plugs. II. Clinical studies. J Reprod Med 23:69, 1979

19. Richart RM, Neuwirth RS, Taylor HC Jr: Experimental studies of fallopian tube occlusion. In Richart RM, Prager DJ (eds): Human Sterilization. Springfield, IL, Charles C Thomas, 1972

20. Richart RM, Neuwirth RS, Bolduc LR: Single-application of a fertility regulating device: Description of a new instrument. Am J Obstet Gynecol 127:86, 1977

21. Rimkus V, Semm K: Hysteroscopic sterilization, a routine method? Int J Fertil 22:121, 1977

22. Schroeder C: Über den Ausbau und die Leistungen der Hysteroskopie. Arch Gynaekol 156:407, 1934

23. Sciarra JJ, Butler JC, Speidel JJ: Hysteroscopic Sterilization. New York, Intercontinental Medical Book Corporation, 1974

24. Sheares BH: Sterilization of women by intra-uterine electro-cautery of the uterine cornu. J Obstet Gynaecol Br Emp 65:419, 1958

25. Siegler AM: Hysterosalpingography, 2d ed. New York, Medcom Press, 1974

26. Sugimoto O: Hysteroscopic sterilization by electrocoagulation. In Sciarra JJ, Butler JC, Speidel JJ (eds): Hysteroscopic Sterilization. New York, Intercontinental Medical Book Corporation, 1974

27. Thompson HE, Dafoe CA, Moulding TS, et al: Evaluation of experimental methods of occluding the uterotubal junction. In Duncan GW, Falb RD, Speidel JJ (eds): Female Sterilization, p 107. New York, Academic Press, 1972

28. Zipper JA, Stachetti E, Medel M: Human fertility control by transvaginal application quinacrine on the fallopian tube. Fertil Steril 21:581, 1970

Hysteroscopic Tubal Sterilization with Electrocoagulation and Thermocoagulation ■

53

Kees Wamsteker

Transcervical electrocoagulation of the intramural segment has promised to become an important application of hysteroscopy, and different distending media have been used by Lindemann and Mohr, Quiñones and associates, Sugimoto, and Neuwirth and colleagues.[2,5-8] This chapter presents my results with hysteroscopic sterilization using electrocautery and thermocautery.

MATERIALS AND METHODS

In the Woman's Clinic of the University Hospital, Leiden, The Netherlands, 57 women underwent hysteroscopy with electrocautery for sterilization of the intramural part of the tube (Fig. 53-1). A 7-mm hysteroscope* with carbon dioxide distention and the Lindemann vacuum cervical adaptor (Fig. 53-2) were used. Carbon dioxide insufflation was accomplished with the Hysteroflator 1000.† The coagulation probe had an insulated tip of 1 mm and a 5-mm coagulation electrode. An electrical current of 16 watts was applied for 90 sec/tube (Fig. 53-3). All procedures were performed during the proliferative phase. General anesthesia was used in the 51 patients who had simultaneous laparoscopic tubal coagulation done 2.5 cm from

the uterine serosal surface. Six patients were sterilized only by hysteroscopy under local anesthesia with a paracervical block (8 ml of 1% lidocaine in each uterosacral ligament). Hysterosalpingography was performed 3 mo after sterilization. In patients with successful hysteroscopic sterilization, hysterosalpingography showed round cornual areas without tubal opacification (Fig. 53-4). In patients who underwent unsuccessful hysteroscopic procedures, the intramural segment was filled (Fig. 53-5).

In a second study hysteroscopic thermocauterization of the intramural part of the tubes was done as an outpatient procedure under local anesthesia in 11 women. A thermocoagulator† was used to apply a temperature of 90°C for 90 sec/tube. Occlusion of the intramural segment was evaluated by hysteroscopy in 7 and by hysterosalpingography in 4 women 3 mo postoperatively. In some patients with patent tubal ostia at hysteroscopy, thermocauterization was repeated and control hysteroscopy was performed after another 3 mo.

RESULTS

Of the 57 patients who underwent hysteroscopy by electrocautery, hysteroscopic sterilization could not be accomplished in 6. Perforation of the myometrium with the coag-

* K.G. Storz, Tuttlingen, West Germany.
† K. G. Wiest, West Berlin, West Germany.

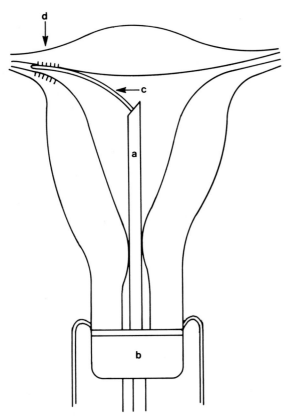

FIG. 53-1. Hysteroscopic sterilization is shown with intramural cauterization of the tube. *a* = hysteroscope; *b* = vacuum cervical adapter; *c* = coagulation probe; *d* = electrode in the intramural part of the tube.

ulation probe occurred twice, and the tubal orifices were obscured in four patients. Hysterosalpingography was not possible in nine instances because eight patients failed to return and one had had laparoscopic coagulation too close to the uterus.

Of the 42 women suited for the procedure, only 24 (57%) had both tubes occluded intramurally. Thirteen (31%) had unilateral intramural occlusion, and five others (12%) showed bilateral intramural patency (Table 53-1). Hysterosalpingograms of the six patients who had no associated laparoscopic coagulation showed bilateral intramural occlusion in only three, but two patients became pregnant more than a year after the operation. Of the 11 patients treated with thermocoagulation, none showed bilateral intramural occlusion, four had unilateral occlusion, and seven others had bilateral patency on follow-up hysterography (Table 53-2).

COMMENT

Transcervical intramural electrocoagulation under hysteroscopic control gave poor results in other series. Most authors have found that the overall results do not answer their expectations.[1-4,6,8] Factors contributing to failure are

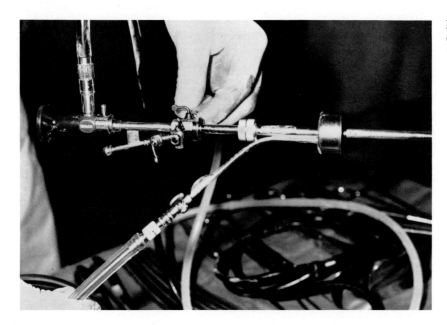

FIG. 53-2. A 7-mm Storz operation hysteroscope with vacuum cervical adapter.

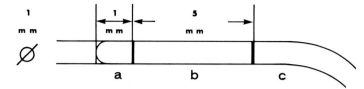

FIG. 53-3. Distal part of the coagulation probe. *a* = isolated tip; *b* = coagulation electrode; *c* = isolated flexible conduction wire.

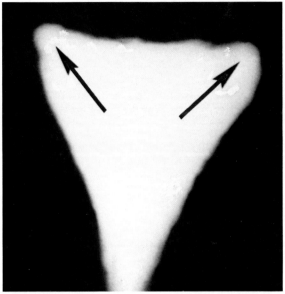

FIG. 53-4. Hysterosalpingogram after successful intramural sterilization shows round cornual areas without intramural opacification (*arrows*).

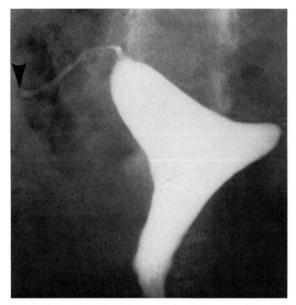

FIG. 53-5. Hysterosalpingogram after unsuccessful intramural sterilization reveals partial tubal filling to isthmus (*arrows*).

Table 53-1

RESULTS OF HYSTEROGRAPHY IN 42 PATIENTS 3 MO AFTER HYSTEROSCOPIC INTRAMURAL ELECTROCOAGULATION WITH HIGH-FREQUENCY CURRENT

HYSTEROSALPINGOGRAPHY	TOTAL		WITH LAPAROSCOPIC COAGULATION		WITHOUT LAPAROSCOPIC COAGULATION
	No. of patients	%	No. of patients	%	No. of patients
Both tubes occluded intramurally	24	57	21	58	3
Unilateral intramural occlusion	13	31	13	36	
Bilateral intramural patency	5	12	2	6	3
Total	42	100	36	100	6

Table 53-2

RESULTS OF HYSTEROSCOPIC THERMOCAUTERIZATION IN 11 PATIENTS (90 C, 90 SEC/TUBE)

NO. OF PATIENTS	NO. OF CAUTERI-ZATIONS	FOLLOW-UP STUDY	PATENCY
3	2	Hysteroscopy	Unilateral
1	1	Hysteroscopy	Unilateral
2	2	Hysteroscopy	Bilateral
1	1	Hysteroscopy	Bilateral
4	1	Hysterosal-pingography	Bilateral

the possibility of recanalization of the initially occluded tube and potential serious complications such as undetected myometrial perforation and thermal intestinal injury. The search for a reliable, safe, and simple hysteroscopic method to sterilize women continues.

REFERENCES

1. Darabi KF, Richart RM: Collaborative study on hysteroscopic sterilization procedures. Preliminary report. Obstet Gynecol 49:48, 1977
2. Lindemann HJ, Mohr J: CO_2 hysteroscopy: Diagnosis and treatment. Am J Obstet Gynecol 124:129, 1976
3. March CM, Israel R: A critical reappraisal of hysteroscopic tubal fulguration for sterilization. Contraception 11:261, 1975
4. Neubueser D, Bailer, P, Bosselmann K: Erfahrungen über die hysteroskopischen Tubensterilisation mit der Hockfrequenz und der Thermomethode. Geburtshilfe Frauenheilkd 37:809, 1977
5. Neuwirth RS, Levine RU, Richart RM: Hysteroscopic tubal sterilization. Am J Obstet Gynecol 116:82, 1973
6. Quiñones RG, Alvarado DA, Ley E: Hysteroscopic sterilization. Int J Gynaecol Obstet 14:27, 1976
7. Sugimoto O: Hysteroscopic sterilization by electrocoagulation. In Sciarra JJ, Butler JC, Speidel JJ (eds): Hysteroscopic Sterilization, p 107. New York, Intercontinental Medical Book Corporation, 1974
8. Wamsteker K: Hysteroscopie. Thesis, University of Leiden, The Netherlands, 1977

Intratubal Devices in Rats: An Experimental Model ■

54

Lothar W. Popp
Siegfried Schulz
Hans J. Lindemann

Hysteroscopic implantation of plugs into the intramural portion of the human fallopian tubes could have the advantage of temporary sterilization.[10,12] The unanswered clinical problems with tubal plugs include reliability, safety, and applicability, the effect of prolonged use on the endosalpinx, the type of materials used for the plug, and reversibility. Some proposed intratubal devices are shown in Figure 54-1.

The cornua of rats were selected as an experimental model (Fig. 54-2). Despite their similarity in length and lumen, human fallopian tubes and the uterine cornua of rats are different organs with different functions. However, the force of expulsion in the uterine cornua of the rat is estimated as being even higher than that in human fallopian tubes, and the rat seemed a good model in which to evaluate plug fixation and test blockade of sperm migration. In rats, plugs cannot be inserted hysteroscopically, and insertion was done at laparotomy.

MATERIALS AND METHODS

Six groups of rats, each containing 5 females and 1 male, were kept under identical conditions for 24 wk. All rats were the same breed and age; all were proved fertile. The male rats were rotated among the groups every few weeks (Fig. 54-3).

Group 1 rats did not undergo surgery. In group 2, all female rats underwent laparotomy and cornuotomy on both sides. The cornuotomy was closed with one suture, as in all the following procedures. The aim was to find out how much this manipulation decreased fertility. In group 3, dilating cylindric plugs were implanted without any additional fixation. In group 4, suitable cylindric plugs were inserted in the cornual lumina and fixed with two ligatures. In group 5, transversely perforated plastic devices of the same shape were fixed with metal splints. The plugs in the rats in group 6 were hooked like a walking stick through the cornual wall with a thick wire. Figure 54-4 shows the plugs in their original size. The results after 24 wk of normal reproductive conditions are tabulated in Table 54-1.

RESULTS

Group 1 rats had a total of 11 litters with 106 young rats (average, 10 a litter). The first litters occurred between 6 and 10 wk. In group 2, the average number of young rats in a litter was re-

(*Text continues on p. 250*)

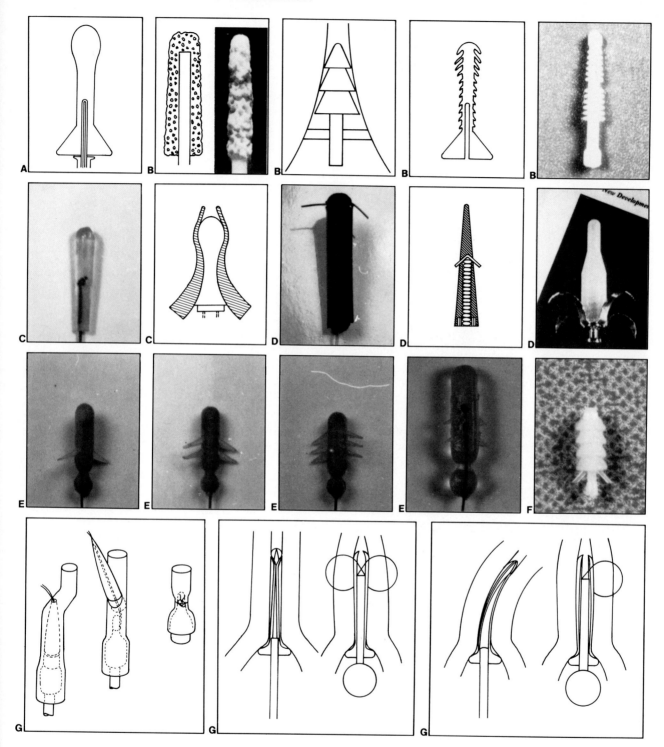

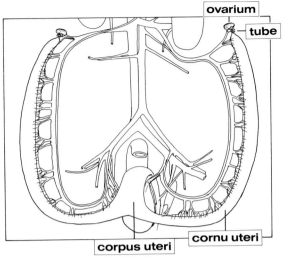

FIG. 54-2. Rat uterus. The long cornua uteri are a good model for the isthmic portion of human fallopian tubes.

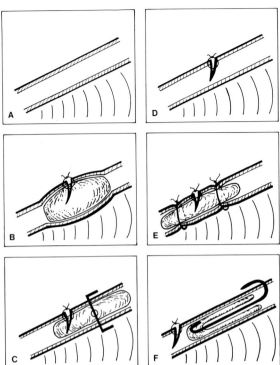

FIG. 54-3. Experimental plan. The cornuotomy and the different types of plugs are demonstrated. (A) First control group, without surgery. (B) Second control group, with cornuotomy. (C) Expanding device. (D) Device with two ligations. (E) Device with a transverse splint. (F) "Claw" device.

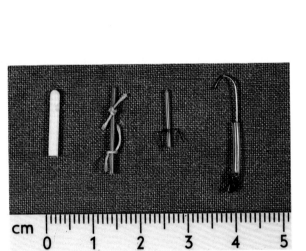

FIG. 54-4. Experimental intratubal devices used in the study.

◁ **FIG. 54-1.** A survey of intratubal devices and the principles of fixation. (A) Insertion without any additional fixation. Bleier.[1] (B) Corrugation of plug surface. (*Left to right*) Craft (porous), Sugimoto (Christmas tree pattern), Bleier, Bleier (fishbone pattern).[1,7,13] (C) Swelling after insertion. (*Left to right*) Brundin (hydratization), Popp (inflation).[29] (D) Fixation with spines. (*Left to right*) Chargoy-Vera, Brueschke and colleagues, Hosseinian and colleagues.[4,5,8] (E) Combination. Brundin (hydratization plus anchoring protrusions; the *far right* shows its swollen state). (F) Combination. Bleier (a solid pin is surrounded by a soft and corrugated cover with two spines).[3] (G) Fixation by tubal wall penetration. (*Left*) Cimber (penetration and fixation through ligation; laparotomy is necessary). (*Center and right*) Popp (the wall-penetrating "claw" fixes the device; a dowel effect and a corrugated surface can also help in fixation).[6,11]

Table 54-1

RESULTS AFTER 24 WK OF NORMAL REPRODUCTIVE CONDITIONS

GROUP	SURVIVING RATS	NO. OF LITTERS	NO. OF YOUNG RATS	YOUNG RATS IN LITTER	FIRST LITTER POSTOPERATIVELY (WK)
1	5	11	106	10	6–10
2	4	10	66	7	5–12
3	4	7	46	7	10–17
4	2	0	0	0	10 and 15
5	3 (of 4)	4	17	4	9–19
6	4	4	18	4	11–15

duced from 10 to 7, but the first litters were born at the same time as those in group 1. The number and the size of the litters in group 3 were reduced, but the number of rats in each litter was equal to that in group 2. In group 3 the first litters were 5 wk late. In group 4, only 2 rats survived and no young were born. Two rats died of late pregnancy complications after 10 and 15 wk, respectively. The results of groups 5 and 6 are very similar; the number and size of litters were reduced, and the first litter was delayed 5 wk.

DISCUSSION

These results are extremely poor. In group 3 rats, no plug was found at the time of the second operation. Three rats had normal pregnancies in both cornua. In one rat a decayed embryo was found in one cornu; the other uterine horn was normal. In group 4 rats, all ligations but no plugs or intact pregnancies were found. In one rat a decayed fetus was found in the right cornu distal to the ligation. In another, two decayed fetuses were found in the left horn distal to the ligations. Two rats died earlier or similar pregnancy complications. In group 5 rats, no plug or splints were found. One rat was pregnant in both cornua, two had severe adhesions, and one had a decayed fetus in the left horn. In a rat in group 6, both devices were found in place. This rat was not pregnant. A second nonpregnant rat had a normal right cornu and a left conglomerate tumor. Two other rats were pregnant in both cornua. No other plug was found.

REFERENCES

1. Bleier W: Deutsches Patentamt, München, Offenlegungsschrift 2 328 175: Tuben-Occlusivpessar und Vorrichtung zum Setzen des Tuben-Occlusivepessars, 1973
2. Brundin JO, Borell US: The Patent Office, London, 1,460,077: Contraceptive device, 1974
3. Brundin J: Intra-tubal devices. In Hafer ESE, Van Os WAA (eds): on Medicated IUDs and Polymeric Delivery Systems, Amsterdam, 1979
4. Brueschke EE, Fadel HE, Mayerhofer K, et al: Transcervical tubal occlusion with a steerable hysteroscope: Implantation of devices into extirpated human uteri. Am J Obstet Gynecol 127:118, 1977
5. Chargoy-Vera J, Zapata-Sanchez G, Rangel-Malagamba S, et al: Dispositivo intratubario. Presented at the VIII World Congress of Gynecology and Obstetrics, Mexico, 1976
6. Cimber HS: United States Patent 3,680,542: Device for occlusion of an oviduct, 1972
7. Craft IL: Uterotubal ceramic plugs. In Sciarra JJ, Droegemueller W, Speidel JJ (eds): Advances in Female Sterilization Techniques, p 176. Hagerstown, Harper & Row, 1976
8. Hosseinian AH, Lucero S, Kim MH: Hysteroscopic implantation of uterotubal junction blocking devices. In Sciarra JJ, Droegemuller W, Speidel JJ (eds): Advances in Female Sterilization Techniques, p 169. Hagerstown, Harper & Row, 1976
9. Popp LW: Deutsches Patentamt, München, Offenlegungsschrift 25 37 620: Tuben-Ballon-Pessar (TBP), 1975
10. Popp LW: Contraception by means of reversible tubal occlusion (film). Presented at the VIII World Congress of Gynecology and Obstetrics, Mexico, 1976
11. Popp LW: Deutsches Patentamt, München, Offenlegungsschrift 29 13 036: Krallenpessar zur Temporären Infertilisierung der Frau durch den reversiblen Verschluss der Eileiterlumina, 1979
12. Sciarra JJ: Hysteroscopic approaches for tubal closure. In Zatuchni GI, Labbok MA, Sciarra JJ (eds): Research Frontiers in Fertility Regulation, p 270. Hagerstown, Harper & Row, 1980
13. Sugimoto O: Hysteroscopic reversible sterilization. In Diagnostic and Therapeutic Hysteroscopy, p 208. Tokyo, Igaku–Shoin, 1978

Experiences with the P Block, A Hydrogelic Tubal Blocking Device ■

55

Jan O. Brundin

Extensive efforts were devoted to the oviduct as a potential target for birth control during the 1960s and 1970s. Experiments were mainly confined to the search for various pharmacologic means to disrupt or modify oviductal function in transporting ascending sperms and descending zygotes.

Since the mammalian oviduct shows very specific properties, it seemed that disruption of oviductal functions would be possible. The scant noradrenergic innervation of the ampulla, in contrast to abundant noradrenergic nerve endings in the isthmoampullary junction and isthmus, was a possible target for achieving pharmacologic birth control. For instance, retention of ova in the uterine part of the ampulla was ascribed to a constrictive action at the isthmoampullary junction based on the noradrenergic innervation.[5] Since neural influence on a series of reproductive events from central functions like gonadotrophin-releasing mechanisms through functions in the ovary had been clearly demonstrated, a noradrenergic role for the control of oviductal function was believed important.[4,5,14,21,31] The role of the sympathetic division of the autonomic nervous system has been extensively studied in this respect to elucidate the role of noradrenergic innervation for ovum transport.[25]

Various attempts to deplete the noradrenergic transmitter substance, norepinephrine, from the oviduct were studied together with ovum transport in various mammals. Reserpine-induced depletion of the norepinephrine stores of a rabbit oviduct caused retention of ova in the isthmus, which could also be provoked by estrogen treatment.[3] Pretreatment with reserpine also caused delay or arrest of mouse ova in the oviduct and interruption of implantation in the rat.[1,8] Moreover, pretreatment with monoamine oxidase (MAO) inhibitor, leading to high norepinephrine concentrations in the rabbit isthmus, identically accelerated ovum transport.[2] Depletion of the norepinephrine stores with 6-hydroxydopamine had varying effects in different species. When administered intraperitoneally to mice, this drug did not prevent a normal pregnancy rate.[19] Although this drug is an abortifacient in the rat, it completely prevents pregnancy in the rabbit.[7,24]

The human oviduct contains both alpha and beta receptors for the noradrenergic response.[4,26] Its predominant alpha receptors change during ovum transport to increased beta-receptor activity that is presumably caused by increased progesterone in the circulation after ovulation.[10,11,16,22,27] Also, the cellular effects upon the adenosine 3':5'-cyclic phosphate (cyclic AMP) in the intracellular tissue are influenced by beta-adrenergic receptors. Prostaglandins F and E influence the cyclic AMP content of the cell and are involved in the presynaptic release of norepinephrine from the noradrenergic nerve endings.[30]

Pharmacologic influence on oviductal function in the human being involves sequelae in other systems, and therefore such agents are probably not useful for contraception. Women desiring a simple method of contraception tend to resist prolonged use of pharmacologically active substances. Consequently, efforts are being directed toward mechanical oviductal occlusion.

TRANSUTERINE TUBAL OCCLUSION

Applying substances to obstruct the tubes transcervically is not new. The first attempts, silver nitrate applications in the cornual region, were described in 1849. These attempts were followed by electric cautery, a technique later successfully used by Prudnikoff and Dickinson.[12,20,28] In a later series, permanent sterilization was obtained in 80% to 89% of the cases; Lindemann more recently did a similar study.[17,23,29] However, serious complications were reported with electrosurgery (see Chap. 39 for a review of transcervical methods of sterilization.)[18] Special instruments were designed for blind application of substances to obstruct the uterine cornu, but even with fluoroscopic control of the application, results were not as good as with the hysteroscopic technique.[9,13]

CHARACTERISTICS OF THE OCCLUSIVE MATERIAL

The occlusive material must be applicable through the hysteroscope if the physician is to observe its exact position. The working channel of the hysteroscope is a limiting factor. Since most hysteroscopes used for intrauterine surgery are equipped with a 2-mm working channel, the applicator cannot exceed that diameter. The applicator is restricted from any refined design such as deflectable distal ends involving space-consuming manipulative mechanisms. The direction of flexible instruments for intrauterine surgery could be varied using an Albaran bridge in the end of the hysteroscope. This equipment allows only minor corrections. To prevent infection, the occlusive material and device must be sterilized without a change in their occlusive potential. The material must minimally damage the surrounding tissues and should have no delayed untoward effects. The material and the device must be easy to insert into the oviductal lumen to minimize the risk of uterine or tubal perforation. Since tubal contractions vary during the menstrual cycle, sperm migration between the occlusive material and the oviductal wall may occur if complete obstruction is not achieved.

THE P-BLOCK

By combining unique physical and chemical characteristics, hydrogels fulfill the criteria listed above.

CHEMICAL CHARACTERISTICS

The hydrogelic compound is a polymeric product containing methacrylate and polyvinylpyrrolidone, constituting a viscous fluid to which liquid nylon 6 has been added, dissolving in the hydrogel. Thus, the basic compound does not contain any additional chemical constituents to elute from the final product, which is characterized by many free hydroxyl groups along a polymeric chain.

PHYSICAL CHARACTERISTICS

This hydrogelic liquid containing liquid nylon 6 can be injected into a mold to produce any kind of hydrogelic body. Polymerization can be achieved either by heat or by gamma radiation. The presence of nylon 6 in the hydrogelic solution reinforces the final product by nylon 6 needles, rendering a fixed memory of shape to the final compound. The swelling capacity of the final product can be varied by changing the amount of liquid nylon 6 in the initial solution. Any hydrogelic body, thus produced, is stiff in the dry state but softens on implantation because the free hydroxyl groups absorb water molecules. In addition to softening the hydrogelic body, this process causes it to swell. After complete hydration, the compound is wider, longer, and softer but has the same shape as the initial dry hydrogelic body. The hydrogelic tubal blocking device, called the *P-block,* consists of a prefabricated skeleton of nylon 6 on which a hydrogelic body has been anchored. The prefabricated skeleton continues into a short indicator tail that, after insertion in the intramural part of the oviduct, protrudes through the tubal orifice and hangs down into the uterine cavity.

PREVIOUS EXPERIENCE

The intratubal, hysteroscopically applicable, occlusive device was in use in my clinic from September 1979 until September 1981 with small variations (Mark 1 to 6). The device was inserted with a flexible forceps into the intramural part in about 60 volunteers applying for nonsurgical, permanent sterilization. Despite a high degree of acceptance among users retaining their plugs, the number of expelled plugs was unacceptably high. Expulsion of the plug was followed by an intrauterine pregnancy in seven women. Surgical sterilization combined with legal abortion in six instances revealed that one oviduct had expelled its P-block. One pregnant patient went to term uneventfully. In two patients the P-block was found in the abdominal cavity. Microscopic examination of the excised intramural segment showed minimal invasion of round cells but no giant cell formation or atypias in the endosalpingeal cells, even on the side with the P-block *in situ.* Fibroblasts had grown into the surface porosities of the P-block with capillary infiltration. The microscopic picture showed a negligible foreign-body reaction even after 20 mo.[6] Maximal microscopic observation time with

P-blocks *in situ* is 34 mo. No extrauterine pregnancy has been recorded.

A NEW INSERTION TECHNIQUE FOR THE P-BLOCK

Because of the high incidence of expulsions, pregnancies, and perforations, a modification of the P-block and the technique for inserting it became mandatory. The modified P-block, Mark 7, was tried during the last quarter of 1981 (Fig. 55-1). P-blocks were mainly expelled because they were inappropriately positioned in the intramural segment. To increase access for adequate cannulation of this tubal segment, a beta$_2$-receptor stimulant was given to the patient during hysteroscopy. If 0.25 mg of terbutaline was injected intravenlusly as the hystero-

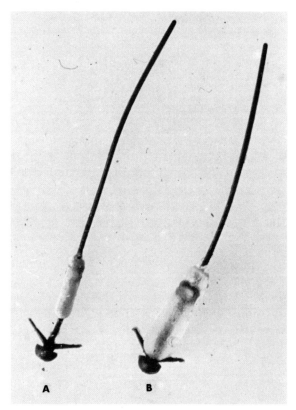

FIG. 55-1. P-block, Mark 7. (*A*) P-block in the dry state before insertion. (*B*) Hydrated P-block after insertion.

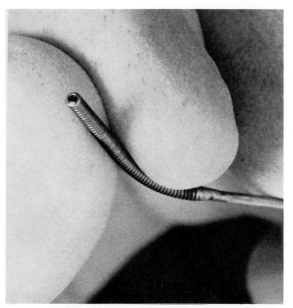

FIG. 55-2. Flexible, hollow tip of stainless steel wire plunger used for intramural deposition of P-block, Mark 7.

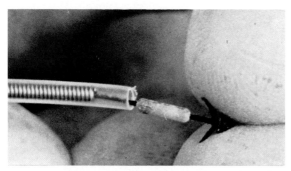

FIG. 55-3. Fingertips flapping retention wings of P-block, Mark 7, used for introduction into insertion catheter that also contains flexible plunger tip.

scope was slowly inserted into the uterine cavity, a pneumometra was more easily achieved. The uterine tubal orifice seemed to widen during this procedure, facilitating its cannulation. The beta$_2$-receptor stimulant facilitated observation of the direction of the intramural, luminal pathway. A stiff end of an intratubal device upon which force would be applied to insert the tubal blocking device could easily leave the lumen and penetrate the myosalpinx

and myometrium even if gentle pressure were exerted. This risk can be avoided by constructing a soft, flexible end with a round tip that will easily follow the course of the intramural lumen. A flexible plunger will automatically reduce the force that can be exerted as the oviduct is cannulated.

The tail of the P-block, Mark 7, is introduced into the hollow end of the flexible plunger (Fig. 55-2). The nylon wings of the P-block that prevent early expulsion are situated immediately below the rounded front of the P-block. They are flapped together and inserted into the applicator that also contains the plunger (Fig. 55-3). When ready for use the catheter has a rounded, smooth end (Fig. 55-4). The Albaran bridge permits the surgeon to apply the P-block in the right position without interrupting hysteroscopy (Fig. 55-5).

APPLICATION CAPACITY OF THE P-BLOCK (MARK 7)

Patients requesting a nonabdominal method of sterilization and who agreed to an early abortion in case of failure were offered the P-block, Mark 7, at Danderyd Hospital during the last quarter of 1981. The pilot study included 22 patients. When possible, insertion was scheduled for the postmenstrual phase and done as an outpatient procedure with local anesthesia. Carbon dioxide hysteroscopy was used. Patients left the hospital within 1 hr of the attempted insertion. The results are shown in Table 55-1. Bilateral, intramural, tubal applications of the P-block were achieved in almost half the women. Occasionally only one oviduct was cannulated because the tubal orifices were too narrow or the intramural segments too sharply bent. In one patient an intramural myoma distorted the shape of the tubal orifice (Table 55-2).

When expulsions occurred with earlier models of the P-block, they took place during the first menses after insertion. Currently patients are advised to continue their previous contraceptive methods until the check-up hysteroscopy verifies bilateral retention of

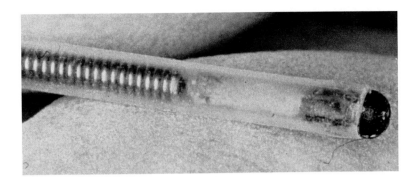

FIG. 55-4. P-block, Mark 7, loaded into plunger and insertion catheter, is ready for hysteroscopic application.

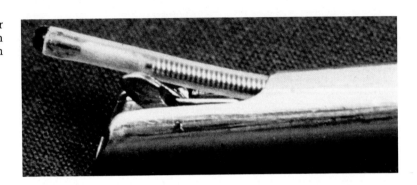

FIG. 55-5. Insertion catheter for P-block, Mark 7, protrudes through end of hysteroscope and rides on Albaran bridge.

P-blocks. No expulsion was recorded after acceptable insertion of P-block, Mark 7. Moreover, no pregnancies have been recorded in this group.

COMMENTS

Although experience with previous models of the P-block should not have encouraged further attempts to construct a retainable intramural tubal blocking device, the degree of satisfaction with the P-block, Mark 7, among patients who are retaining it is encouraging. Retention of the P-block in the intramural segment is free of side-effects. No pain, discomfort, or dyspareunia has been recorded, and menses remain unaffected. The diameter of this P-block seems crucial. When insertion fails because of a narrow orifice, a P-block of smaller diameter should be used. Similarly, a too sharply bent intramural segment requires a thinner insertion device and P-block to permit entrance into the oviductal lumen; the flexi-

Table 55-1
P-BLOCK (MARK 7) INSERTION ATTEMPTS FROM SEPTEMBER THROUGH DECEMBER 1981 IN 22 PATIENTS

Total	22
Bilateral success	10
Unilateral success	4
Anatomic reasons for failure	11
Uterine perforation	1

Table 55-2
CAUSES FOR FAILURE IN 11 PATIENTS

Ostia too narrow	5
Angulated intramural segment	5
Ostium obstructed by myoma	1

ble-tipped inserter permits it to follow a sharply curved intramural lumen. Inspection of the tubal orifice during an early phase of each hysteroscopy can predict whether a small or a normal sized P-block is needed. The smaller size, now under construction, will enhance the value of this method as an alternative to abdominal methods of sterilization.

REFERENCES

1. Bennett JP, Kendle KE: The effect of reserpine upon the rate of egg transport in the fallopian tube of the mouse. J Reprod Fertil 13:345, 1967
2. Bodkhe RR, Harper MJK: Mechanism of egg transport: Changes in the amount of adrenergic transmitter in the genital tract of normal and hormone treated rabbits. In Segal SJ, Crozier R, Corfman PA et al (eds): The Regulation of Mammalian Reproduction, p 364. Springfield, Charles C Thomas, 1972
3. Bodkhe RR, Harper MJK: Changes in the amount of adrenergic neurotransmitter in the genital tract of untreated rabbits and rabbits given reserpine or iproniazid during the time of egg transport. Biol Reprod 6:288, 1972
4. Brundin J: Distribution and function of adrenergic nerves in the rabbit fallopian tube. Acta Physiol Scand (Suppl 259) 66, 1965
5. Brundin J: Pharmacology of the oviduct. In Hafez ESE, Blandau RJ (eds): The Mammalian Oviduct, p 251. Chicago, University of Chicago Press, 1969
6. Brundin J, Sandstedt B: Longterm toxicity of hydrogelic occlusive device in the human oviductal isthmus. (in press)
7. Castrén O, Airaksinen M, Saarikoski S: Decrease of litter size and fetal monoamines by 6-hydroxy dopamine in mice. Experientia 29:576, 1973
8. Chatterjee A, Harper MJK: Interruption of implantation and gestation in rats by reserpine, chlorpromazine and ACTH: Possible mode of action. Endocrinology 87:966, 1970
9. Corfman PA, Taylor HC Jr: An instrument for transcervical treatment of the oviducts and uterine cornua. Obstet Gynecol 27:880, 1966
10. Coutinho EM, Maia H, Adeodato-Filho JA: Response of the human fallopian tube to adrenergic stimulation. Fertil Steril 21:590, 1970
11. Coutinho EM, de Mattos CER, da Silva AR: The effect of ovarian hormones on the adrenergic stimulation of the rabbit fallopian tube. Fertil Steril 22:311, 1971
12. Dickinson RL: Simple sterilization of women by cautery stricture at the intrauterine tubal openings, compared with other methods. Surg Gynecol Obstet 23:203, 1916
13. Erb RA: Silastic: A retrievable custom-molded oviductal plug. In Sciarra JJ, Droegemuller W, Speidel JJ (eds): Advances in Female Sterilization Techniques, p 259. Hagerstown, Harper & Row, 1976
14. Ferrando G, Nalbandov AV: Direct effect on the ovary of the adrenergic blocking drug dibenzyline. Endocrinology 85:38, 1969
15. Froriep R: Zur Vorbeugung der Notwendigkeit des Kaiserschnitts und der Perforation. Notiz Geb Natur Heilk 11:9, 1849
16. Higgs GW, Moawad AH: The effect of ovarian hormones on the contractility of the rabbit oviductal isthmus. Can J Physiol Pharmacol 52:74, 1974
17. Hyams MN: Sterilization of the female by coagulation of the uterine cornu. Am J Obstet Gynecol 28:96, 1934
18. Israngkun CH, Phaosavasdi S: Hysteroscopic sterilization: Complications in 269 cases. In Sciarra JJ, Droegemuller W, Speidel JJ (eds): Advances in Female Sterilization Techniques, p 148. Hagerstown, Harper & Row, 1976
19. Johns A, Chlumecky J, Paton DM: Role of adrenergic nerves in ovulation and ovum transport. Lancet 2:1079, 1974
20. Kocks J: Eine neue Methode der Sterilisation der Frauen. Zentralbl Gynaekol 2:617, 1878
21. Lasbhsetwar AP: Evidence for the involvement of a catecholaminergic pathway in gonadotrophin secretion for implantation in rats. J Reprod Fertil 33:545, 1973
22. Levy B, Lindner HR: The effects of adrenergic drugs on the rabbit oviduct. Eur J Pharmacol 18:15, 1972
23. Lindemann HJ: Transuterine tubal sterilization by CO_2 hysteroscopy. In Sciarra JJ, Butler JC, Speidel JJ (eds): Hysteroscopic Sterilization, p 61. New York, Intercontinental Medical Book Corporation, 1974
24. MacDonald EJ, Airaksinen M: The effect of 6-hydroxy dopamine on the oestrous cycle and fertility of rats. J Pharm Pharmacol 26:518, 1974
25. Marshall JM: Effects of catecholamines on the smooth muscle of the female reproductive tract. Ann Rev Pharmacol 13:19, 1973
26. Nakanishi H, Wood C: Effects of adrenergic blocking agents on human fallopian tube motility in vitro. J Reprod Fertil 16:21, 1968
27. Pauerstein CJ, Fremming BD, Hodgson BJ, et al: The promise of pharmacologic modifications of ovum transport in contraceptive development. Am J Obstet Gynecol 116:161, 1973
28. Prudnikoff YV: Artificial sterilization of women by means of electrocoagulation. Thesis, Imperial Academy of Medicine, St. Petersburg, 1912
29. Sheares BH: Sterilization of women by intra-uterine electro-cautery of the uterine cornu. J Obstet Gynaecol Br Emp 65:419, 1958
30. Stjärne L, Brundin J: Frequency–dependence of ^{3}H-noradrenaline secretion from human vasoconstrictor nerves: Modification by factors interfering with alpha or beta adrenoceptor or prostaglandin E_2 mediated control. Acta Physiol Scand 101:199, 1977
31. Virutamasen P, Hickok RL, Wallach EE: Local ovarian effects of catecholamines on human chorionic gonadotropin-induced ovulation in the rabbit. Fertil Steril 22:235, 1971

Hysteroscopic Sterilization with Formed-in-Place Silicone Rubber Plugs: Basic Process and Instruments ∎

56

Robert A. Erb

Early mention of the concept of formed-in-place silicone rubber plugs was made by Braley and Helmer and by Corfman and Taylor.[1,2] Experimental studies in rabbits were reported by Hefnawi and colleagues and in women by Rakshit.[15,16-18]

Erb has worked actively since 1970 on developing instruments, materials, and techniques to make the procedure practicable.[8-10] Among his specially developed items are the obturator tip, guide assembly for remote delivery of the liquid silicone and release of the cured plug system; non-air-entraining mixer–dispenser to permit rapid mixing of viscous materials, fluid-flow actuator, and pump for dextran 70 (Hyskon). Research efforts from 1971 to 1975 were sponsored by the Contraceptive Development Branch, National Institutes of Health, Bethesda, MD; descriptions of instruments, materials, and animal experiments were published by Erb and associates.[11-13] Davis and colleagues published further studies on rabbits and rhesus monkeys.[3-7] Adaptation of the basic procedure as a hysteroscopic method began in 1975, with components miniaturized to permit passage of the guide assembly through the operating channel of a standard hysteroscope.[14] Reed and De Maeyer conducted the pioneering clinical studies beginning in 1978, which have since been expanded, under the sponsorship of RSP Laboratories, Inc. in Stamford, Connecticut, to a multicenter, 1000-patient clinical study program.[19-22]

The purpose of this chapter is to describe the basics of an approach to female tubal sterilization that uses formed-in-place silicone rubber plugs. The method involves introducing catalyzed liquid silicone polymer into the oviduct through an obturator tip to which the formed plug becomes bonded. The procedure is done with conventional operating hysteroscopes. This approach has several attractive features:

It is nonincisional
It is done in the office under local anesthesia
It damages the oviduct less than other tubal sterilization methods
Tubal patency can be restored without surgery

The potential for reversibility exists, but this has not yet been demonstrated in women. Clinical studies are continuing in several institutions; the results were presented by several of the participating investigators at the First World Congress of Hysteroscopy held in Miami, Florida in January, 1982.

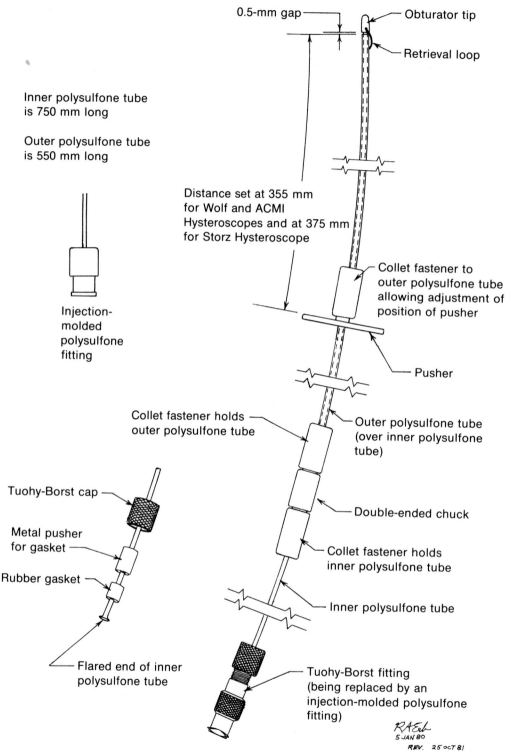

0.5-mm gap

Obturator tip

Retrieval loop

Inner polysulfone tube
is 750 mm long

Outer polysulfone tube
is 550 mm long

Distance set at 355 mm
for Wolf and ACMI
Hysteroscopes and at 375 mm
for Storz Hysteroscope

Collet fastener to
outer polysulfone tube
allowing adjustment of
position of pusher

Pusher

Injection-
molded
polysulfone
fitting

Collet fastener holds
outer polysulfone tube

Outer polysulfone tube
(over inner polysulfone
tube)

Tuohy-Borst cap

Double-ended chuck

Metal pusher
for gasket

Collet fastener holds
inner polysulfone tube

Rubber gasket

Inner polysulfone tube

Flared end of inner
polysulfone tube

Tuohy-Borst fitting
(being replaced by an
injection-molded polysulfone
fitting)

R A Erb
5 JAN 80
REV. 25 OCT 81

FIG. 56-1. Guide assembly.

THE GUIDE ASSEMBLY

The guide assembly is the system conveying the liquid silicone composition through the operating channel of the hysteroscope, and it provides communication to and obturation (sealing) at the tubal ostium. It also allows remote release of the preformed tip (and its bonded plug) from other parts of the assembly. The guide assembly consists of six main parts: obturator tip, inner polysulfone tube, outer polysulfone tube, pusher, double-ended chuck, and a Luer fitting (Fig. 56-1).

The obturator tip is a very important member. By its sealing action at the tubal ostium and by its participation in the release step, it allows the remotely actuated formation of the plug. Because the bonded tip is larger in diameter than the oviductal lumen at the isthmus, it prevents intraperitoneal expulsion of the plug. The retrieval loop permits nonincisional removal of the plug if desired (e.g., to replace improperly formed plugs or to restore tubal patency).

The basic obturator tip, approximately 2 mm in diameter and 5 mm long, is molded of Dow Corning Silastic 382 Medical Grade Elastomer (75%) and spherical silver powder (25%), with an embedded multifilament polyester retrieval loop. The silver powder is a radiopaque agent.

Because of variations in anatomy, other tips have also been molded (Fig. 56-2). The E-1 (Erbone) tip is the basic tip presently supplied with the guide assembly. The R-1 and C-1 tips were configurations requested by clinical investigators Reed and Cooper. The E-1 and C-1 tips will pass through a 2.3-mm operating channel; with E-2, E-3 and R-1 tips, the hysteroscope must be withdrawn, the replacement tip installed on the protruding guide, and the hysteroscope reinserted.

The inner polysulfone tube is 750 mm long with an inside diameter of 1 mm. It has an at-

FIG. 56-2.   Standard and special obturator tips.

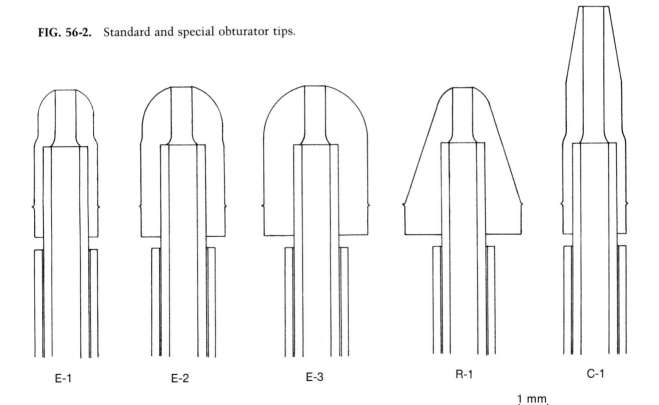

E-1   E-2   E-3   R-1   C-1

1 mm

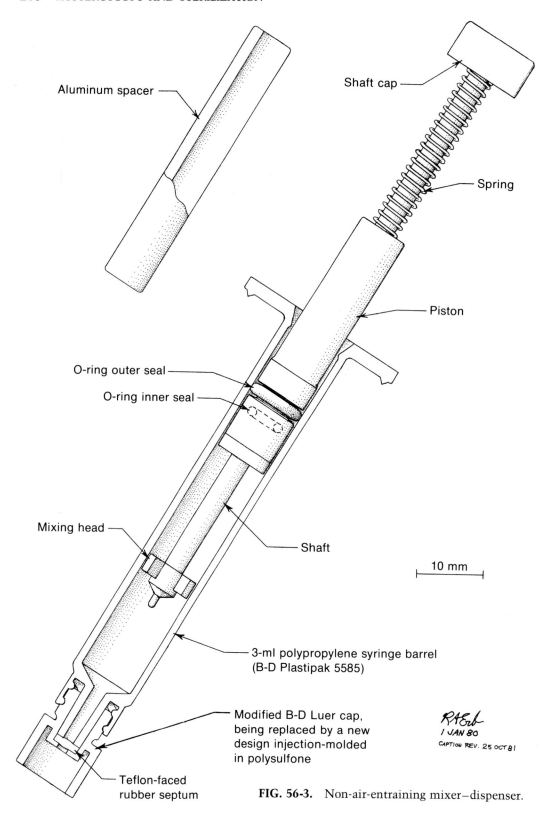

Aluminum spacer

Shaft cap

Spring

Piston

O-ring outer seal

O-ring inner seal

Mixing head

Shaft

10 mm

3-ml polypropylene syringe barrel
(B-D Plastipak 5585)

Modified B-D Luer cap,
being replaced by a new
design injection-molded
in polysulfone

Teflon-faced
rubber septum

RAErb
1 JAN 80
CAPTION REV. 25 OCT 81

FIG. 56-3.   Non-air-entraining mixer–dispenser.

tached Luer fitting at one end and a transverse thread or ringed constriction at the other to prevent tail formation and to promote cutoff of the cured silicone for release. The outer polysulfone tube (550 mm long) provides the release function by the sliding arrangement with the inner tube. The inner and outer tubes are initially held in fixed relation by a double-ended collet device (double-ended chuck), injection molded of polysulfone, through which the inner tube passes completely.

A pusher, attached to the outer tube with a collet fastener, allows the hysteroscopist to put an axial force on the guide and obturator tip, controlled with one finger. This is also injection molded of polysulfone; polysulfone is used throughout the guide assembly because it can be sterilized with steam and is strong and transparent. The guide assembly is supplied, packaged and sterilized, to clinical investigators.

THE MIXER-DISPENSER

The non-air-entraining mixer–dispenser is an important element of the specialized instruments developed for the plug-forming proce-dure (Fig. 56-3). It permits thorough mixing of a small quantity of catalyst with a viscous material in a short time (35 sec), without entraining any air, and then allows the catalyzed material to be dispensed directly, again without entraining any air.

The piston, mixing head, and shaft cap are injection molded of polysulfone. In use, the stannous octoate catalyst is added with a 0.1-ml gastight syringe with a hypodermic needle through the septum cap. The mixing head is moved back and forth for 45 double strokes with quarter turns. The spacer is inserted to convert the system for the dispensing function.

THE FLUID-FLOW ACTUATOR

The flow of the catalyzed silicone composition through the guide assembly cannot be accomplished by direct hand holding of the mixer–dispenser syringe because of the high viscosity of the fluid (about 10,000 times the viscosity of water), the narrow diameter, the length of the inner polysulfone tube, and the short time before flow is stopped by gelling (about 3 min after catalyst is added). Figure 56-4 shows the

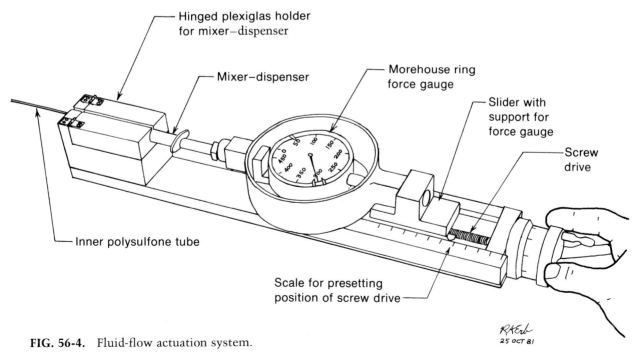

FIG. 56-4. Fluid-flow actuation system.

system presently used. It has a manually actuated screw drive with a driven-force gauge pressing on the mixer–dispenser piston. The force gauge permits setting the pressure during flow. The plug is formed during a coasting phase. When the hysteroscopist sees the silicone reach the obturator tip, the screw drive turning is stopped; liquid spring action in the silicone and other elastic behavior in the system cause the coasting. The force gauge allows the decay pressure to be followed to ensure that the plug cures under pressure. Curing under pressure is important for properly holding open and filling the cross-section of the oviductal lumen.

THE PUMP FOR DEXTRAN 70

The hysteroscopic fluid found most effective for distending the uterine cavity has been 32% dextran 70,000 in 10% aqueous glucose solution. A device for automatically pressurizing the dextran 70 has been designed; it contributes to making the tubal occlusion a two-person procedure (hysteroscopist and assistant). The pump consists of a support stand for a 50-ml disposable syringe and a weight for the piston that provides 150-mm Hg nominal pressure in the liquid. A light touch on the weight can provide a pressure increment when this is needed for observation.

MISCELLANEOUS COMPONENTS

A special sealing cap has been made for the operating channel of the hysteroscope. It is molded of Dow Corning MDX 4-4210 silicone rubber and has three sealing rings rather than the usual one. The aim of the design is to avoid damage to the delicate obturator tip that passes through the seal while maintaining sealing action against the outer polysulfone tube.

An enlarging sheath for the hysteroscope has been fabricated to be used in patients in whom a patulous cervix causes excessive leakage of the dextran 70. This sheath has a sliding O-ring seal and will enlarge the diameter of

Wolf or Storz operating hysteroscope from 7 mm to 9 mm.

An aspirator tube has been designed and used to remove debris. It consists of a 750-mm piece of the larger diameter polysulfone tubing, flared at one end and attached to a Tuohy–Borst fitting. It is used with a 30-ml disposable syringe.

MATERIALS

The materials (designated as Composition A) used to form plugs consist of Silastic 382 Medical Grade Elastomer, 68%; Dow Corning 360 Medical Fluid (20 centistoke grade), 17%; and spherical silver powder (−400 mesh), 15%. These are the same materials used in animal studies with rabbits and rhesus monkeys. The Silastic 382 base material has been used for more than 20 yr in humans. The 360 medical fluid is incorporated as a viscosity reducer, and the silver powder enables the clinical team to ascertain by x-ray study whether bilateral plugs have formed properly.

The catalyst is stannous octoate (Dow Corning Catalyst M), added in a quantity equal to about 1.5% of the Silastic 382 present. The curing reaction, producing a snappy rubbery solid in 5 min, involves cross-linking of the silicone polymer. No sensible heat is generated in the reaction.

The Composition A is supplied to the clinical investigators in mixer–dispensers that have been filled and degassed in a high-efficiency particle attenuation (HEPA)-filtered hood. The mixer–dispensers are packaged with the spring compressed (to reduce vacuum bubbles in cold storage by maintaining positive internal pressure) and stored and used at −15°C.

PROCEDURE

To proceed, attach the guide assembly, while it is in its sterile bag, to a 3-ml syringe containing 1:10,000 methylene blue solution (1% methylene blue diluted 1:100 in physiologic saline solution). Feed the guide through the dextran

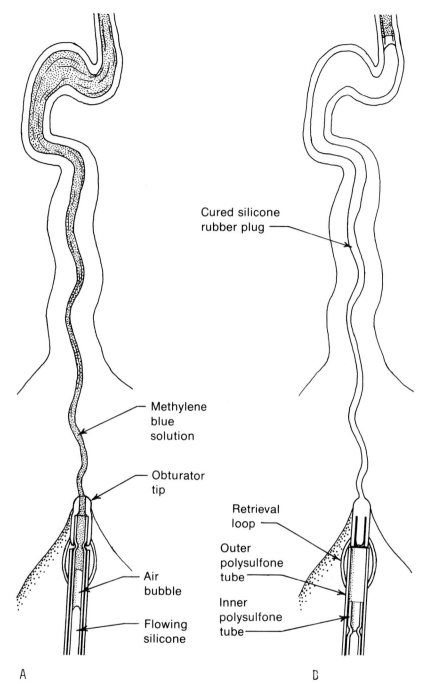

FIG. 56-5.   Sequence in plug-forming procedure. (*A*) Silicone flow.
(*B*) Release.

70–lubricated sealing cap after the end of the hysteroscope is in the uterine cavity. The methylene blue solution is used as a current tracer to locate the tubal ostium. Its more important function is with the "push test," with the obturator tip seated in the tubal ostium. No resistance to flow indicates that communication with a patent tubal lumen has occurred; no reflux shows good obturation. At this point, proceed with plug formation as follows:

1. Remove the mixer–dispenser from the freezer.
2. Add catalyst through the septum cap, and start a stopwatch.
3. Mix: 45 double strokes, ending at 35 to 40 sec.
4. Insert the spacer, remove the Luer cap, and expell a 0.4-ml sample onto a test plate to follow the cure outside the body.
5. Remove the Luer fitting on the guide assembly from the methylene blue syringe and attach it to the mixer–dispenser.
6. Place the mixer–dispenser in the holder on the fluid-flow apparatus, and turn the screw drive to reach and maintain a force of between 290 N and 305 N.
7. Sample the consistency of the material on the test plate with a probe to follow the transition from "long" (strands forming), to "short," to gelling (flow stops here, at about 3 min), to a soft slow-recovery rubber, to a snappy rubber (at about 4 min 45 sec).
8. When the silicone comes into view (usually an air bubble gets between it and the methylene blue solution), tell the assistant to stop the screw drive (Fig. 56-5A). The stopwatch time should be about 2 min.
9. Record the time when pressure decay stops (when flow stops); turn the drive, if necessary, to prevent the decay force from dropping below 50 N.
10. When a snappy cure is achieved, accomplish release by loosening the rearward collet and withdrawing the inner polysulfone tube (Fig. 56-5B). Withdraw the outer polysulfone tube to leave the finished plug

in place. Repeat the procedure on the other side.

The procedure requires that the assistant have special skills, including learning to work efficiently with the materials and instruments under tight time constraints. Identifying tubal ostia and achieving sealing and alignment of the obturator tip with the uterotubal junction are crucial. Efforts have continued at The Franklin Institute in Philadelphia with the support of other investigators to improve instruments and methods.

ACKNOWLEDGMENTS

My work was conducted under the sponsorship of RSP Laboratories, Inc. My special thanks is given to Doretta L. Erb, R.Ph., Research Scientist I, Franklin Research Center, for her preparation of thousands of individual items for the clinical test program since 1978 and for her active support of the overall development from its inception.

REFERENCES

1. Braley SA, Helmer JD: Method for sterilization of males. United States Patent 3,422,813, Jan. 21, 1969
2. Corfman PA, Taylor HC Jr: An instrument for transcervical treatment of the oviducts and uterine cornua. Obstet Gynecol 27:880, 1966
3. Davis RH, Erb RA, Kyriazis GA, et al: Fallopian tube occlusion in rabbits with silicone rubber. J Reprod Med 14:56, 1975
4. Davis RH, Erb RA, Schneider HP, et al: Chronic rabbit and rhesus monkey fallopian tube occlusion with polymer. Fed Proc 34:339, 1975
5. Davis RH, Moonka DK, Platt HA, et al: Chronic occlusion of the rabbit fallopian tube with silicone rubber. Reprod Obstet Gynecol 6:142, 1978
6. Davis RH, Platt HA, Moonka DK, et al: Chronic occlusion of the monkey fallopian tube with silicone polymer. Obstet Gynecol 53:527, 1979
7. Davis RH, Moonka DK, Platt HA, et al: Chronic occlusion of the rabbit fallopian tube with silicone polymer. Gynecol Obstet Invest 10:281, 1979
8. Erb RA: Method and apparatus for non-surgical reversible sterilization of females. United States Patent 3,805,767, April 23, 1974; reissue 29,345, Aug. 9, 1977
9. Erb RA: Silastic: A retrievable custom-molded oviduc-

tal plug. In Sciarra JJ, Droegemuller W, Speidel JJ (eds): Advances in Female Sterilization Techniques, p 259. Hagerstown, Harper & Row, 1976

10. Erb RA: Apparatus and method for the hysteroscopic non-surgical sterilization of females. United States Patent 4,245,623, Jan. 20, 1981

11. Erb RA, Davis RH, Balin H, et al: Device and technique for blocking the fallopian tubes: A method for reversible contraceptive sterilization. In Schima ME, Lubell I, Davis JE, et al (eds): Advances in Voluntary Sterilization, p 336. Proceedings of the Second International Conference. Amsterdam, Excerpta Medica, 1974

12. Erb RA, Davis RH, Kyriazis GA, et al: Device and technique for blocking the fallopian tubes. Contemp Obstet Gynecol 3:92, 1974

13. Erb RA, Davis RH, Kyriazis GA, et al: System and technique for blocking the fallopian tubes. Adv Plann Parent 9:42, 1974

14. Erb RA, Reed TP: Hysteroscopic oviductal blocking with formed-in-place silicone rubber plugs. I. Method and apparatus. J Reprod Med 23:65, 1979

15. Hefnawi F, Fuchs A, Laurence KA: Control of fertility by temporary occlusion of the oviduct. Am J Obstet Gynecol 99:421, 1967

16. Rakshit B: Intratubal blocking device for sterilization without laparotomy. Calcutta Med J 65:90, 1968

17. Rakshit B: Attempts at chemical blocking of the fallopian tube for female sterilization. J Obstet Gynaecol India 20:618, 1970

18. Rakshit B: The scope of liquid plastics and other chemicals for blocking the fallopian tube. In Richart RM, Prager DJ (eds): Human Sterilization, p 213. Springfield, IL, Charles C Thomas, 1972

19. Reed TP, Erb RA: Hysteroscopic oviductal blocking with formed-in-place silicone rubber plugs. II. Clinical studies. J Reprod Med 23:69, 1979

20. Reed TP, Erb RA: Tubal occlusion with silicone rubber: An update. J Reprod Med 25:25, 1980

21. Reed TP, Erb RA, DeMaeyer J: Tubal occlusion with silicone rubber: Update 1980. J Reprod Med 26:534, 1981

22. Reed TP, Erb RA: Hysteroscopic female sterilization with formed-in-place silicone rubber plugs. In Phillips JM (ed): Endoscopic Female Sterilization—A Comparison of the Methods, p 143. Downey, CA, American Association of Gynecologic Laparoscopists, 1983

Methods for Improving Tubal Ostial Observation, Obturation, and Perfusion with the Hysteroscope ■

57

Theodore P. Reed, III
Robert A. Erb
Jay M. Cooper

Concern has been expressed on many occasions about physicians' ability to observe and obturate the fallopian tubal ostia with the hysteroscope. For tubal occlusion with formed-in-place silicone rubber plugs under hysteroscopic control, it is essential to locate, obturate, and perfuse fallopian tubes for sterilization.[1,3,4] Success depends on three basic factors, namely, patient selection, doing the procedure in the early proliferative phase of the cycle, and special instruments.

MATERIALS AND METHODS

PATIENT SELECTION

Patients are screened for hysteroscopy after a careful history is taken, with attention paid to previous pelvic infection or pelvic surgery (*e.g.*, ruptured appendicitis, ectopic pregnancies, endometriosis, the use of an intrauterine device [IUD], infected abortion, or postpartum uterine infection). Patients in these categories are evaluated by hysterosalpingography before hysteroscopy is attempted.

On physical examination, a pelvic mass or fixed uterine retroversion either contraindicates the attempt at hysteroscopic sterilization or a hysterosalpingogram is advised preoperatively. With retroversion, frequently tubes cannot be obturated and sterilization is not possible. The symphysis pubis and rami prevent proper angulation of the scope and access to the tubal ostia.

INSTRUMENTS

Before starting tubal obturation and perfusion the uterine cavity is aspirated. The aspirator (designed by Erb) is inserted through the operating channel of the scope, and the uterine cavity is cleansed in a few moments using the attached 30-ml syringe for suction (Fig. 57-1). The physician can selectively manipulate the instrument in the uterine cavity and remove small pedunculated endometrial fragments. Occasional cornual occlusion seen on hysterosalpingography and hysteroscopy is caused by small polypoid endometrial fragments directly over the tubal ostium. These can be aspirated and obturation, perfusion, and occlusion subsequently achieved.

A memory curve in the guide assembly is quite helpful in many cases. This is done by removing the hysteroscope from the uterine cavity with the guide assembly in place through the operating channel. At two points, approximately 1 cm and 2 cm from the obturator tip, the operator kinks or bends the guide assembly

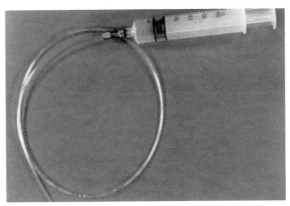

FIG. 57-1. Aspirator: standard 30-ml syringe; polysulfone tubing with Tuohy–Borst fitting for syringe.

Hamberger suggests that it relieves tubal spasm as well.[2] In patients who required a repeat hysteroscopy, naproxen sodium was used; patients reported that they were much more comfortable than during the first operation.

Glucagon has been used to relieve tubal spasm. When both tubal ostia are seen and a guide assembly is introduced into the uterus, both tubes are obturated with the guide assem-

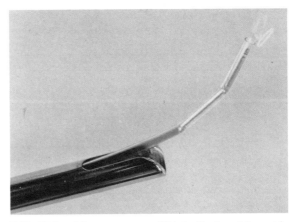

FIG. 57-2. Memory curve ("kinks") placed in guide after guide has been placed through operating channel of the hysteroscope.

and then pulls the guide assembly back into the operating channel and reinserts the scope and guide assembly (Fig. 57-2). When the guide assembly is pushed out of the operating channel, the guide often enters easily in "laterally" placed fallopian tubes (Fig. 57-3). A hysteroscope with a deflector on the operating channel also is helpful with this problem.

Enlargement or elongation of the obturator tips is important. Two of the tips (designed by Erb) are enlarged cylinders similar to the standard type, being 3 mm to 4 mm in diameter (Fig. 57-4). The Reed modification is a cone-shaped tip approximately 4 mm at its base and slightly less than 2 cm at its apex. The third modification (Cooper) is an elongated tip that bends around and enters some laterally placed tubes rather easily with or without a curve in the guide assembly.

MEDICATIONS USED IN TUBAL PERFUSION AND OBTURATION

Drugs inhibiting prostaglandin synthesis alleviate uterine cramping and appear to inhibit tubal smooth muscle contraction. These medications are used before hysterosalpingograms to relieve pain and overcome tubal spasm. Naproxen sodium (Anaprox), 550 mg, given 1 hr preoperatively, seems to make patients more comfortable. A recent report by Lindblom and

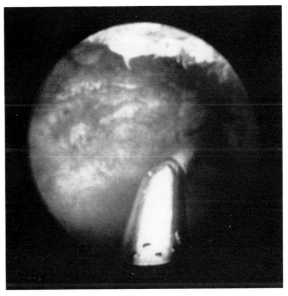

FIG. 57-3. Curved guide is seen with obturator tip in tubal opening.

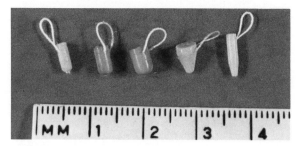

FIG. 57-4. Various sizes and shapes of obturator tips include standard E 1 tip.

bly and perfused with the push test of methylene blue.[3] If good perfusions are obtained, one tube is occluded with silicone rubber. The second tube often shows resistance on the repeat methylene push test, and a slight reflux of methylene blue results. The patient may report some discomfort during this push test. One unit (1 mg) of glucagon is given intravenously; the operator waits for 6 to 7 min; perfusion with methylene blue becomes easy; and occlusion can be accomplished without difficulty. Twenty patients underwent this technique, and successful sterilizations resulted in 17 instances.

RESULTS

Of 297 patients, including all patients who applied for the operation (accepted or not), proper plug formation was accomplished in 79%. Of the 252 patients on whom the procedure was attempted, 85% had proper plug formation. As of Dec. 1, 1981, in the cooperative study 792 patients were considered for sterilization; 755 operations were attempted, with successful results in 576 (75%). The number of total woman-months without contraception and with proper plugs is now 2405 mo; no pregnancies occurred to date in this group, and 6 patients were not followed. One hundred and thirty patients did not receive proper plugs on the first attempt, but 77 (55%) received proper plugs bilaterally after another procedure.

COMPLICATIONS

Minor bleeding occurred in 10% of women, and 3 patients who developed chronic pain 12 to 18 mo after the procedure were relieved by removal of the plugs. No major complications have been reported. Eleven pregnancies were associated with failure to achieve proper bilateral plug formation.

REFERENCES

1. Erb RA, Reed TP: Hysteroscopic oviductal blocking with formed-in-place silicone rubber plugs. I. Method and apparatus. J Reprod Med 23:65, 1979
2. Lindblom B, Hamberger L: Copper and contractility of the human fallopian tube. Am J Obstet Gynecol 141:398, 1981
3. Reed TP, Erb RA: Hysteroscopic oviductal blocking with formed-in-place silicone rubber plugs. II. Clinical studies. J Reprod Med 23:69, 1979
4. Reed TP, Erb RA: Tubal occlusion with silicone rubber: An update. J Reprod Med 25:25, 1980

Hysteroscopic Sterilization by Silastic Plugs ◼ 58

Michael S. Baggish

A method of sterilization under hysteroscopic control in which liquid silicone polymer and a catalyst, which solidify (cure) *in situ,* are instilled into the fallopian tubes has been described by Reed and Erb.[1] The purpose of this chapter is to describe the technique in 41 procedures performed at Mount Sinai Hospital, Hartford, CT. A panoramic hysteroscope with an operating channel and 32% dextran 70 (Hyskon) are used to distend the uterine cavity. An assistant is trained to prepare the silicone mixture and deliver it through a fluid-flow activator into the oviduct.

MATERIALS AND METHODS

Each woman is given a detailed, informed consent form indicating that the procedure is experimental and that long term-data on conception control are unknown. Patients almost always prefer to have the procedure done in the office with local anesthesia rather than in the operating room. The patient is informed that the gynecologist cannot ascertain before hysteroscopy whether sterilization can be done. The early proliferative phase of the menstrual cycle is the best time to do the operation.

A plastic syringe containing 50-ml of dextran 70 is placed in a pump and attached by a Silastic tube to the intake channel of the hysteroscope sheath (Fig. 58-1). Air is pushed out of the system by placing pressure on the syringe. A prepackaged paracervical block set containing a 22-gauge spinal needle and 1% carbocaine (Mepivacaine) with 1:200,000 epinephrine is used. Pratt dilators, up to 23 Fr, dilate the endocervical canal as indicated. A single hinged speculum, open on one side, may be removed once the hysteroscope is in place so as not to cause patient discomfort. The special equipment consists of a guide assembly (Fig. 58-2) through which both methylene blue and liquid silicone are delivered; it is fitted at its terminal extremity with a hollow silicone plug (Fig. 58-3). Methylene blue is drawn up into a 5-ml syringe and attached to the guide assembly. Silicone is prepackaged and kept frozen in a special mixing syringe. The silicone catalyst is drawn up in an airtight tuberculin syringe (Fig. 58-4). A small sampling dish, which will contain some of the catalyzed silicone polymer, allows observation of the curing process. A fluid-flow activator is a precise pressure-gauged pump for driving and monitoring silicone flow into the oviduct (Fig. 58-5).

To proceed, place the patient in the lithotomy position in comfortable leg and foot stirrups. A ledge is fitted to the operating table to support and steady the operator's arms. Prepare

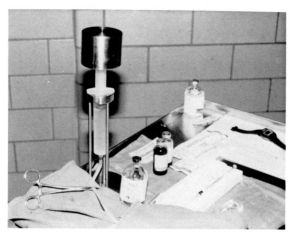

FIG. 58-1. A dextran 70 (Hyskon) pump facilitates uterine distention.

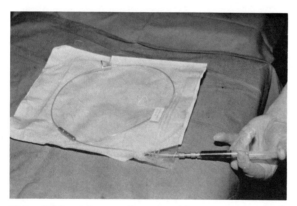

FIG. 58-2. The guide assembly transmits both methylene blue and liquid silicone.

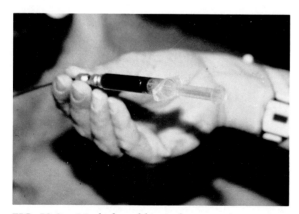

FIG. 58-3. Methylene blue is drawn up in a syringe and attached to the guide assembly.

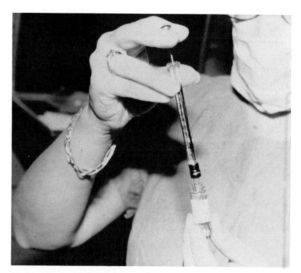

FIG. 58-4. Catalyst is drawn up in an airtight tuberculin syringe.

the perineum and vagina with povidone-iodine (Betadine), and attach a single-tooth tenaculum to the cervix. Place anesthetic blocks into the parametria laterally and into the uterosacral ligaments. Sound the uterus, insert the hysteroscope with or without previous dilatation into the cervical canal, and pump dextran 70 into the uterine cavity. By following the flow of dextran 70, the tubal ostia are discerned (Fig. 58-6). The size, shape, and position of the ostia vary. If the ostia are too lateral, cannulation will be difficult and aligning the axes of the oviduct and cannula may not be possible. Sometimes during the secretory phase the ostia are difficult to locate and become plugged with small endometrial fragments caught in the dextran 70 flow.

Advance the guide assembly, which is inserted into the operating sheath, once the ostium is located (Fig. 58-7). Line up the guide assembly cannula with the tubal orifice and cannulate the ostium (Fig. 58-8). Asks the assistant for a light tap of methylene blue to check for a tight fit and to ascertain whether there is free flow of liquid, indicating that the correct axis has been attained (Fig. 58-9). If everything is in order, administer a sustained injection of methylene blue. If there is no resistance, continue the procedure; if there is resistance, readjust the cannula. Secure the hysteroscope and cannula in place; an arm rest is essential. Instruct the assistant to mix the silicone and catalyst, and inject the air-free catalyst into the silicone syringe as a stopwatch is started. The two components are mixed by moving the syringe plunger in and out while rotating the syringe with each plunge (Fig. 58-10). When mixing has been completed, a small amount of the mixture is spilled into the sampling dish. The silicone syringe replaces the methylene blue syringe on the guide assembly. Deftly place the syringe containing the silicone catalyst into the fluid-flow activator and accurately record the time as the assistant brings the pressure on the syringe up to 300 mm Hg (Fig. 58-11). Carefully watch the transparent cannula for the silicone flow. First a tiny tinged air bubble appears and then the stark white silicone enters the tube. The assistant should relieve pressure on the fluid-flow activator and record time and pressure readings as the gauge falls, at the lowest stabilized pressure, and the time interval elapsed. The silicone in the test dish is tested to ascertain its degree of solidification and elasticity as it cures (Fig. 58-12). When the silicone becomes very elastic (usually between 6 and 6½ min) the fluid as-

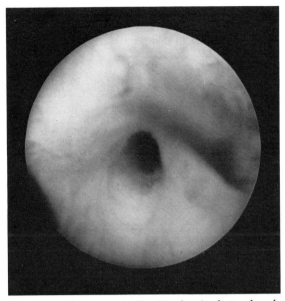

FIG. 58-6. Dextran 70 (Hyskon) distends the uterus, enabling the tubal ostium to be located.

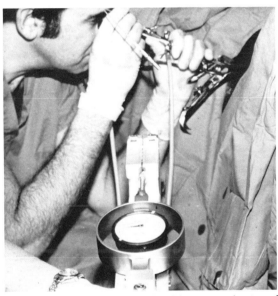

FIG. 58-7. The guide assembly; cannula is advanced toward the tubal ostium.

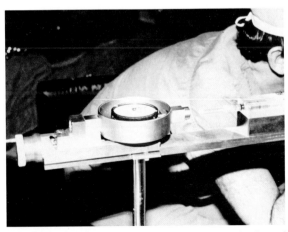

FIG. 58-5. A fluid-flow activator pumps the liquid silicone through the guide assembly into the tube.

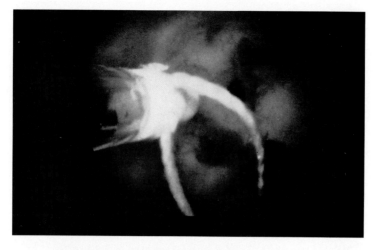

FIG. 58-8. The cannula is approaching the tubal ostium.

FIG. 58-9. Methylene blue is injected to check resistance and tightness of fit.

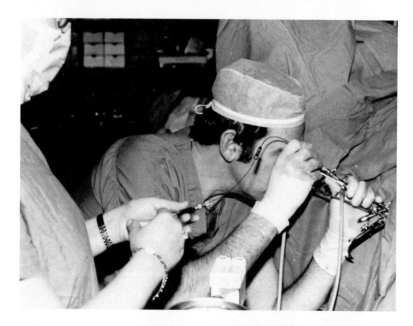

FIG. 58-10. A test sample of silicone is spilled into the sampling dish.

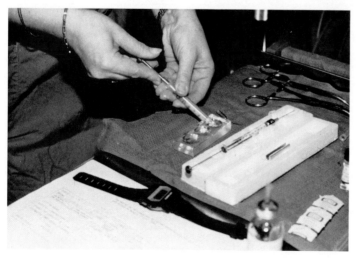

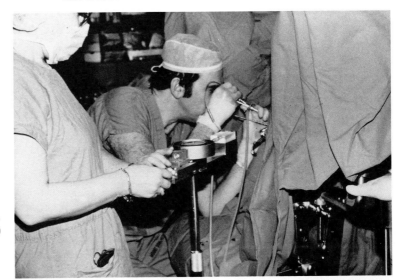

FIG. 58-11. Pressure in the fluid-flow activator is increased to 300 mm Hg.

FIG. 58-12. The silicone sample has stiffened.

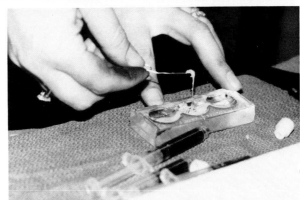

sembly is separated from the plug. The assistant performs this maneuver, and the physician removes the assembly and observes the *in situ* plug. The procedure is repeated on the opposite ostium (Fig. 58-13). Instruments are withdrawn, and the patient is sent to the radiology department for a pelvic x-ray film to decide whether the plugs appear normal (Fig. 58-14). The silicone plug bonds to the intraluminal solidified silicone and forms a single unit.

COMMENT

The advantages of formed *in situ* silicone plugs are that their placement is an outpatient procedure using local anesthesia, no incisions are required, there is minimal patient discomfort,

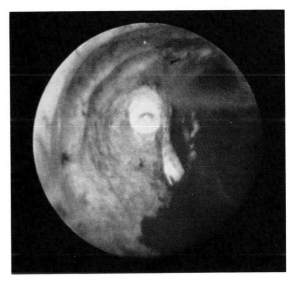

FIG. 58-13. The formed plug is seen *in situ*.

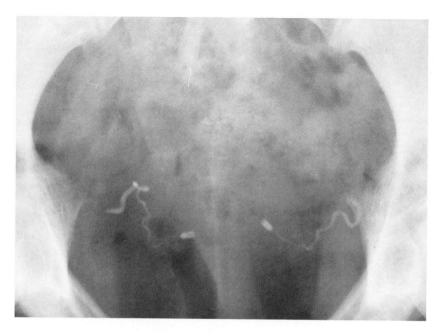

FIG. 58-14. A postoperative roentgenogram shows the plugs in proper position.

and the procedure may be reversible. The main disadvantages include the need for better instruments, standardization of silicone and catalyst, a fixed mixing procedure in a single container, and the performance of hysteroscopy before a decision can be made on the feasibility of sterilization.

REFERENCE

1. Reed TP, Erb RA: Hysteroscopic oviductal blocking with formed-in-place silicone rubber plugs. II. Clinical studies. J Reprod Med 23:69, 1979

Hysteroscopic Sterilization with Silicone Rubber: A Review of 3½ Years' Experience

59

Joris F.D.E. De Maeyer

Tubal occlusion with silicone rubber through a hysteroscopic method was mainly made possible by the preliminary laboratory work of Erb.[1-4] In April 1978 I started its clinical application, and later Reed and Erb described their findings.[5-8] The purpose of this chapter is to report my results from April 1978 until October 1981 on 67 patients.

MATERIALS AND METHODS

The technique has been described previously.[1-4] The essential step is to mix a liquid silicone mass with a catalyst just before using it. The mass coagulates into a rubbery substance in 4½ to 6 min. Within this time, the liquid silicone is delivered into the tube through the working channel of the hysteroscope, where the silicone coagulates. An intratubal plug is made. Applying this technique to the two tubes results in sterilization. The coagulation process is always checked on a small glass plate. The uterus is distended with carbon dioxide or with dextran 70 (Hyskon) in 10% glucose. Initially the procedure was done under general or epidural anesthesia. Currently, only local anesthesia is used (a paracervical block); if necessary, supplementary intracervical injections are used. The operation takes 25 to 35 min and is an outpatient procedure. As a control for plug formation, methylene blue perfusion (2 ml to 5 ml) is given immediately before the silicone is injected. Pelvic x-ray films are taken immediately after the operation and at 3 mo and 1 yr postoperatively. Hysterosalpingograms are not done, since they gave little significant information. Patients underwent a repeat hysteroscopy after 2 yr to evaluate the position of the plug.

RESULTS

Of 67 patients, 5 were excluded because of hysteroscopic problems that made applying the silicone impossible. Four of these patients were among the initial eight. Two patients showed obstruction during the test with methylene blue and were thus excluded, although silicone was instilled; poor plug formation resulted. These findings demonstrate the prognostic value of the methylene blue test. Bilateral complete occlusion succeeded in 75% of patients. Together with patients having a natural occlusion on one side, this gives a success rate of 78% (47 patients). Bilateral occlusion was not achieved in 13 women because of a faulty plug on one side in 12 and failure to place 1 plug in 1. All 44 patients whose operations were successful used this method as their only contraception (Figs. 59-1 and 59-2).

After 3½ years, 53 patients are still using the method, including the 9 with unilateral faulty plugs. One patient had a hysterectomy, another expelled a normal plug, and one patient requested supplementary laparoscopic

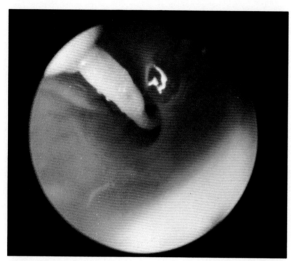

FIG. 59-1. Silastic plug was in place for more than 2 yr.

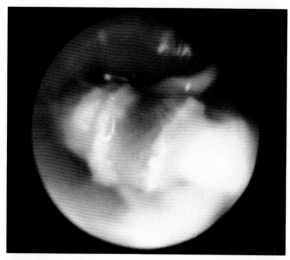

FIG. 59-2. Closeup of silicone plug in right tubal ostium.

sterilization. Plugs have been used as contraception for 1093 mo overall. Four patients became pregnant; three of the pregnancies, including a tubal gestation, occurred after the initial 12 operations. Three of these patients expelled plugs, and one had a slow coagulation of the silicone with abnormal plug formation.

One hundred and six normal plugs were placed, including the two that were expelled. Twenty-one abnormal plugs included 17 expulsions. In 92 attempts, general anesthesia was used in 16 patients and epidural anesthesia in 5. The other 71 operations were done under local anesthesia.

COMPLICATIONS

Abnormal vaginal bleeding occurred or persisted in seven patients, and slight postoperative infectious morbidity was noted in two women. Minor inflammatory changes were seen in tissue sections taken in a few patients. Two perforations occurred—one of the uterus and one of the tube. Two silastic intramural injections were noted, and one patient had syncope under local anesthesia during a dextran 70 injection.

COMMENT

Formed *in situ* silicone plugs can be successfully inserted for sterilization by hysteroscopy. Bilateral normal plugs resulted in 78% of patients during the development of the method, and these results will improve. Fewer patients will require reoperation, and this operation causes minimal additional risk to hysteroscopy. The improperly formed plug could have an anticonceptional effect but more likely would be spontaneously expelled. In this series, the method has proved effective, with no poststerilization pregnancy in any patient with adequate bilateral plugs.

REFERENCES

1. Erb RA: Method and apparatus for non-surgical reversible sterilization of females. United States Patent 3,805,767, April 23, 1974; reissued 29, 345, Aug. 9, 1977
2. Erb RA: Silastic: A retrievable custom-molded oviductal plug. In Sciarra JJ, Droegemuller W, Speidel JJ (eds): Advances in Female Sterilization Techniques, p 259. Hagerstown, Harper & Row, 1976
3. Erb RA: Apparatus and method for the hysteroscopic non-surgical sterilization of females. United State Patent 4,245,623, Jan. 20, 1981
4. Erb RA, Reed TP: Hysteroscopic oviductal blocking with formed-in-place silicone rubber plugs. I. Method and apparatus. J Reprod Med 23:65, 1979
5. De Maeyer JFDE: Die hysteroskopische Sterilisation mit Silastic-Plugs. In Lindemann HJ (ed): Keitumer Kreis. Proceedings of the Colloquium on Questions of Hysteroscopy held in Keitum/Sylt, May 2–4, 1980
6. De Maeyer JFDE: Een nieuwe methode van definitieve contraceptie. Patient Care 3:31, 1980
7. Reed TP, Erb RA: Hysteroscopic oviductal blocking with formed-in-place silicone rubber plugs. II. Clinical studies. J Reprod Med 23:69, 1979
8. Reed TP, Erb RA, De Maeyer JFDE: Tubal occlusion with silicone rubber: An update 1980. J Reprod Med 26:534, 1981

60

Hysteroscopic Tubal Sterilization and Formed-in-Place Silicone Rubber Plugs: Cause, Significance, and Prevention of Abnormal Plugs ■

Jay M. Cooper
Richard Houck

Hysteroscopic tubal sterilization with formed *in situ* silicone plugs is under study in eight medical centers, and more than 700 patients have undergone the sterilizing procedure. Twelve pregnancies have been reported.[1,5]

No two patients have identical plugs because of the unique method in which plugs are formed (Fig. 60-1), but hysteroscopic and radiologic characteristics allow appropriate analysis. A normal plug has a dumbbell configuration with a thick obturator tip at the uterotubal ostium, a thin intramural portion, and a bulbous distal portion. A properly formed plug cannot migrate into either the uterine or the peritoneal cavity (Fig. 60-2).

ABNORMAL PLUGS

Abnormal plugs can be characterized as refluxed, intravasated, discontinuous, foreshortened, or slowly cured. Of these five types, the refluxed plug is the most common (Fig. 60-3A). Its identification depends on its hysteroscopic and radiologic appearance. Most commonly, a refluxed plug results from the physicians' inability to obtain a parallel axis between the obturator tip and the tubal ostium. It can occur because the patient or operator moves inappropriately or because the operator fails to apply

adequate pressure on the obturator tip during the instillation and flow of the liquid silicone. An unusually patulous tubal ostium can prevent a proper seal between the obturator tip and the ostium, tubal spasm can prevent proper "seating" of the obturator tip, or the uterus can be inadequately distended with dextran 70 (Hyskon) because of a patulous cervix or inadvertent uterine perforation. The refluxed plug is not likely to be retained because an inadequate volume of silicone has flowed into the tube at a reduced pressure. Migration into the uterine cavity is likely, and the plug should be replaced (Fig. 60-3B).

The second type of abnormal plug, less frequently encountered, results from intravasation of silicone into the myometrium. The most common cause is improper alignment between the obturator tip and the tubal ostium. Often, there is no hysteroscopic evidence that such a plug has formed. Sometimes unusual resistance to the flow of methylene blue solution is encountered before silicone infusion. Inadequate uterine distention can be implicated. The postoperative x-ray film will show silicone in a myometrial outpouching adjacent to the tubal ostium (Fig. 60-4). Obviously ineffectual and radiologically abnormal, such a plug should be replaced.

To minimize the incidence of refluxed and

intravasated plugs, the curve of the catheter should be altered to the correct alignment and parallel axis at the tubal ostium. Alternate tip designs can accommodate different diameters of tubal ostia. The C-1 (Cooper-1) tip has increased length and flexibility, allowing greater success in properly cannulating laterally placed tubal ostia and in patients with tubal spasm. A specially designed sheath to increase the diameter of the hysteroscope is available to minimize leakage of dextran 70 through the cervix, and glucagon can be administered intravenously to counteract tubal spasm.[2]

The discontinuous plug (Fig. 60-5A) results from improper mixing of silicone and catalyst or abnormal operation of the infusion pump or catheters used to deliver silicone. During hys-

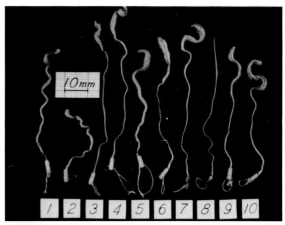

FIG. 60-1. No two plugs are identical because of the unique method in which they are formed. Except for No. 8, each is normal.

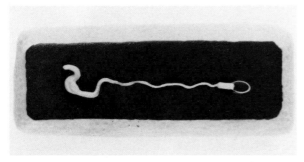

A B

FIG. 60-2. (A) Normal plug. (B) Normal plugs seen on an immediate postprocedure roentgenogram.

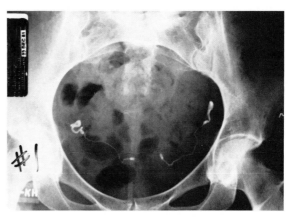

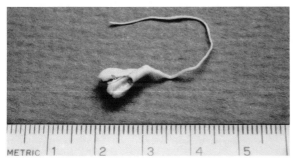

A B

FIG. 60-3. (A) Refluxed or ejected plug. (B) Roentgenogram shows partial intrauterine migration of plug (arrow).

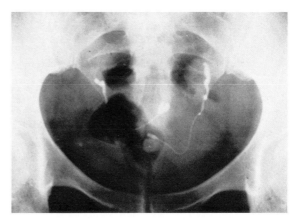

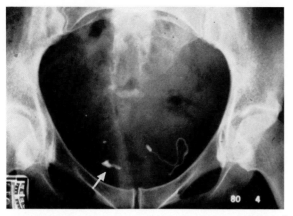

FIG. 60-4. Roentgenogram shows intravasation of plug (*arrow*).

teroscopy a peculiar starting and stopping activity of the infusing silicone is noted. Inappropriate movement by the patient or physician during silicone infusion may result in loss of plug continuity. The x-ray film will then show discontinuity between the obturator tip and the distal portion of the plug. Close scrutiny of the postoperative x-ray film may be necessary. Strict adherence to proper technique in mixing and dispensing silicone and minimizing patients' anxiety and discomfort significantly diminish the formation of abnormal plugs.

The fourth abnormal plug appears foreshortened (Fig. 60-5*B* and *C*). It results from tubal disease or, most often, an inadequate vol-

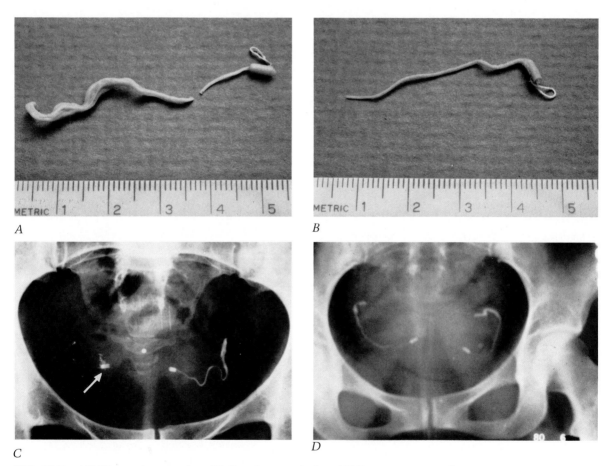

FIG. 60-5. (*A*) Discontinuous plug. (*B*) Foreshortened plug. (*C*) Roentgenogram shows foreshortened plug (*arrow*). (*D*) Roentgenogram shows slowly cured plugs.

ume of silicone. A quick cure precipitated by the addition of an excessive amount of catalyst to the liquid silicone, or slow delivery of the syringe containing silicone to the infusion pump, is generally noted.

The slowly cured plug has no typical x-ray or hysteroscopic appearance, as illustrated by postoperative x-ray film of normal plugs (Fig. 60-5D). The operation had been uncomplicated except that curing the silicone was not noted until 7 min after mixing silicone with the catalyst. Six months postoperatively the patient became pregnant. At her request, therapeutic abortion and bilateral salpingectomy were performed. Histologic examination showed no tubal damage or salpingitis. The left plug was ovoid and did not fill the tubal lumen properly. When curing is not completed within 6 min, there is potential loss of intratubal pressure from the liquid silicone, with collapse of the plug into an ovoid. This is the only patient with radiologically normal plugs who conceived.[5]

RESULTS

We have inserted tubal plugs in 308 women, in 365 operations, from November 1980 through December 1981. The average age was 38.2 yr, and patients had had an average of 2.35 pregnancies and 1.75 deliveries. The operations were performed during the follicular phase of the menstrual cycle, at average day 11.07. The mean duration of the operation was 35.36 min. No patient had a serious complication or has become pregnant.

Bilateral normal plugs were placed in 257 (85%); in 5 instances a normal plug was placed in the single functional tube. The operation was not completed in 43 women, 23 of whom did not return for a repeat procedure; in 3, unilateral faulty plugs were identified.

DISCUSSION

The major factor preventing successful hysteroscopic tubal sterilization is inability to cannulate the tubal ostia properly. The maneuver requires special training and experience in hysteroscopy. Either hysteroscopic or radiologic evidence can almost always distinguish between normal and abnormal plugs. Correct interpretation of the pelvic x-ray film minimizes the need for hysterosalpingography. Regardless of the hysteroscopic or x-ray impression, slowly cured plugs (more than 6 min to form) or quickly cured plugs (less than 4.5 min to form) should be removed and replaced with normal plugs. Migration of a normal plug is rare, but an x-ray film at 3 mo postoperatively is necessary to confirm proper continuity and plug placement. Pregnancies have not occurred in patients with normally formed plugs. The anatomic variation of the intramural segment sometimes creates a difficulty that precludes successful cannulation and formation of adequate plugs.[3,6] No structural arrangement or sphincter seems to separate the extramural segment from the uterine cavity.[4] The three myometrial layers continue with the myosalpinx and may cause tubal closure by contraction. Initial experience with glucagon has led us to suggest its use in alleviating spasm at the uterotubal junction.

Preoperative treatment with hormonal or pharmacologic agents may make the proximal tubal segment more amenable to consistent cannulation. Improvements in endoscopic instruments, the sterilization procedure, and the materials used should make tubal occlusion with silicone plugs a reliable method in more than 95% of women desiring transcervical sterilization.

REFERENCES

1. Erb RA, Reed TP: Hysteroscopic oviductal blocking with formed-in-place silicone rubber plugs. I. Method and apparatus. J Reprod Med 23:65, 1979
2. Gerlock AJ: Oviduct response to glucagon during hysterosalpingography. Radiology 119:727, 1976
3. Hermstein A, Neustadt B: Über den intramuralen Tubenteil. Z Geburtshilfe Gynaekol 88:43, 1924
4. Pauerstein CJ: The Fallopian Tube: A Reappraisal, p 16. Philadelphia, Lea & Febiger, 1974
5. Reed TP, Erb RA: Tubal occlusion with silicone rubber plugs. An update. J Reprod Med 25:25, 1980
6. Sweeney WJ Jr: The interstitial portion of the uterine tube: Its gross anatomy, course, and length. Obstet Gynecol 19:3, 1962

Will the Hysteroscopic Silicone Tubal Plug Become a Widely Accepted Technique? ■

61

Franklin D. Loffer
Patricia S. Loffer

Preparation in learning hysteroscopy in order to locate the uterotubal ostia consistently is essential before the physician places plugs into the tubes.

MATERIALS AND METHODS

Between June 1981 and January 1982, 55 patients underwent hysteroscopic sterilization. Nine required a second operation, seven because only a single plug was inserted during the initial attempt and two because abnormal plugs had to be replaced.

The technique has been adequately described.[1] All operations were done in an office setting using a paracervical block of 1% lidocaine with 1 : 100,000 epinephrine. Two patients received 5 mg of diazepam, and 13 required meperidine hydrochloride, 25 mg intravenously (IV). Most patients received 500 mg of tetracycline before and for 3 doses after the procedure because it is technically difficult to do this procedure in a sterile field. Later in the series patients received naproxen sodium, 550 mg, given 1 hr preoperatively to decrease tubal spasm and uterine cramping. Glucagon, 1 mg IV, was used in three women to overcome tubal spasm, but it did not seem to help.

RESULTS

The time from vaginal preparation until the operation was completed in 55 patients ranged from 24 to 120 min. Although the average time decreased from 55.6 to 49.3 min in the patients examined later in the series, the mean time remained at 45 min. Only two successful operations lasted more than 70 min. Spending more than 75 min is seldom helpful when problems are encountered; office scheduling is made difficult by the unpredictable length of the operation.

Bilateral plugs (normal and abnormal) were successfully inserted on the first attempt in 47 (85.5%) of 55 patients; 8 had only a single plug inserted. The most common cause of failure was inability to inject silicone into the tube in six patients. Three of these patients had transient, natural tubal spasm; one had a blocked tube. These problems are not preventable and probably will always account for failure. The cause for failure in one other patient is unknown but could have been spasm or blockage. The other three failures relate more to physician inexperience. In one patient, spasm was caused by unnecessary manipulation of the tube. The loss of intrauterine pressure in another patient could have been prevented if proper equipment had been available. The final failure was related to a lost screw in the fluid-flow actuator.

Seven of the eight women who had only one good plug underwent a second operation, of which five received plugs, two did not, and one did not undergo a second operation. One of the failures resulted from previous pelvic inflammatory disease (PID) and a blocked tube proved on laparoscopy. The cause of the other failure is unknown. Including the second procedure in seven women, bilateral plugs were eventually inserted into 52 (96.3%) of 54 patients. There is a difference between inserted plugs and normal plugs, and the above figures relate only to inserted plugs. Abnormal plugs appear related to improper technique from inexperience. Seven abnormal plugs occurred in five patients; four were found in three patients on postoperative x-ray study. Three abnormal plugs were found in 2 other patients on the 3-mo x-ray film. All abnormal plugs occurred during the first procedure. Two patients with abnormal plugs had successful reinsertions at a second operation, and three others have not yet undergone a second attempt.

The success of inserting bilateral normal plugs after one procedure as measured by the postoperative and 3-mo follow-up x-ray film was 76.4% (42 of 55 patients) (Table 61-1). The success for bilateral normal plugs improved to 94.3% (50 patients of 53) when a second procedure was done. An overall rate for normal plugs after two procedures was 90.9% (50 patients of 55), including 3 women who have not had a second procedure and 2 others in whom the operation failed.

Five patients were identified with abnormal plugs; one did not have distal enlargement of the tubal plug; three had a missing tip unilaterally; and one had missing tips bilaterally. One unilateral missing tip was detected on the immediate postoperative x-ray film, and another was found by the patient on a menstrual pad 48 hr after insertion. The other unilateral and the bilateral missing plugs were noted on 3 mo x-ray study. The abnormal plugs probably occurred because too much silicone was used in the test plate and the insertion pressure dropped when the syringe ran out of silicone, a

Table 61-1
INSERTION RATE FOR BILATERAL NORMAL PLUGS AFTER 1 PROCEDURE IN 55 PATIENTS

TYPE OF PLUG	PATIENTS	
	No.	%
Bilateral normal plugs	42	76.4
Unilateral normal plug (opposite plug missing)	8	14.5
Unilateral abnormal plug (opposite plug normal)	3	5.5
Bilateral abnormal plugs	2	3.6
Total	55	100

totally preventable problem. In these cases the tip is expelled vaginally and the remainder of the plug passes into the abdominal cavity by tubal contractions.

Bilateral inadequate enlargement of the distal end of the tubal plug occurred because too much catalyst was used and the silicone gelled before an adequate distal tip was achieved. These plugs were expelled vaginally. This problem did not recur but does point out a technical problem in dealing with these materials. Although no pregnancies have been reported, and the number of women and the total months without contraception are few, the experiences of others suggest that a patient with bilateral normal plugs is adequately sterilized.[4]

DISCUSSION

The most uncomfortable part of the operation is the injection of the local anesthesia. A preoperative anesthetic gel can be used on the vaginal mucosa to decrease the pain of injection. Cervical dilation was needed in one third of patients, and both tubal ostia were identified in all patients. To achieve a clear field, mucus was aspirated in two thirds of the operations. No significant problems were encountered because of endometrial bleeding. In two operations a problem with maintaining intrauterine pressure occurred because of a patulous cervical canal. One of the two patients had one plug fail on the first occasion, but successful insertion was obtained at a second procedure. No significant complications were noted in this series.

The syringe filled with silicone must have the precise amount of catalyst added and carefully mixed. The materials must be maintained at a specific temperature for proper curing. The amount of catalyst recommended by the supplier is not always consistent across the United States. These problems can be overcome, but they make the procedure difficult to accomplish unless there is a team approach. The assistant in the procedure is critical. Few gynecologic procedures require as much expertise from an assistant.

The guide assembly is good, but the ability to place it in parallel axis with the tube is often difficult. Parallel axis refers to aligning the guide assembly so that an unobstructed outflow of fluid can pass from the syringe into the guide, out of the silicone tip, and through the fallopian tube. The assistant, not the physician, must decide if a free flow is obtained. Better instruments are needed to increase the success and decrease the time involved in inserting bilateral plugs. The primary problem is to be able to curve the guide easily at its tip to reach the lateral tube. This could be achieved either by having control over the curve of the guide or by the ability to bend the guide by an adjustment on the hysteroscope. Current equipment, patterned after urologic instruments, does not yet solve the problem.

Despite the experimental aspect of this procedure, patient acceptance is good. Patients perceive the procedure as an effective and permanent contraceptive technique that does not require an incision and is easily done under local anesthesia in the office. The lack of an incision is especially appealing to some patients. The use of IV analgesics, tranquilizers, and topical anesthetic agent to the vaginal mucosa has been helpful.

Is the operation reversible? There is no basis yet for a prediction. It may be, however, since no tube is destroyed and there is no evidence of damage to the endosalpinx. If shown to be reversible, it will become a major method of family planning. Patients would be able to use this procedure instead of the prolonged use of birth control pills or intrauterine devices. Plugs can be removed by pulling the proximal tip off the formed plug. This can be done easily through the hysteroscope. The distal enlarged part of the plug can be flushed or will migrate by peristalsis into the peritoneal cavity. Hysteroscopic methods of sterilization are not suited for all women, since some will have recognized tubal occlusion.[2,3]

The anatomic landmarks in hysteroscopy are not as clear as in laparoscopy, and a new endoscopic skill must be learned. The procedure also requires a special table, additional equipment and supplies, and a well-trained assistant. Better instruments are needed to improve the feasibility of inserting bilateral plugs and to decrease the incidence of tubal spasm and thus reduce the causes for failure. Some patients and physicians will be reluctant to use this method of sterilization because of its limitations.

REFERENCES

1. Erb RA: Hysteroscopic sterilization with formed-in-place silicone rubber plugs: Basic process and instruments. In Siegler AM, Lindemann HJ (eds): Hysteroscopy: Principles and Practice. Philadelphia, JB Lippincott, 1983
2. Loffer FD, Pent D: Risks of laparoscopic fulguration and transection of the fallopian tubes. Obstet Gynecol 49:218, 1977
3. Loffer FD, Pent D: Pregnancy after laparoscopic sterilization. Obstet Gynecol 55:643, 1980
4. Reed TP, Erb RA, Cooper JM: Methods for Improving Tubal Ostial Observation, Obturation, and Perfusion with the Hysteroscope. In Siegler AM, Lindemann HJ (eds): Hysteroscopy: Principles and Practice. Philadelphia, JB Lippincott, 1983

HYSTEROSCOPY IN PRACTICE   VII

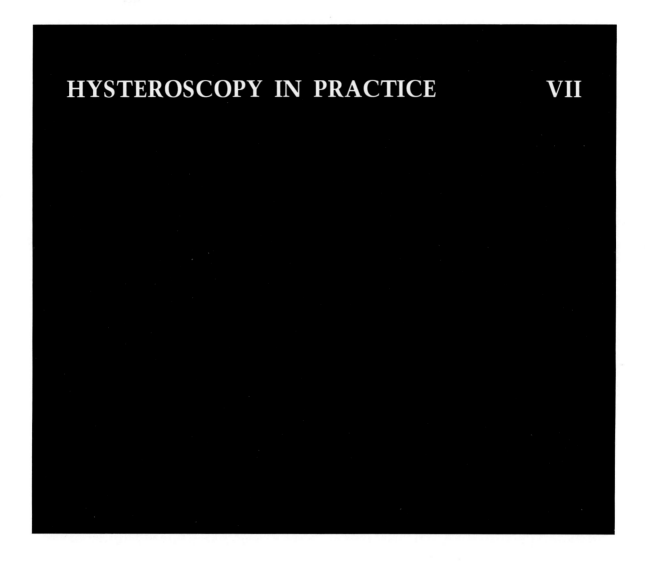

Hysteroscopy can be learned by most obstetricians and gynecologists, but it does require additional training and experience. The technique should be accepted as clinically effective for general use in gynecology. The authors who have contributed chapters in this section are experienced physicians who are also well-known laparoscopists. The routine technique is described with precision by Herendael, whose chapter contains the essentials of the procedure.

Roland, an experienced gynecologist aware of the possible complications from even this minor procedure, urges careful selection of patients to avoid sequelae that would discourage the use of hysteroscopy. Gamerre and Porto, and Lübke, were among the first in Europe to use carbon dioxide hysteroscopy. Proliferative, secretory, and atrophic endometria are distinguishable on hysteroscopic examination, as are adenomyosis and endometrial hyperplasia. These authors also correctly emphasize the need for histologic confirmation of suspicious lesions. They have no qualms about using this hysteroscopic procedure to search for endometrial adenocarcinoma.

Sellner presents important information about hysteroscopy that he gives to his patients preoperatively. It is probably a good idea to educate patients in this manner.

Semm and Riedel believe that there are relatively few indications for hysteroscopy other than for basic research in embryoscopy. They claim that endocrinologic assays, curettage, and laparoscopy can solve most gynecologic problems for which other physicians advocate the addition of hysteroscopy. Despite their disclaimer, Semm and Riedel describe the results of hysteroscopy in 147 patients who were examined because of abnormal bleeding during 1980. In addition, hysteroscopy was used to remove occult intrauterine devices (IUDs) in infertile women, in the search for intrauterine adhesions, and to evaluate uterine malformations.

An Introduction to Routine Hysteroscopy ■ 62

Bruno J. van Herendael

The aim of this chapter is to introduce the technique of hysteroscopy to operating room nurses and hospital staff, including the problems of hysteroscopy for the beginner and its pitfalls during working conditions.

The Hysteroflator is designed for hysteroscopy.[5] Dials indicate the amount of gas in the reservoir, the flow rate, and the intrauterine pressure. The absorption of carbon dioxide in human blood is precisely known.[3,4,6] The intrauterine pressure varies between 50 mm Hg and 80 mm Hg. The major difference between an ordinary insufflator and the Hysteroflator is the interdependence of flow rate and intrauterine pressure.

The apparatus also has a device to maintain suction on the cervical adaptor cups. These metal adaptors have two openings; one is in the cup so that a vacuum can be made between the cup and the cervix, and the second is larger and lies in the center. A large trocar is brought through this opening into the dilated cervix. Once the cup and trocar are in place, the vacuum is created, the trocar is removed, and the hysteroscope takes its place. Suction cups are not always necessary, but during the learning process their use is advisable. The hysteroscope consists of a fiberoptic, a metal tube, and a sheath with or without an Albaran lever; the fiberoptic light is attached to the telescope.

The procedure is as follows: Provide local anesthesia as a paracervical nerve block. Do not use a hysterometer to measure the length of the uterus because it could cause uterine bleeding. Gently dilate the cervix with dilators from 7 mm to 8 mm. The aim is not to dilate the internal os but to leave this dilatation to the pressure of the insufflated gas.

Resist the temptation to push the hysteroscope blindly through the internal os, because uterine perforation can result. One problem for a beginner occurs after the hysteroscope is in the cavity because very often there appears to be a red haze. Experience will allow the physician to avoid this problem, which is caused mostly by too hastily passing the scope through the cervical canal. Pushing the hysteroscope back and forward (trombone playing) (Fig. 62-1) is a typical maneuver used by the beginner; it causes annoying intrauterine gas bubbles. The remedy is to wait until the working pressure is built up, even if it takes 2 to 3 min. Plan more time for the initial hysteroscopies; let the operating room nurse look through the hysteroscope.

Do not take photographs of the first few procedures alone. An assistant should stabilize the camera and the apparatus, thereby improving the sharpness of hysteroscopic pictures once the instrument is within the uterine cavity.

Inspect the fundus, the anterior and the pos-

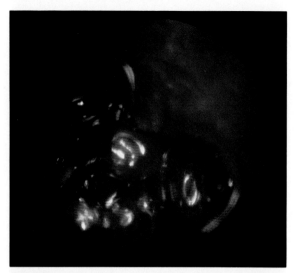

FIG. 62-1. "Trombone playing" causes gas bubbles.

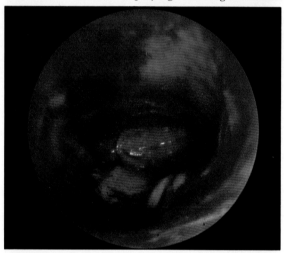

FIG. 62-2. General view of the uterine cavity through the dilated cervix.

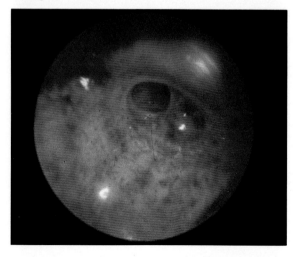

terior walls, and the lateral wall (Fig. 62-2). Locate the cornua and the tubal ostia (Fig. 62-3). Move the instrument as little as possible by turning it on its own axis while keeping the axis of the scope in the axis of the uterine cavity. Most patients have a slight uterine torsion, so that the ostia will not lie on a horizontal line. The right ostium will be situated under the horizontal line and the left one will be slightly elevated. Then, slowly withdraw the scope. Inspect the anterior and side walls by rotating the scope on its axis. Inspecting the posterior wall can be difficult because of blood pooling in the most dependent portion. This pool of blood usually is an artifact.[1] Next, inspect the isthmus by rotating the scope. Inspecting the endocervical canal is easy and should not be overlooked. In the first few operations, resist the temptation to bring auxiliary instruments through the working channels during the procedure because gas will escape and the pneumometra will collapse; it is sometimes difficult to restore. Do 25 diagnostic explorations before embarking on surgical hysteroscopy.[9]

After mastering the technique for exploration, try the biopsy forceps before the next step of cutting and coagulation.[8] Use the instruments initially in a patient who has had a tubal ligation because the uterus is easier to inflate and a more constant working pressure can be maintained throughout the procedure. Put the auxiliary instrument in the work channel before slipping the hysteroscope into the uterus, thus reducing the possibility that gas will escape.

Hysteroscopy on the infertile patient requires attention to certain details. Look mainly for adhesions between anterior and posterior walls but also for small adhesive formations at the tubal ostia.[7] Every strand of tissue seen in the uterus is not an adhesion by definition because strands of hyperplastic endometrium are

FIG. 62-3. View of the left tubal ostium; note the depth of the cornu. Under the ostium to the right an air bubble is visible. There is a distinct margin between the uterine cavity and the horn.

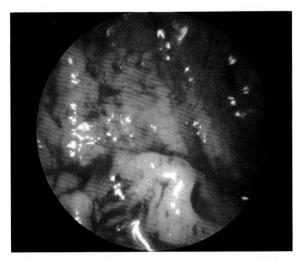

FIG. 62-4. Hyperplastic endometrium just before menstruation; a strand of endometrium is seen at the six o'clock position.

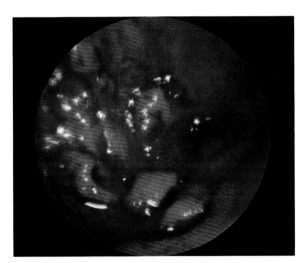

FIG. 62-5. At the posterior wall of the uterine cavity to the right, a hyperplastic endometrial fragment mimics polyps.

found lying in the uterus (Figs. 62-4 and 62-5).[2] Every biopsy calls for pathologic examination. Look for major defects such as myomas (Fig. 62-6), polyps (Fig. 62-7), and septa.[5,9] Atrophic

---

FIG. 62-6. (*A*) Large submucous myoma has normal vascular pattern in upper right corner; note the left tubal ostium. The position of the ostium is distorted by the myoma. (*B*) The back of the uterine cavity is distorted by the myoma. (*C*) Large myoma on the posterior side in an atrophic endometrium. Tubal ostium is visible on the left.

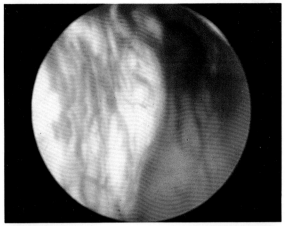

A

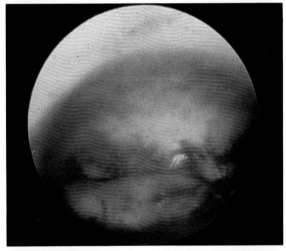

B

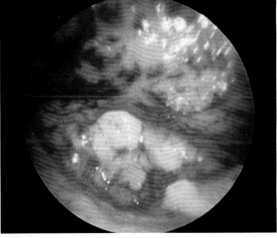

C

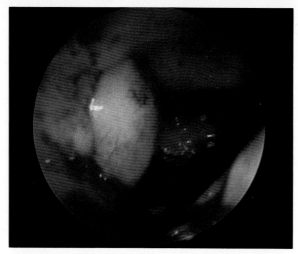

FIG. 62-7. A polyp is visible at the border between the cervix and the uterine cavity.

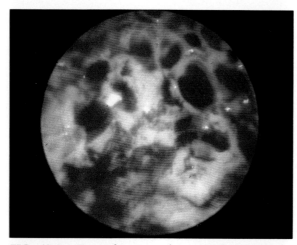

FIG. 62-8. Typical aspect of an atrophic endometrium.

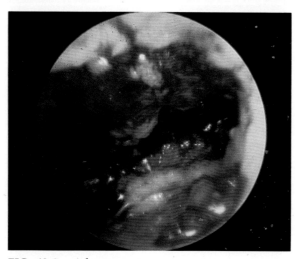

FIG. 62-9. Adenomyosis.

endometrium (Fig. 62-8) and adenomyosis (Fig. 62-9) can be differentiated.

A very important finding is the flap–valve mechanism at the tubal ostia. If the tube is patent, carbon dioxide passes through the tube into the abdominal cavity. Observe *in vivo* the phenomenon of persufflation. Every tube has a pressure gradient. As the working pressure in the uterus becomes greater than this gradient, the carbon dioxide passes through the tube to the abdominal cavity. The tubal ostium opens, a portion of the intramural segment becomes visible, and, after a few seconds when the gas has escaped the cavity, the ostium again collapses. Sometimes the actual passage of gas bubbles through the tubal ostia can be observed. This phenomenon is observed best if the cervical seal is tight, and cervical adaptors are thus helpful. If the tubes seem blocked, the more experienced hysteroscopist can attempt a tubal catheterization. The golden rule in hysteroscopy is patience and gentleness.

REFERENCES

1. Englund F, Ingelman-Sundberg B, Westin B: Hysteroscopy in diagnosis and treatment of uterine bleeding. Gynaecologia 143:217, 1957
2. Levine RU, Neuwirth RS: Simultaneous laparoscopy and hysteroscopy for intrauterine adhesions. Obstet Gynecol 42:441, 1973
3. Lindemann HJ: Pneumometra für die Hysteroskopie. Geburtshilfe Frauenheilkd 33:18, 1973
4. Lindemann HJ, Gallinat A: Physikalische und physiologische Grundlagen der CO_2-Hysteroskopie. Geburtshilfe Frauenheilkd 36:729, 1976
5. Lindemann HJ: Atlas der Hysteroskopie. Stuttgart, Gustav Fischer Verlag, 1980
6. Lindemann HJ, Mohr J, Gallinat A, et al: Der Einfluss von CO_2-Gas während der Hysteroskopie. Geburtshilfe Frauenheilkd 36:153, 1976
7. March CM, Israel R: Intrauterine adhesions secondary to elective abortion: Hysteroscopic diagnosis and management. Obstet Gynecol 48:422, 1976
8. Mettler L, Semm K, Rimkus V: Conclusions d'une experimentation sur la sterilisation thermique transuterine. Gynaecologia 27:383, 1976
9. van der Pas H, van Herendael BJ: Atlas on Hysteroscopy. (in press)

Hysteroscopy for Diagnosis and Therapy ■ 63

Marc Gamerre
Roberto Porto
Henri Serment

Hysteroscopy provides the physician with a direct view of the uterine cavity. Its goals are to confirm or to exclude a diagnosis, to evolve a therapy, and to verify the results of treatment. The physician can search for a suspected intrauterine lesion because of signs and symptoms or evaluate suggestive shadows seen on hysterography. In addition, the topography and extent of gross intrauterine lesions can be ascertained and directed biopsies are possible. By examining the uterine cavity endoscopically, the physician can check the results of surgical correction of selected uterine malformations and monitor synechiae. After curettage for abnormal uterine bleeding, symptoms may either persist or recur. Using a hysteroscope, the surgeon can look for a persistent intrauterine tumor missed with the curet or a new lesion.

MATERIALS AND METHODS

At the Clinique Obstétricale et Gynécologique at the Hôpital de la Conception, Marseille, France, at least two hysteroscopic examinations are performed each week. The technique includes the use of a cervical cap, hysteroscopes of different diameters, and a variety of operating instruments. Once the cannula is centered on the cervix, it is fixed in place with

suction. The hysteroscope is inserted into the cannula until it reaches the endocervical canal. The cavity is distended with carbon dioxide with a maximal flow rate of 30 ml/min. The intrauterine pressure usually remains under 150 mm Hg. As the cervical canal opens because of the flow of gas, uterine exploration begins. The isthmic canal is seen, and the endometrial cavity slowly comes into view. When the endoscope is turned slowly and gently with the fingers, the lateral horns and tubal ostia slowly come into view. Sometimes they appear to open and close, and their patency is suggested by the passage of carbon dioxide. At the uterotubal junction, a mucosal fold sometimes is observed. It has been described as the *pretubal sphincter* that Siegler finds in nearly 60% of hysterograms.[1]

The normal endometrium has a smooth, orange, velvety surface that is thin in the proliferative phase and undulating and thicker in the secretory phase. In menopausal women the endometrium appears atrophic because the mucosa appears flat, thin, and fragile, often conforming to the relief of the underlying myometrium. The tubal ostia are prominent, resembling the configuration seen after curettage; occasionally endometrial atrophy can be the cause of bleeding in postmenopausal women.

Hysteroscopy can be safely performed even in the presence of some uterine bleeding, provided that the insufflation proceeds slowly, the physician is patient, and the end of the hysteroscope is kept clean by gently touching its tip on the endometrium.

INTRAUTERINE ABNORMALITIES

Although uterine malformations can be detected by hysteroscopy and hysterography, laparoscopy is absolutely necessary for their precise evaluation. Hysteroscopy cannot distinguish a bicornuate from a septate uterus, since the thickness of the septum is not diagnostic of either condition. Therefore, hysterography, hysteroscopy, laparoscopy (Figs. 63-1 to 63-4), and even sonography are all indicated in the evaluation of fundal malformation.

Postraumatic intrauterine adhesions are seen clearly during a hysteroscopic examination, and the physician can ascertain their direction, origin, and insertion (Figs. 63-5 to 63-7). Some of them are removable during hysteroscopy, but the lateral, fibromuscular adhesions require excision by the Musset technique. Synechiae caused by tuberculous endometritis produce a narrow, tubular cavity that corresponds to the classic hysterogram showing a "nightcap" or "fingerlike" configuration. Pseudosynechiae are thin, white, "veillike" structures easily disrupted on contact with the end of the hysteroscope. They are very common and do not have any clinical significance (Fig. 63-8).

Endometrial hyperplasia causes the endometrium to appear scalloped, thickened, congested, and sometimes polypoid. It may be diffused or localized, and confirmation with histologic examination is always required (Fig. 63-9). Adenomyosis produces small openings in the endometrium caused by projections of the mucosa into the myometrium. They are discernible on hysteroscopy and correspond to the diverticuli seen on hysterography (Fig. 63-10).

Polyps appear as small, oval, soft, pedunculated growths with smooth surfaces. Pseudopolyps (mucous polyps) have a similar configuration but are easily disrupted by contact with the endoscope. Submucous myomas are sessile or pedunculated, firm, whitish, generally smooth, and larger than polyps (Figs. 63-11 to 63-13). Malignant lesions appear as craggy, irregular growths, often with hemorrhagic, necrotic surfaces. Localized or diffused, they can involve the entire cavity, and although their appearance is quite typical, tissue study is mandatory for confirmation (Figs. 63-14 and 63-15). Endocervical extension can be delineated.

Hysterography, hysteroscopy, and tissue biopsy or curettage enable a physician to arrive more adequately at a proper diagnosis, thereby resulting in the most appropriate therapy. Hysterography remains the basic nonoperative procedure for exploring the uterine cavity.

REFERENCES

1. Siegler AM: Hysterosalpingography, 2d ed, p 125. New York, Medcom Press, 1974

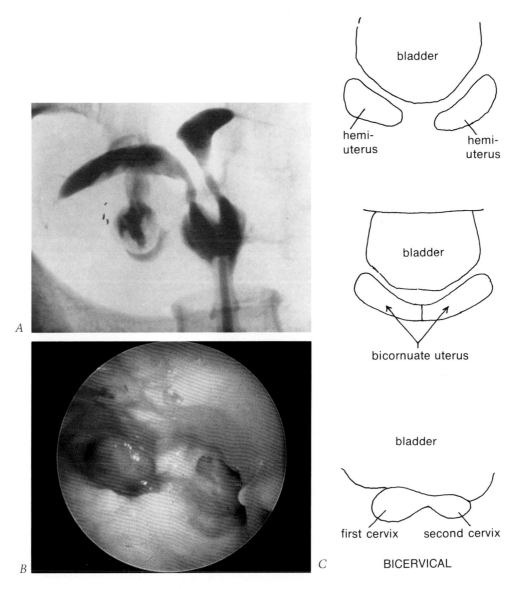

FIG. 63-1. (A) Congenital uterine malformation is revealed on hysterography as a possible septate uterus with two horns and one cervix. Note cervical suction cup surrounding the single cervix. (B) This radiologic finding was confirmed at hysteroscopy. (C) Sonograms at different levels show the configuration of a bicornuate uterus.

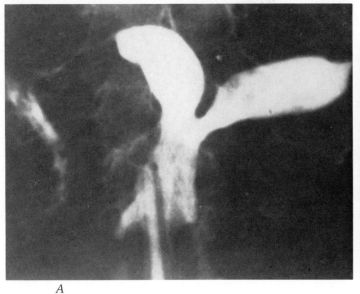

A

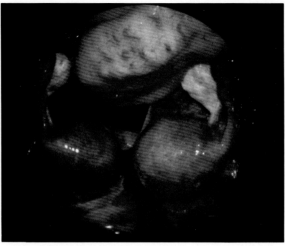

B

FIG. 63-2. (A) This hysterogram shows a single cervix and two fairly equal-sized horns with rounded inner borders suggesting a bicornuate uterus. (B) At laparoscopy the diagnosis was confirmed.

FIG. 63-3. (A) Hysterogram reveals a unicornuate uterus. An intravenous pyelogram (IVP) is essential to search for the contralateral kidney. (B) Hysteroscopy proved that only one horn was present and no other abnormality caused the failure of the contralateral horn to opacify.

A B

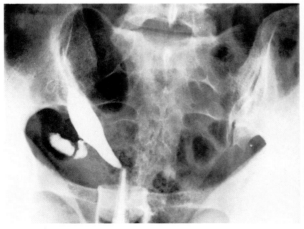

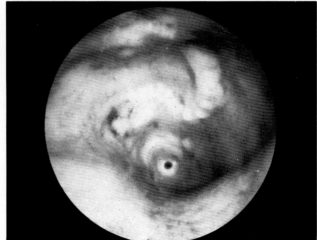

A B

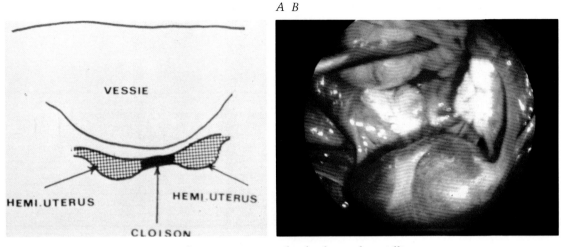

FIG. 63-4. (*A*) Sonogram of a septate uterus clearly shows the midline septum separating the two horns. (*B*) At laparoscopy the external serosal surface shows the characteristic small midline indentation.

A B

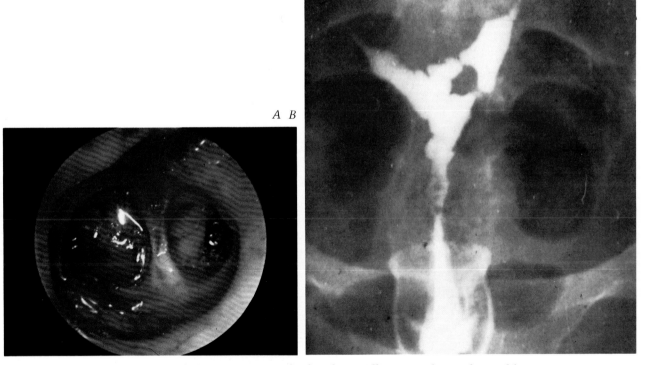

FIG. 63-5. (*A*) Hysteroscopy disclosed a midline synechiae, almost like a septate uterus. (*B*) The hysterogram revealed multiple, central, and peripheral irregularities, suggesting severe adhesions.

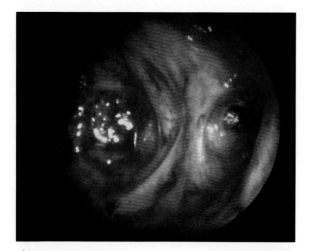

A

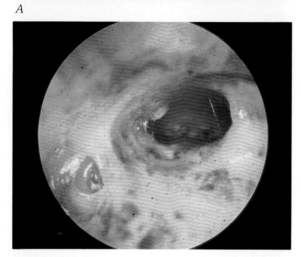

B

FIG. 63-6. Other hysteroscopic views confirm the presence of thick fibromuscular adhesions.

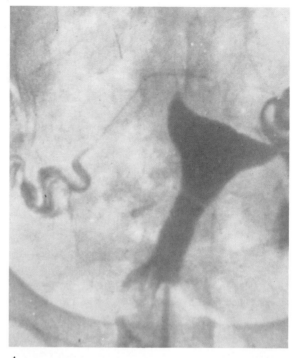

A

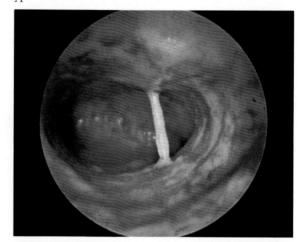

B

FIG. 63-7. (*A*) Hysterogram disclosed an apparent separation of the upper and lower parts of the uterine cervix. (*B*) This appearance was caused by a thin pseudoadhesion.

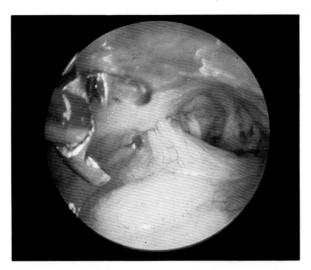

FIG. 63-8. An attempt was made to cut an intra-uterine adhesion with scissors introduced through an accessory channel of the hysteroscope.

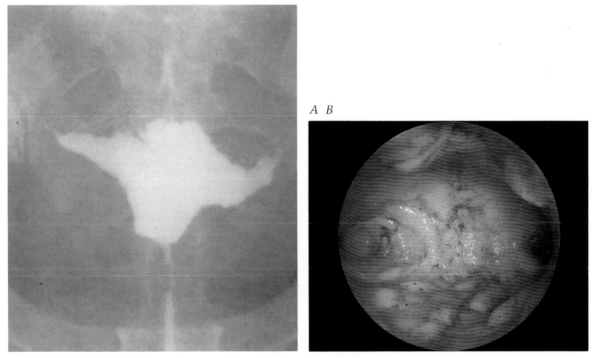

A B

FIG. 63-9. (*A*) Hysterogram shows a uterine fundus with a very irregular sawtoothed border. (*B*) At hysteroscopy the endometrial surface was corrugated; a biopsy specimen showed endometrial hyperplasia.

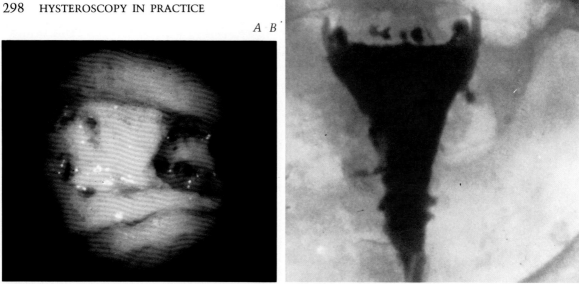

FIG. 63-10. (*A*) Glandular openings are seen in the myometrium. (*B*) Hysterography reveals intravasation of contrast material into the myometrium, caused by adenomyosis.

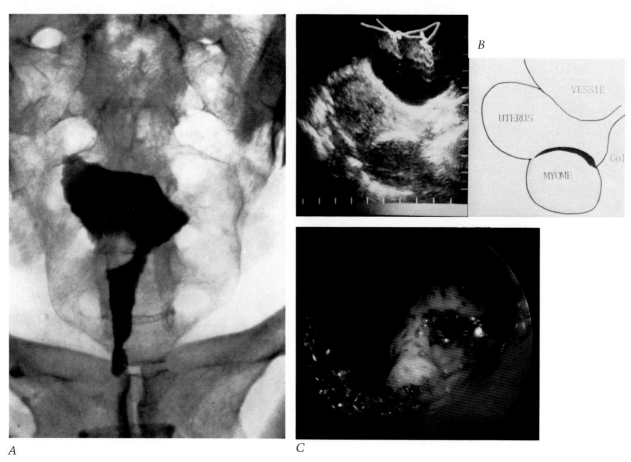

A   *C*

FIG. 63-11. (*A*) Hysterogram reveals an oval filling defect in the lower uterine segment extending from the uterine wall to beyond the center of the cavity. (*B*) Sonogram discloses a solid mass in the lower segment. (*C*) Hysteroscopy confirms the presence of a large myoma.

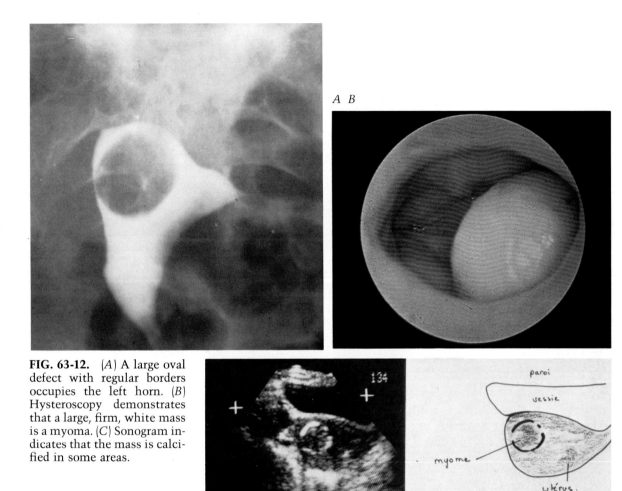

FIG. 63-12. (*A*) A large oval defect with regular borders occupies the left horn. (*B*) Hysteroscopy demonstrates that a large, firm, white mass is a myoma. (*C*) Sonogram indicates that the mass is calcified in some areas.

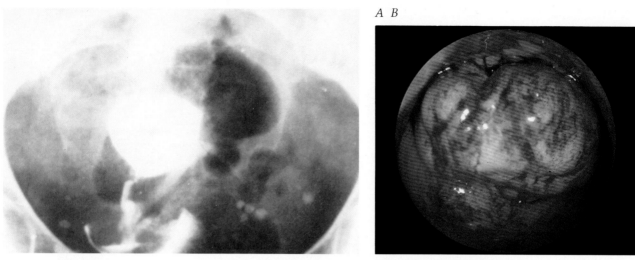

FIG. 63-13. (*A*) Hysterogram shows a regular uterine outline on the follow-up film, but a lacuna is seen. (*B*) Subsequent hysteroscopy shows a large submucous myoma.

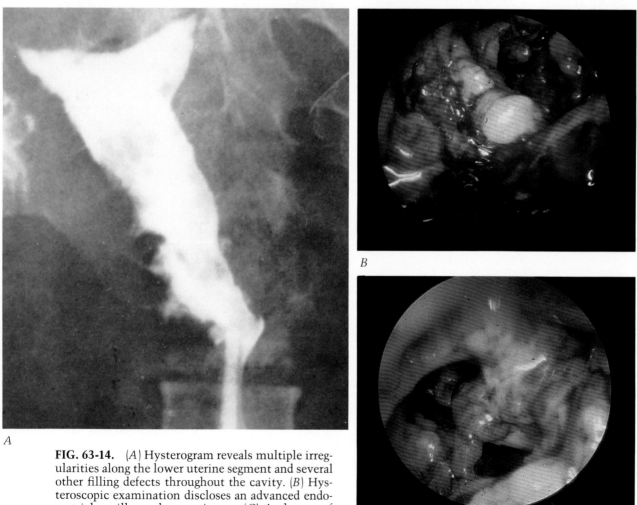

FIG. 63-14. (*A*) Hysterogram reveals multiple irregularities along the lower uterine segment and several other filling defects throughout the cavity. (*B*) Hysteroscopic examination discloses an advanced endometrial papillary adenocarcinoma. (*C*) A closeup of the same lesion.

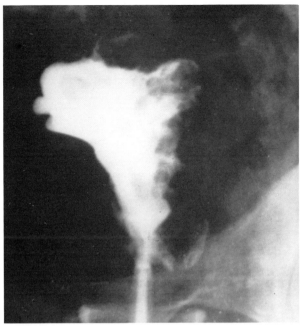

A

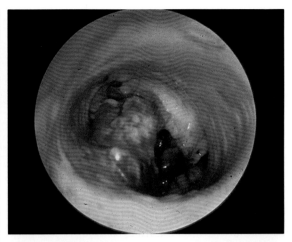

B

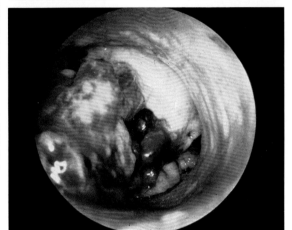

C

FIG. 63-15. (A) Another hysterogram shows a characteristic, motheaten appearance. This proved to be caused by a nodular, endometrial adenocarcinoma. (B) The lower segment and the endocervical canal are free of carcinoma. (C) A closeup. (D) In the extirpated specimen, exact tumor location is demonstrable.

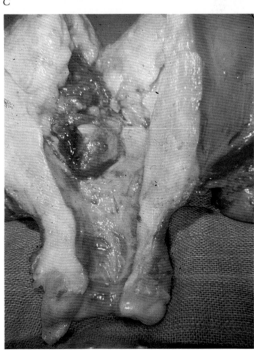

D

Importance of Hysteroscopy as a Clinical Method for Examination ■

64

Friedhelm Lübke

Lindemann published his first report on carbon dioxide hysteroscopy in 1971, describing an endoscopic examination of the uterine cavity and the endocervical canal.[2] Previously von Mikulicz-Radecki and Freund had made several pioneering experiments in this field, but technical difficulties prevented adequate examination.[6] Hysteroscopy has not yet succeeded as a clinical method because its value is only achieved with a good deal of experience, and histologic confirmation of the observations made endoscopically are often lacking.[1,4,5]

MATERIALS AND METHODS

Since 1972, I have performed 2660 hysteroscopic examinations in combination with curettage. Patients' ages ranged from 17 to 84 yr. In each examination special attention was given to the uterine cavity, the tubal ostia, the endometrial surfaces, the internal os, and the endocervical canal. The indications for the most recent hysteroscopic operations were as follows:

Abnormal uterine bleeding (dysfunctional, climacteric, or postmenopausal), 424 patients (36%)
Sterilization, 237 patients (20.2%) (Sterilization by hysteroscopy no longer performed because of a failure rate of 7%)
Investigation of infertility, 213 patients (18.2%)
Suspicious smear or cervical polyp, 168 patients (14.3%)
Other indications, unspecified, 62 patients (5.2%)
Removal of intrauterine devices (IUDs), 18 patients (1.5%)
Indications not documented, 53 patients (4.1%)

The observations were classified as follows by gross appearance:

Normal. No pathologic changes were seen in the uterine cavity, the endometrium, the tubal orifice, or the cervix.
Adhesions. Adhesions or sails of synechiae were noted between the anterior and posterior sidewall or uterine fundus.
Polypoid. Thick-walled, irregular, or protruding alterations of the endometrium were found.
Polyp. Pedunculated tumors of endometrial origin were noted.
Submucous myoma. White, prominent, bulgings of the myometrium were seen under the endometrium.
Endometrial adenocarcinoma. Irregular, partly polypoid, prominent, sometimes ulcerated tissue was detected.

Sometimes it is difficult to classify the endoscopic result under the aforementioned categories. Proliferative and secretory endometria, endometritis, and endometrial atrophy cannot be detected on hysteroscopy. An endoscopic

302

diagnosis of a submucous myoma is not easily confirmed by the specimen produced from a curettage. A tissue diagnosis must ultimately confirm endometrial polyps or adenocarinoma.

RESULTS

Hysteroscopic diagnoses were compared with histologic findings in tissues obtained by curettage in 478 patients (Table 64-1). Among the 142 patients with normal hysteroscopic appearances, 28 were found to have endometrial atrophy, 3 had endometritis, 3 had polyps, and 1 had endometrial adenocarcinoma *in situ*. Polypoid changes were diagnosed by hysteroscopy in 212 patients; histologically, 35 had glandular cystic hyperplasia, 14 had polyps, 10 had endometrial atrophy, and 2 had endometrial adenocarcinomas. Adhesions were seen by hysteroscopy in 15 instances but were not confirmed in the histologic examinations, 4 had glandular cystic hyperplasia, and 2 had endometrial polyps. The hysteroscopic diagnosis of endometrial polyps was confirmed histologically in 10 of 33 patients; 4 had glandular cystic hyperplasia, 1 had endometrial atrophy, and 1 had an endometrial adenocarcinoma. The hysteroscopic diagnosis of submucous my-

omas was confirmed histologically in only 5 of 28 instances; 4 patients had polyps and 2 had adenocarcinomas. Thus, six endometrial adenocarcinomas were missed by hysteroscopy, one being *in situ* and not seen macroscopically. Hysteroscopic appearances suggested adenocarcinoma in nine instances, and all were confirmed histologically; all but one was missed in the curettage but found in the extirpated uterus. Hysteroscopy was unsuccessful in 39 instances because of technical difficulties; two of the women had adenocarcinomas. The curettages were done blindly, and presumably some of the failures of histologic confirmation occurred because curettage missed the affected foci.

Some significant misinterpretations of the hysteroscopic appearances occurred in the subgroup of 106 women with postmenopausal bleeding. Of 13 endometrial adenocarcinomas, 6 were not detected, 2 because of technical difficulties, and 4 were seen but not recognized (Table 64-2).

DISCUSSION

Histologic diagnosis cannot be replaced by hysteroscopy. Nevertheless, diagnostic hyster-

Table 64-1

HYSTEROSCOPIC AND HISTOLOGIC FINDINGS COMPARED IN 478 PATIENTS

HYSTEROSCOPY \ HISTOLOGY	PROLIFERATIVE PHASE	SECRETORY PHASE	ATROPHY	ENDOMETRITIS	GLANDULAR CYSTIC HYPERPLASIA	ENDOMETRIAL ADENOCARCINOMA	POLYP	SUBMUCOUS MYOMA	WITHOUT HISTOLOGIC FINDING	TOTAL
Normal	62	12	28	3	10	1†	3	1	22	142
Polypoid endometrium	121	23	10		35	2	14	3	4	212
Adhesions	5	1	1		4		2	1	1	15
Polyps	11	6	1		4	1	10			33
Submucous myoma	6	1	5	1	1	2	4	5	3	28
Carcinoma suspected			1*			8				9
Technical difficulties	13	2	8		2	2	4	1	7	39
Total	218	45	54	4	56	16	37	11	37	478

* Histologic verification by operation.
† Carcinoma *in situ*.

Table 64-2

HYSTEROSCOPIC AND HISTOLOGIC FINDINGS IN 106 PATIENTS WITH POSTMENOPAUSAL BLEEDING

HYSTEROSCOPY \ HISTOLOGY	PROLIFERATIVE PHASE	SECRETORY PHASE	ATROPHY	SUBMUCOUS MYOMA	POLYP	GLANDULAR CYSTIC HYPERPLASIA	ENDOMETRIAL ADENOCARCINOMA	ENDOMETRITIS	WITHOUT HISTOLOGIC FINDING	TOTAL
Cavity										
Normal	7		17		2	5			2	33
Submucous myoma			4			1	1			6
Adhesion			1	1	2	1				5
Endometrium										
Polypoid changes on the surface, isolated or diffuse	5		4		4	14	2			29
Polyps	1				5	3	1			10
Carcinoma suspected			1				7			8
Technical difficulties			4		1					5
Failures	2		3		2		2		1	10
Total	15		34	1	16	24	13		3	106

oscopy has its value in selected instances. In the patient with hypermenorrhea, a submucous myoma can be recognized and secure the indication for a hysterectomy or myomectomy. In instances of dysfunctional or postmenopausal bleeding, the hysteroscopic finding of a normal cavity supports the diagnosis of a negative tissue diagnosis. The location and extension of endometrial carcinoma can be ascertained by the endoscopic observation and the appropriate type of therapy given. If the tumor has invaded the cervix, radical vaginal or abdominal hysterectomy is indicated. If the malignancy is confined to the corpus, a total hysterectomy is sufficient. In women with unexplained uterine bleeding, polyps missed on curettage can be precisely located on hysteroscopy and directed biopsy or removal performed. The search and removal of "misplaced" IUDs is easily done through hysteroscopy. Hysteroscopy is used to evaluate the endocervical canal before a hysterectomy for recurrent bleeding resistant to therapy to exclude or recognize an endocervical carcinoma. In infertile patients, the cavity can be searched for anomalies and synechiae.

There are few risks in hysteroscopy. The uterus can be perforated; 12 perforations occurred in my series. Ascending infections are possible, although none was found among my patients. When a pressure-controlled Hysteroflator is used, carbon dioxide insufflation presents no risks.[3] Higher gas pressure or flow to insufflate the cavity should never be used.

REFERENCES

1. Hindenburg HJ: Die Hysteroskopie als klinische Routinemethode. III. Presented at the Europäischer Kongress of Endoskopie (EECO), Berlin, June 14–17, 1981
2. Lindemann HJ: Eine neue Untersuchungsmethode für die Hysteroskopie. Endoscopy 4:194, 1971
3. Lindemann HJ: Komplikationen bei der CO_2-Hysteroskopie. Arch Gynaekol 219:257, 1975
4. Lübke F: Erste Erfahrungen mit der Hysteroskopie. Geburtshilfe Frauenheilkd 34:387, 1974
5. Lübke F: Kritische Bemerkungen zur Hysteroskopie. II. Presented at the Europäischer Kongress of Endoskopie (EECO), Konstanz, April 16–19, 1975
6. Mikulicz-Radecki F von, Freund A: Ein neues Hysteroskop und seine praktische Anwendung in der Gynäkologie. Geburtshilfe Gynaekol 92:13, 1927

The Value of Hysteroscopy and Its Limitations ■

65

Maxwell Roland

Attempts to look into the endometrial cavity date back about a century. In 1950, Norment introduced a hysteroscope similar to that used in cystoscopy and used water as the distending medium. The disadvantage was the high pressure required to distend the endometrial cavity, and, during prolonged procedures, patent tubes permitted too much water to enter the pelvis. The presence of blood in the endometrial cavity caused the water to become cloudy and made observation difficult.

MATERIAL AND METHODS

Fifty-six women underwent hysteroscopic examination because of a preoperative diagnosis of endometrial polyps in 22, Asherman's syndrome in 9, and submucous myoma in 7 and to assess proximal tubal obstruction in 16. In two instances the uterus was examined for possible endometrial carcinoma. The technique used for these examinations was either the contact or the panoramic hysteroscope. Local anesthesia was used in some procedures, but hysteroscopic examination combined with laparoscopy was performed under general anesthesia.

COMMENT

I prefer general anesthesia for patients who undergo combined laparoscopy and hysteroscopy.

Local anesthesia may be employed for women who require only hysteroscopy. My current indications for hysteroscopy are to search for causes of abnormal uterine bleeding, to evaluate the findings of an abnormal hysterosalpingogram or curettage, to localize endometrial polyps or submucous myomas, to study the involvement of the endometrial cavity with synechiae, and to identify more precisely the spread and extent of endometrial carcinoma. Its therapeutic potential includes the possibility of polypectomy, targeted biopsy, lysis of intrauterine adhesions, dilatation of tubal ostia, and possibly a method for tubal sterilization. Thus far, poor success rates, delayed effectiveness, and complications preclude its general acceptance as a method of tubal sterilization. Combined with laparoscopy, it provides additional information so that the most efficacious management of pelvic abnormalities can be developed.

Hysteroscopy should not be done in the presence of acute or chronic salpingitis, endometritis, pregnancy, or more than minimal uterine bleeding. A history of recent uterine perforation is another contraindication. Physicians should be aware of the possible complications from hysteroscopy so that they can select patients carefully. Attention to details is important. One serious complication will discourage the use of a potentially valuable procedure.

Hysteroscopy in a Suburban Community Hospital ■ 66

H. Ascher Sellner

This chapter reports on 51 patients who had hysteroscopy and curettage under general anesthesia in a suburban community hospital. A hysteroscope (21 Fr) with an operating channel was used with 30 ml to 50 ml of dextran 70 to distend the cavity. Whenever possible, the opertion was done during the proliferative phase. Hysteroscopy was occasionally repeated to verify the removal of polyps and submucous fibroids. The main indications for hysteroscopy were premenopausal abnormal uterine bleeding in 41 patients, postmenopausal bleeding in 7, and infertility in 3 others. No intraoperative or postoperative complications occurred. Definite lesions were seen at hysteroscopy in 20 (39%) of 51 patients, and these were confirmed at pathologic examination in 11 (55%). Although nine women had definite submucous myomas, sufficient tissue was obtained to verify the diagnosis in only two patients.

TECHNIQUE

Hysteroscopy should be a relatively easy operation to add to the repertoire of the gynecologist. Postgraduate courses are available for educating the physician, and the instruments required, other than the hysteroscope, are min-

imal. Each patient receives a description of the operation, and none of the 51 patients expressed any hesitancy regarding the operation. After a course in hysteroscopy and extensive reading of texts and atlases, even the beginner will find that lesions that might otherwise have been missed can be identified. Endometrial polyps and submucous fibroids not detected by hysterosalpingogram or curettage are sometimes located by hysteroscopy. As experience increases, the accuracy of hysteroscopic diagnosis will improve. The ease of application and minimal morbidity of this operation should make it routine for patients needing curettage for abnormal uterine bleeding. Patients should not have to travel to special medical centers, and there is no reason to delay its use until after the patient has had one or more curettages.

PATIENT INFORMATION ON HYSTEROSCOPY

Hysteroscopy employs a long narrow tube about ¼" in diameter to look inside of the uterus. It is generally performed along with dilatation and curettage. A dilatation and curettage scrapes out the uterine cavity to find whether polyps or other growths are present. When hysteroscopy is done with dilatation and curettage, the physician has a better chance to find abnormalities and to correct them.

Reasons to do hysteroscopy include abnormal uterine bleeding, previous uterine surgery, a "lost" intrauterine device (IUD), abnormal hysterosalpingogram (x-ray film of the uterine cavity), infertility, and tubal sterilization. The hysteroscope is used to find cervical or uterine polyps, fibroids, "lost" IUDs, retained placental tissue, cancer of the cervix and uterus, and uterine adhesions. Hysteroscopy can prevent unnecessary surgery such as hysterectomy by finding abnormalities missed by a dilatation and curettage. It can also find correctable causes of infertility such as uterine adhesions and septae.

Hysteroscopy is not a painful procedure. It can be done in the office, sometimes with local anesthesia. The hysteroscope is inserted, and a thick sugar solution (dextran) is put into the uterus to spread the uterine walls apart so that they may be seen. The procedure resembles the cystoscopic examination for the urinary bladder.

Hysteroscopy for Diagnosis and Therapy in Gynecology ■

Asghar Afsari

Hysteroscopy is an adjunct to diagnostic dilatation and curettage, enabling observation of the uterine cavity and directed endometrial biopsy. Technical instrumental developments have followed other endoscopic procedures. Modern hysteroscopic technique and its revival of interest is due to the effort and work of investigators such as Edström and Fernström, Rubin, Lindemann, and Quiñones.

My technique for hysteroscopy includes a hysteroscope whose outer diameter is 5 mm and a sheath with three channels. The inflow and outflow channels are for flushing the uterine cavity; one operative channel is for introducing ancillary operative instruments such as probes, coagulators, scissors, biopsy forceps, and hooks. A fiber light-transmitting cable connects the hysteroscope to the light source. A weighted speculum, cervical tenaculum, uterine sound, and graduated dilators are also needed (Fig. 67-1). Dextran 70 (Hyskon), a 32% dextran solution with a 70,000 molecular weight in 10% dextrose, is used to distend the cavity. A clear, plastic syringe is needed, to which is attached clear, intravenous tubing.

The uterine cavity is surrounded by a thick myometrium, and in the nonpregnant woman the normal cavity can hold 4 ml to 6 ml of fluid. For thorough observation, the cavity should be adequately distended. The endometrium bleeds easily from slight trauma, but constant pressure created by the distending medium creates a hemostatic mechanism, facilitating a clear operative field. The media used for hysteroscopy, their advantages, disadvantages, and many of their particular characteristics have been described elsewhere in this book. The endocervical canal, internal os, uterine cavity, fundus, and tubal ostia are systematically examined. Polyps, submucous myomas, uterine septa, and missing IUDs can be located. Endometrial carcinoma appears as a vegetative, cauliflower growth, and involvement of the endocervix can be identified. A histologic diagnosis is always needed for confirmation.

Documentation of the findings can be accomplished through the use of a schematic drawing or, perhaps, intraoperative photography. The complications and contraindications from hysteroscopy are described elsewhere in this book.

In the future, hysteroscopy may enable improvement in the management of infertility and in the diagnosis and treatment of intrauterine abnormalities, including the staging of endometrial carcinoma before therapy. It is already a useful adjunct to hysterography, curettage, and endometrial biopsy. Ambulatory sterilization by a hysteroscopic method is a distinct possibility. Direct observation of the uterine cavity by hysteroscopy and directed biopsy is superior to a diagnostic curettage.

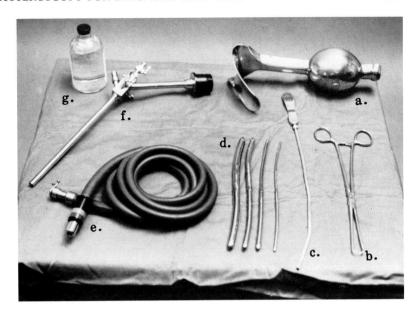

FIG. 67-1. Instruments used for hysteroscopic examinations include a = weighted speculum, b = tenaculum, c = sound, d = dilators, e = fiberoptic cord, f = operating hysteroscope, g = dextran 70 (Hyskon).

Kurt Semm
Hans-Harald Riedel

At the University of Kiel, hysteroscopy is performed primarily with the patient under general anesthesia. Hysteroscopy requires an aseptic technique, and we advise control of vaginal flora with appropriate local antibiotics. Urinalysis and sedimentation rates are done uniformly.

Concern for uterine perforation should make the surgeon proceed with care during cervical dilatation. To proceed, sound the uterus before hysteroscopic manipulation. Before performing hysteroscopy, thoroughly disinfect the vulva, vagina, and cervix, followed by gentle cervical dilatation to Hegar 8; insufflate carbon dioxide at 100 ml/min. The total amount of carbon dioxide should never exceed 1000 ml because shoulder pain can occur postoperatively for several days.[4]

As the carbon dioxide is insufflated, insert the hysteroscope into the external os; the cervical canal will begin to open (Fig. 68-1). Under visual control advance the instrument into the uterine cavity, and the tubal ostia will come into view (Fig. 68-2). The hysteroscope is specially designed with a self-cleaning device in front of the lens to provide for a windshield-wiper effect (Fig. 68-3).

Carbon dioxide is insufflated by maintaining a constant volume using variable pressure or a preselected pressure at approximately 50 mm Hg at a maximal carbon dioxide gas volume of 100 ml/min (Fig. 68-4).[2,8,9] The flow of gas automatically stops when the preselected pressure is reached. Since the minimal required pressure for opening the uterine cavity is lower than for tubal opening, any flow of carbon dioxide into the abdomen is prevented, even in a patient with patent tubes. For tubal distention a minimal pressure of 70 mm Hg is necessary. To prevent carbon dioxide flow into the fallopian tubes, the gas pressure is limited to 100 mm Hg. Even if the entire gas volume entered the bloodstream, it would not constitute any danger for the patient. The human body tolerates 200 ml carbon dioxide gas/min by insufflation with intravascular resorption.[2]

During tubal insufflation for diagnostic purposes using the Universal Insufflator according to Fikentscher and Semm and the atraumatic flexible cervical adaptor, vascular injury is uncommon.[1] Trauma by dilatation of the cervical canal can occur, and opened blood vessels are especially prone to assimilate gas being insufflated into the cavity. Hysteroscopy with carbon dioxide insufflation in uncontrolled amounts and pressures would be dangerous for the patient.

Hysteroscopy can be used to remove tubal polyps before performing microsurgical tubal operations in cases of sterility and tubal occlu-

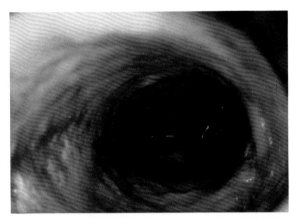

FIG. 68-1. The endocervical canal is seen as carbon dioxide is insufflated.

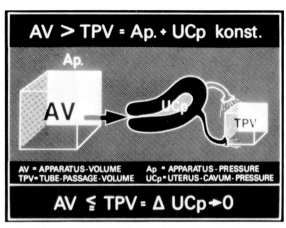

FIG. 68-4. Formula for carbon dioxide hysteroscopy.

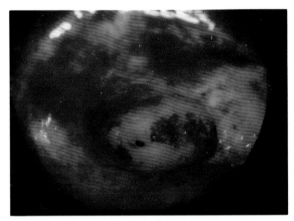

FIG. 68-2. The right tubal ostium is visible.

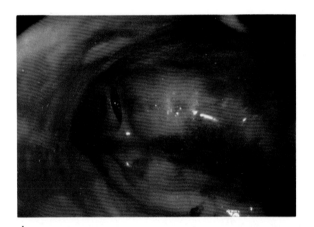

A

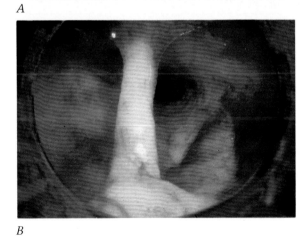

B

FIG. 68-5. Intrauterine synechiae (*A, B*).

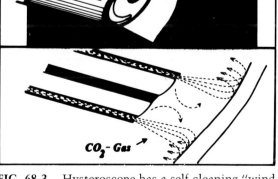

FIG. 68-3. Hysteroscope has a self-cleaning "windshield-wiper" effect.

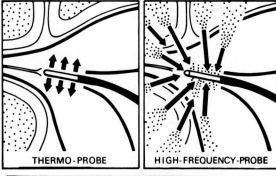

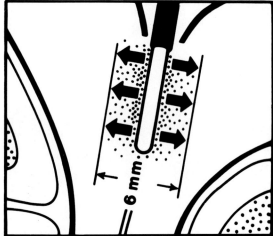

FIG. 68-6. (*A*) Comparison of electrosurgical techniques for hysteroscopic sterilization. (*B*) Special thermoprobe is inserted into the ostium.

Table 68-1
EVALUATION OF 50 PATIENTS STERILIZED USING ENDOCOAGULATION FOR HYSTEROSCOPIC STERILIZATION*

No success; bilateral patency: 19 (38%)

Partial success, unilateral occlusion: 11 (22%)

Success, bilateral occlusion: 20 (40%)

* Complications: two perforations with thermosound (clinically silent), and nine undesired pregnancies.

sion and to diagnose intrauterine adhesions (Fig. 68-5) and uterine malformations. In 1980, 147 patients were examined for abnormal uterine bleeding, and 6.1% showed malignant tumors that were confirmed histologically.[6] At × 8 magnification the course of small blood vessels could be traced. The following factors sion should be evaluated in the study of intrauterine tumors: atypical vascular patterns, surface changes, zone between normal and abnormal areas, degree of necrosis, changes in color, and consistency.

In 1974 Rimkus and Semm used the endocoagulation technique to sterilize 50 patients hysteroscopically.[3,7,8] The Thermo-Probe (Wisap) has a diameter of 1.5 mm. It was inserted 10 mm into the intramural segment with a coagulation temperature between 140 C and 160 C. The low current is produced by the coagulation unit. Temperature and period of heating and the cooling period or a technical fault is indicated by a special sound from the coagulation unit (Fig. 68-6). After a coagulation period of 30 sec, a lack of activity of the tissue enzymes in a cylinder 10 mm long with a diameter of 10 mm was found. All sterilizations were thus performed under constant conditions.

When the patency of the tubes was examined by hysterosalpingography 3 mo later, both tubes were open in 38% of patients, 22% had unilateral occlusion, and 40% were closed bilaterally. Nine patients became pregnant postoperatively. Since the results were in agreement with the pregnancy rate of nearly 20% cited in the world literature, it was decided not to apply this type of sterilization technique (Table 68-1).[5] In addition, thermointestinal injuries can occur if the tubal probe inadvertently perforates the intramural segment and juxtaposed intestine become coagulated (Fig. 68-7).

Contact hysteroscopy has been used for research to observe the fetus during the first trimester in selected instances (Fig. 68-8).[10]

There are relatively few indications for which carbon dioxide hysteroscopy is used in gynecology at the University of Kiel except for basic research in embryoscopy. Abnormal uterine bleeding is evaluated by endocrinologic assay and uterine curettage, since hysteroscopy alone rarely discovers the cause. The detection of occult intrauterine devices (IUDs) by ultrasonic localization and their subsequent recovery is easy, but hysteroscopy is sometimes a necessary operation (Fig. 68-9). For sterility,

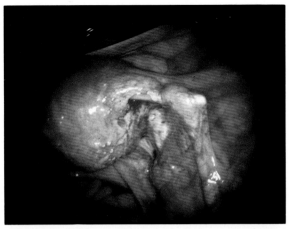

FIG. 68-7.   The uterotubal junction was perforated during laparoscopy.

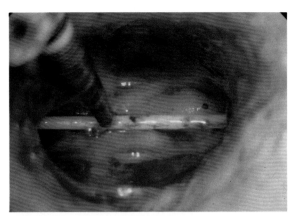

FIG. 68-9.   Copper-T is intrauterine and can be removed under hysteroscopic control.

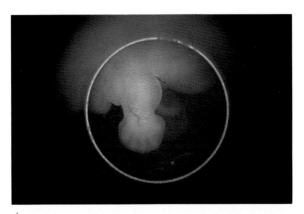

A

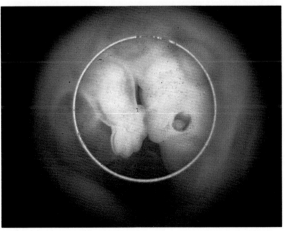

B

FIG. 68-8.   Contact hysteroscopy. (*A*) Fetal hand. (*B*) Fetus.

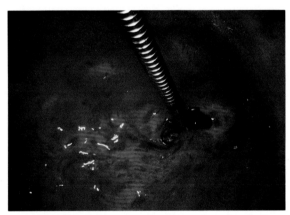

FIG. 68-10.   Endometrial biopsy is done under hysteroscopic control.

the procedure is done in conjunction with pelviscopy. Only in patients with secondary sterility and repeated abortions does hysteroscopy have a potential value in the search for intrauterine adhesions and congenital uterine malformations. For performing tubal sterilizations, hysteroscopy is particularly inadequate. Endometrial biopsy is feasible under hysteroscopic control (Fig. 68-10).

REFERENCES

1. Fikentscher R, Semm K: Physikalische Grundlagen zur utero-tubaren Persufflation. Arch Gynaekol 188:184, 1956

2. Lindemann HJ: Eine neue Untersuchungsmethode für die Hysteroskopie. Endoscopy 4:194, 1971

3. Rimkus V, Semm K: Hysteroscopic sterilization using carbon dioxide. In Sciarra JJ, Butler JC, Speidel JJ (eds): Hysteroscopic Sterilization, p 75. New York, Intercontinental Medical Book Corporation, 1974

4. Riedel HH, Semm K: Das postpelviskopische (laparoskopische) subphrenische Schmerzsyndrom. Arch Gynaekol 20:228, 1979

5. Rimkus V, Semm K: Hysteroscopic sterilization, a routine method? Int J Fertil 22:121, 1977

6. Seki M, Riedel H, Viehweg J et al: Ein Vergleich der Flüssigkeits- und CO_2-Hysteroskopie bei Blutungsanomalien im reproduktiven Alter. Arch Gynaekol 232:741, 1981

7. Semm K: Sterilisierung durch Tubenkoagulation der pars intramuralis tubae per Hysteroskopiam. Endoscopy 5:218, 1973

8. Semm K, Rimkus V: Technische Bemerkungen zur CO_2 Hysteroskopie. Geburtshilfe Frauenheilkd 34:392, 1974

9. Semm K: Pelviskopie und Hysteroskopie Farbatlas und Lehrbuch. Stuttgart, Schattauer, 1976.

10. Semm K: Kontakt-hysteroskopische Fetoskopie. Gynaekol Prax 2:369, 1978

Bibliography ■

Adstran K, Femtral I: The diagnostic possibilities of a modified hysteroscopic technique. Acta Obstet Gynecol Scand 49:327, 1970

Agüero O, Aure M, López R: Hysteroscopy in pregnant patients; a new diagnostic tool. Am J Obstet Gynecol 94:925, 1966

Agüero O, Aure M, López R: Histeroscopia en embarazadas. Rev Obstet Ginecol Venez 27:111, 1967

Agüero O, Aure M: La histeroscopía en el diagnóstico de rotura prematura de los membranos. Rev Obstet Ginecol Venez 29:471, 1969

Agüero O, Aure M: Histeroscopía en embarazadas. Ginecol Obstet Mex 27:629, 1970

Ahumada JC, Gandolfo-Herrera R: Histeroscopía. Rev Med Latino Am 21:265, 1935

Albeck V: Application of hysteroscopy and colposcopy in obstetrics. Jydsk Med Selsk Forh 73:98, 1930

American College of Obstetricians and Gynecologists: Technical Bulletin, August 1974

Andersen PK, Stokke DB, Hole P, et al: Carbon dioxide tensions in manually ventilated, prone patients. Anaesthetist 30:610, 1981

Antoine T: Der heutige Stand der Auflichtmicroskopie in der Gynaecologie. Arch Gynaekol 180:62, 1951

Antoine JM, Hamou J, Salat-Baroux J, et al: Contribution à l'étude de la microhystéroscopie. Paris, Thèse, 1980

Aribarg A: Epidural analgesia for laparoscopy. J Obstet Gynaecol Br Commonw 80:587, 1973

Asherman JG: Amenorrhoea traumatica (atretica). J Obstet Gynaecol Br Emp 55:23, 1948

Asherman JG: Traumatic intra-uterine adhesions. J Obstet Gynaecol Br Emp 57:892, 1950

Auberger HQ: Praktische Lokalanasthesie, p 116. Stuttgart, Georg Thieme Verlag, 1974

Aubinais EJ: De l'uteroscopie. J Sect Med Soc Acad Dept Loire-Infer. 39:71, 1863

Autunes CMF, Stolley PD, Rosenheim NB, et al: Endometrial cancer and estrogen use. N Engl J Med 300:9, 1979

Babson SG, Benson RC, Pernoll ML, et al: Management of High-Risk Pregnancy and Intensive Care of the Neonate. St. Louis, CV Mosby, 1975

Baggish MS: Contact hysteroscopy: A new technique to explore the uterine cavity. Obstet Gynecol 54:350, 1979

Baggish MS: Evaluation and staging of endometrial and endocervical adenocarcinoma by contact hysteroscopy. Gynecol Oncol 9:182, 1980

Baggish MS, Barbot J: Contact hysteroscopy for easier diagnosis. Contemp Obstet Gynecol 16:93, 1980

Bailey G, Strub RL, Klein RC, et al: Dextran-induced anaphylaxis. JAMA 200:889, 1967

Bank EB: Erfahrungen mit der Metroskopie. Zentralbl Gynaekol 82:866, 1960

Barbot J: L'hystéroscopie de contact. Paris, Thèse, 1975

Barbot J, Parent B, Doerler B: Hystéroscopie de contact et cancer de l'endomètre. Acta Endoscopy 8:17, 1978

Barbot J, Parent B, Dubuisson JB: Contact hysteroscopy: Another method of endoscopic examination of the uterine cavity. Am J Obstet Gynecol 136:721, 1980

Bartich EG, Dillon TF: Carbon dioxide hysteroscopy. Am J Obstet Gynecol 124:746, 1976

Behrman SJ: Historical aspects of hysteroscopy. Fertil Steril 24:243, 1973

Behrman SJ: Hysteroscopy: An overview. Clin Obstet Gynecol 19:307, 1976

Behrman SJ, Kistner RW: Progress in Fertility, 2d ed, p 91. Boston, Little, Brown & Co, 1968

Belvederi GD, Borghetti G: L'isteroscopia: Tecnica, indicazioni e limiti. Minerva Ginecol 23:770, 1971

Bennett JP, Kendle KE: The effect of Reserpine upon the rate of egg transport in the fallopian tube of the mouse. J Reprod Med 13:345, 1967

Bergquist CA, Rock JA, Jones HW: Pregnancy outcome fol-

315

lowing treatment of intrauterine adhesions. Int J Fertil 26:107, 1981

Beutler HK, Dockerty MB, Randall LM: Precancerous lesions of the endometrium. Am J Obstet Gynecol 86:433, 1963

Beuttner O: Über Hysteroskopie. Zentralbl Gynaekol 22:580, 1898

Blaustein AU: Pathology of the Female Genital Tract, New York, Springer-Verlag, 1977

Bleier W: Deutsches Patentamt, Offenlegungsschrift 2, 328, 175: Tuben-Occlusivpessar und Vorrichtung zum Setzen des Tuben-Occlusivpessars, 1973

Bodkhe RR, Harper MJ: Changes in the amount of adrenergic neurotransmitter in the genital tract of untreated rabbits, and rabbits given Reserpine or proniazid during the time of egg transport. Biol Reprod 6:288, 1972

Bodkhe RR, Harper MJK: Mechanism of egg transport: Changes in the amount of adrenergic transmitter in the genital tract of normal and hormone treated rabbits. In Segal SJ et al (eds): The Regulation of Mammalian Reproduction, p 364. Springfield, IL, Charles C Thomas, 1972

Bonica JJ: Principles and Practice of Obstetric Analgesia and Anesthesia. Philadelphia, FA Davis, 1967

Borell U, Fernström I, Ohlson L: Membrane-like structures in the uterine cavity. A hysterographic study. Acta Obstet Gynecol Scand 49:185, 1970

Bozzini P: Der Lichtleiter oder Beschreibung einer einfachen Vorrichtung und ihrer Anwendung zur Erleuchtung innerer Höhlen und Zwischenräume des lebenden animalischen Körpers. Weimar, Landes-Industrie-Comptoir, 1807

Braley SA, Helmer JD: Method for sterilization of males. United States Patent 3,422,813, Jan. 21, 1969

Brueschke EE, Wilbanks GD: A steerable fiberoptic hysteroscope. Obstet Gynecol 44:273, 1974

Brueschke EE, Archie JT, Wilbanks GD: Hysteroscopy. Am Fam Physician 15:126, 1977

Brueschke EE, Fadel JE, Mayerhofer K, et al: Transcervical tubal occlusion with a steerable hysteroscope: Implantation of devices into extirpated human uteri. Am J Obstet Gynecol 127:118, 1977

Brueschke EE, Wilbanks GD, Zaneveld LJ, et al: Development of a steerable hysteroscope: Studies in the baboon. Am J Obstet Gynecol 123:278, 1975

Brundin JO: Distribution and function of adrenergic nerves in the rabbit fallopian tube. Acta Physiol Scand 66 (Suppl 259):1, 1965

Brundin JO: Pharmacology of the oviduct. In Hafez ESE, Blandau RJ (eds): The Mammalian Oviduct, p 251, Chicago, University of Chicago Press, 1969

Brundin JO: Intra-tubal devices. Presented at the International Symposium on Medicated IUDs and Polymeric Delivery Systems, Amsterdam, 1979

Brundin JO, Borell US: The Patent Office London 1,460,-077: Contraceptive device, 1974

Brundin JO, Sandstedt B: Longterm toxicity of hydrogelic occlusive device in the human oviductal isthmus. (in press)

Buchwald W: Die Verwendung schnell resorbiesbares Gase bei diagnostichen Gasinsufflationen. Fortschr Geb Rontgenstr Nuklearmed Erganzungsband 103:187, 1965

Bumm E: Diskussion über die Endometritis. In Chrobak R, Pfannenstiel I (eds): Verhandlungen der Deutschen Gesellschaft für Gynäkologie, p 524. Leipzig, Breitkopf & Hartel, 1895

Burnett JE Jr: Hysteroscopy-controlled curettage for endometrial polyps. Obstet Gynecol 24:621, 1964

Castrén O, Airaksinen M, Saarikoski S: Decrease of litter size and fetal monoamines by 6-hydroxy dopamine in mice. Experientia 29:576, 1973

Cates W, Ory HW, Rochat RW, et al: The intrauterine device and deaths from spontaneous abortion. N Engl J Med 295:1155, 1976

Charogoy-Vera J, Zapata-Sanchez G, Rangel-Malagamba S, et al: Dispositivo intratubario. Presented at the VIII World Congress of Gynecology and Obstetrics, Mexico, 1976

Chatterjee A, Harper MJ: Interruption of implantation and gestation in rats by Reserpine, chlorpromazine and ACTH: Possible mode of action. Endocrinology 87:966, 1970

Chervenak FA, Neuwirth RS: Hysteroscopic resection of the uterine septum. Am J Obstet Gynecol 141:351, 1981

Choate WH, Just-Viera JO, Yeager GH: Prevention of experimental peritoneal adhesions by dextran. Arch Surg 88:249, 1964

Cibils LA: Permanent sterilization by hysteroscopic cauterization. Am J Obstet Gynecol 121:513, 1975

Cimber HS: United States Patent 3,680,542: Device for occlusion of an oviduct, 1972

Cittadini E, Quartararo P, Perino A: Prospective diagnostiche di una nuova tecnica endoscopia: La colpomicroiscroscopia. Co Fe Se 8:19, 1981

Cittadini E, Perino A, Scarselli G, et al: Diagnosi e trattauento delle neoplasie cervicali intraepiteliali con una nuova tecnica endoscopica la microisteroscopia. Oncol Ginecol 1:48, 1982

Cohen MR, Dmowski WP: Modern hysteroscopy: Diagnostic and therapeutic potential. Fertil Steril 24:905, 1973

Corfman PA, Richart RM, Taylor HC Jr: Response of the rabbit oviduct to a tissue adhesive. Science 148:1348, 1965

Corfman PA, Taylor HC Jr: An instrument for transcervical treatment of the oviducts and uterine cornua. Obstet Gynecol 27:880, 1966

Coutinho EM, de Mattos CER, da Silva AR: The effect of ovarian hormones on the adrenergic stimulation of the rabbit fallopian tube. Fertil Steril 22:311, 1971

Coutinho EM, Maia H, Filho JA: Response of the human fallopian tube to adrenergic stimulation. Fertil Steril 21:590, 1970

Craft IL: Hysteroscopy. Proc R Soc Med 69:144, 1976

Craft IL: Hysteroscopy and laparoscopy. Br J Hosp Med 16:25, 1976

Craft IL: Uterotubal ceramic plugs. In Sciarra JJ, Droegemueller W, Speidel JJ (eds): Advances in Female Sterilization Techniques, p. 176. Hagerstown, Harper & Row, 1976

Cronjé HS, Street B, Van Niekerk WA: The value of hysteroscopy as a gynecological diagnostic procedure. S Afr Med J 59:326, 1981

Cumming DC, Taylor PJ: Combined laparoscopy and hysteroscopy in the investigation of the ovulatory infertile female. Fertil Steril 33:475, 1980

Darabi KF, Richart RM: Collaborative study on hysteroscopic sterilization procedures. Preliminary report. Obstet Gynecol 49:48, 1977

David A, Mettler L, Semm K: The cervical polyp: A new diagnostic and therapeutic approach with CO_2 hysteroscopy. Am J Obstet Gynecol 130:662, 1978

David C: Endoscopie de l'uterus après l'avortement et dans les suites de couches normales et pathologiques. Bull Soc Obstet 10:288, 1907

David C: L'endoscopie utérine. Paris, Thèse, 1908

David C: L'endoscopie utérine: Ses applications au diagnostic et au traitement des affections intra-uterines. Bull Mem Soc Medde Paris 138:91, 1934

Davis RH, Erb RA, Kyriazis GA, et al: Fallopian tube occlusion in rabbits with silicone rubber. J Reprod Med 14:56, 1975

Davis RH, Erb RA, Schneider HP, et al: Chronic rabbit and rhesus monkey fallopian tube occlusion with polymer. Fed Proc 34:339, 1975

Davis RH, Moonka DK, Platt HA, et al: Chronic occlusion of the rabbit fallopian tube with silicone rubber. Reprod Obstet Gynecol 6:142, 1978

Davis RH, Moonka DK, Platt HA, et al: Chronic occlusion of the rabbit fallopian tube with silicone polymer. Gynecol Obstet Invest 10:281, 1979

Davis RH, Platt HA, Moonka DK, et al: Chronic occlusion of the monkey fallopian tube with silicone polymer. Obstet Gynecol 53:527, 1979

De Brux J: Histopathologie Gynecologique. Paris, Masson et Cie, 1971

Dellepiane G, Mossetti C, Russo A: Semeiotica: L'esame ginecologico. Semeiotica: Esami speciali ginecologici. In Trattato Italiano di Ginecologia, Vol 2. Novara, De Agostini, 1966

De Maeyer JFDE: Die hysteroskopische Sterilisation mit Silastic plugs. Keitumer Kreis 2:4, 1980

De Maeyer JFDE: Een nieuwe methode van definitieve contraceptie. Patient Care 3:31, 1980

Désormeaux AJ: De l'endoscope et de ses applications au diagnostic et au traitement des affections de l'uréthre et de la vessie. Paris, Baillière, 1865

Deutschmann C, Lueken RP, Lindemann HJ: Hysteroscopic findings in postmenopausal bleeding. In Siegler AM, Lindemann HJ (eds): Hysteroscopy: Principles and Practice. Philadelphia, JB Lippincott, 1983

Devi PK, Gupta AN: Hysteroscopic removal of intrauterine contraceptive devices with missing threads. Indian J Med 65:5, 1977

Dexeus S, Labastida R, Galera L: Oncological indications of hysteroscopy. Eur J Gynaecol Oncol 2:61, 1982

Dexeus S, Labastida R, Serva X: Value of hysteroscopy in gynecological practice. In Albano V, Cittidini E (eds): Endoscopia Ginecologia. Palermo, Co Fe Se, 1981

Dickinson RL: Simple sterilization of women by cautery stricture at the intrauterine tubal openings, compared with other methods. Surg Gynecol Obstet 23:203, 1916

DiSaia PJ, Creaseman WT: Clinical Gynecologic Oncology, p 38. St. Louis, CV Mosby, 1981

Dmowski WP, Steele RW, Baker GF: Deficient cellular immunity in endometriosis. Am J Obstet Gynecol 141:377, 1981

Dorsey JH, Diggs ES, Baggish MS: Cystourethroscopy with the direct view contact endoscope. Obstet Gynecol 57:115, 1981

Droegemueller W, Greer BE, Davis JR, et al.: Cryocoagulation of the endometrium at the uterine cornua. Am J Obstet Gynecol 131:1, 1978

Droegemueller W, Greer BE, Makowski E: Cryosurgery in patients with dysfunctional uterine bleeding. Obstet Gynecol 38:256, 1971

Droegemuller W, Makowski E, Macsalka R: Destruction of the endometrium by cryosurgery. Am J Obstet Gynecol 110:467, 1971

Drühl S, Lindemann HJ: Sterlitität der Frau: Organische Ursachen. Diagnostik 9:50, 1976

Drühl S, Lindemann HJ, Mohr J: Erste Erfahrungen mit einer neuen Thermosonde für die transuterine Tubensterilization. Arch Gynaekol 219:39, 1975

Dubuisson JB, Barbot J, Henrion R: L'embryoscopie de contact. J Gynecol Obstet Biol Reprod 8:39, 1979

Duplay S, Clado S: Traite D'hystéroscopie. Rennes, Simon, 1898

Edström K: Intrauterine surgical procedures during hysteroscopy. Endoscopy 6:175, 1974

Edström K, Fernström I: The diagnostic possibilities of a modified hysteroscopic technique. Acta Obstet Gynecol Scand 49:327, 1970

Edström K, Fernström I: Delvis ny hysteroskopish metodik med mögjligheter till operativa ingrepp. Nord Med 86:990, 1971

El'Tsov-Strelkov VI, Lebedev NV, Golikova TP: Hysteroscopic potentials with continuous irrigation of the uterine cavity. Akush Ginekol 2:44, 1981

Englund F, Ingleman-Sundberg A, Westin B: Hysteroscopy in diagnosis and treatment of uterine bleeding. Gynaecologia 143:217, 1957

Erb RA, Davis RH, Balin H, et al: Device and technique for blocking the fallopian tubes: A method for reversible contraceptive sterilization. In Schima ME, Lubell I, Davis JE, et al (eds): Advances in Voluntary Sterilization, p. 336. Proceedings of the Second International Conference. Amsterdam, Excerpta Medica, 1974

Erb RA, Davis RH, Kyriazis GA, et al: Device and technique for blocking the fallopian tubes. Contemp Obstet Gynecol 4:92, 1974

Erb RA, Davis RH, Kyriazis GA, et al: System and technique for blocking the fallopian tubes. Adv Plann Parent 9:42, 1974

Erb RA: Silastic: A retrievable custom-molded oviductal plug. In Sciarra JJ, Droegemueller W, Speidel JJ (eds): Advances in Female Sterilization Techniques, p 259. Hagerstown, Harper & Row, 1976

Erb RA: Method and apparatus for non-surgical reversible sterilization of females. United States Patent 3,805,-767, April 23, 1974; reissued 29, 345, Aug. 9, 1977

Erb RA, Reed TP: Hysteroscopic oviductal blocking with formed-in-place silicone rubber plugs. I. Method and apparatus. J Reprod Med 23:65, 1979

Erb RA: Apparatus and method for the hysteroscopic non-surgical sterilization of females. United States Patent 4,245,623, Jan. 20, 1981

Esposito A, Accinelli G: Valore dell' isteroscopia e dell' isterosalpingografia nella diagnosi delle alterazioni della cavita uterina. Atti Ostet Ginecol 11:383, 1965

Esposito A, Accinelli G: Primi rilievi in tema di isteroscopia. Minerva Ginecol 17:483, 1965

Esposito A, Accinelli G: Praktische Anwendung der Hysteroskopie in der Gynaekologie. Zentralbl Gynaekol 88:1676, 1966

Esposito A, Ledda A: L'isteroscopia: Technica ed applicazioni cliniche. Arch Ostet Ginecol 72:155, 1967

Esposito A: Une exploration gynécologique trop negligée: l'Hystéroscopie. Gynecol Pract 19:167, 1968

Fermanian AKH: Diagnosis of submucosal nodules and large polyps by hysteroscopy and hysterography. Zh Eksp Klin Med 14:42, 1974

Ferrando G, Nalbandov AV: Direct effect on the ovary of the adrenergic blocking drug dibenzyline. Endocrinology 85:38, 1969

Fikentscher R, Semm K: Physikalische Grundlagen zur utero-tubaren Persufflation. Arch Gynaekol 188:184, 1956

Fishburne JI Jr, Keith L: Anesthesia. In Phillips JM (ed): Laparoscopy, p 69. Baltimore, Williams & Wilkins, 1977

Fourestier M, Gladu A, Vulmiere J: Perfectionnements à l'endoscopie médicale. Presse Med 60:1292, 1952

Fourestier M, Vulmiere J, Gladu A: Étude technique de l'endoscope medical universel. Sem Med Hop (Suppl) 17:13, 1956

Freund A: Ein neues, mit Kürett verbundenes Uterusendoskop. Geburtshilfe Gynaekol 91:663, 1927

Fritsch K: Über Endocervicoskopie und Colorphotographie in diesem Bereich. Med Bild-Dienst 12:32, 1960

Froriep R: Zur Vorbeugung der Notwendigkeit des Kaiserschnitts und der Perforation. Notiz Geb Natur Heilkunde 11:9, 1849

Fujimori H: Colpomicroscope in the early diagnosis of the cancer of the uterine cervix. Jpn Obstet Gynecol Soc 7:207, 1960

Gallinat A: Metromat—a new insufflation apparatus for hysteroscopy. Endoscopy 3:234, 1978

Gallinat A, Lueken RP, Lindemann HJ: A preliminary report about transcervical embryoscopy. Endoscopy 10:47, 1978

Gallinat A, Lueken RP, Lindemann HJ: Der ambulante Schwangerschaftsabbruch im ersten Trimenon in Parazervikalblockade mit Carticain. Geburtshilfe Frauenheilkd 38:105, 1978

Gallinat A, Lueken RP, Lindemann HJ: Komplikationen mit Intrauterinpessaren. Sexualmedizin 7:215, 1978

Gammelgaard J, Holm HH: Transurethral and transrectal ultrasonic scanning in urology. J Urol 124:863, 1980

Garmanova NV, Dekster LI, Urmancheeva AF, et al: Endoscopic study methods in the diagnosis of the initial forms of cervical cancer in pregnant women. Vopr Onkol 27:72, 1981

Gauss CL: Hysteroskopie. Arch Gynaekol 133:18, 1928

Gentile GP, Siegler AM: Inadvertent intestinal biopsy during laparoscopy and hysteroscopy. A report of two cases. Fertil Steril 36:402, 1981

Gerlock AJ: Oviduct response to glucagon during hysterosalpingography. Radiology 119:727, 1976

Getzen JH, Speiggle W: Anaphylactic reaction to dextran. Arch Intern Med 112:168, 1963

Goldrath MH, Fuller TA, Segal S: Laser photovaporization of endometrium for the treatment of menorrhagia. Am J Obstet Gynecol 140:14, 1981

Goodlin RC: Fetal monitoring. In Iffy L, Kaminetzky H (eds): Principles and Practice of Obstetrics and Perinatology, pp 839–888. New York, John Wiley & Sons, 1981

Gottinger E: Die Endozervikoscopie in der Praxis. Wien Med Wochenschr 118:568, 1968

Gribb JJ: Hysteroscopy: An aid in gynecologic diagnosis. Obstet Gynecol 15:593, 1960

Grode GA, Parkov KL, Falb RD: Feasibility study of the use of a tissue adhesive for the nonsurgical blocking of fallopian tubes. Phase I: Evaluation of a tissue adhesive. Fertil Steril 22:552, 1971

Grozdanov G: Aspects of contact hysteroscopy. Akush Ginekol 19:358, 1980

Grozdanov G: Khisteroskopiia—razviti i sushnost. Akush Ginekol 17:277, 1978

Grozdanov G: Podgotovka i tekhnika na kontaknata khisteroskopiia. Akush Ginekol 19:249, 1980

Gupta AN, Gupta I: Tubal occlusion by hysteroscopic electrocoagulation. Indian J Med Res 64:509, 1976

Gupta I, Devi PK, Gupta AN: Hysteroscopic removal of intrauterine devices with missing threads. Indian J Med Res 65:661, 1977

Gusberg SB, Kaplan AL: Precursors of corpus carcinoma. Am J Obstet Gynecol 87:662, 1963

Gusberg SB: Endometrial cancer. Int Surg Dig 76:497, 1976

Gutenberg I: Hysteroscopy. J Am Obstet Assoc 71:418, 1972

Hahnemann N: Early prenatal diagnosis: A study of biopsy techniques and cell culturing from extraembryonic membranes. Clin Genet 6:294, 1974

Hamant A, Durand E: L'hystéroscopie: Sa technique, ses résultats. Rev Fr Gynecol Obstet 31:1 1936

Hamou JE: Hystéroscopie et microhystéroscopie avec un instrument nouveau: Le microhystéroscope. In Albano V, Cittadini E, Quartararo P (eds): Endoscopia Ginecologica. Palermo, Co Fe Se, 1980

Hamou JE: Microhysteroscopy. Acta Endoscopy 10:415, 1980

Hamou JE: Hystéroscopie et microhystéroscopie avec un instrument nouveau: Le microhystéroscope. Endosc Gynecol 2:131, 1980

Hamou JE, Salat-Baroux J, Coupez F: La microhystéroscopie dans la detection du carcinome intraepithelial. Serment. Entretiens de Bichat, expansion scientifique française, Paris, 1981, p 179

Hamou JE, Salat-Baroux J: Microhystéroscopie. Misesa J Gynecol Obstet 5:25, 1981

Hamou JE: Hysteroscopy and microhysterocopy with a new instrument: The microhysteroscope. Acta Eur Fertil 10:29, 1981

Hamou JE: Microhysteroscopy. A new procedure and its original applications in gynecology. J Reprod Med 26:375, 1981

Haning RV Jr, Harkins PG, Uehling DT: Preservation of fertility by transcervical resection of a benign mesodermal uterine tumor with a resectoscope and glycine distending medium. Fertil Steril 33:209, 1980

Haselhorst G: Unsere Erfahrungen mit der Hysteroskopie. Zentralbl Gynaekol 59:2442, 1935

Hayashi M: Tubal sterilization by cornual coagulation under hysteroscopy. In Richart RM, Prager DJ (eds): Human Sterilization, p 334. Springfield, IL, Charles C Thomas, 1972

Hefnawi F, Fuchs A, Laurence KA: Control of fertility by temporary occlusion of the oviduct. Am J Obstet Gynecol 99:421, 1967

Heineberg A: Uterine-endoscopy, an aid to precision in the diagnosis of intra-uterine disease. Surg Gynecol Obstet 18:513, 1914

Hepp H: Zum Problem des "verlorenen" Intrauterinpessars. Geburtshilfe Frauenheilkd 37:653, 1977

Hepp H, Roll H: Die Hysteroskopie. Gynaekologe 7:166, 1974

Hepp H, Hoffmann G, Kreienberg R, et al: Möglichkeiten und Grenzen der Hysteroskopie unter Diagnostik des Korpuskarzinom. Fortschr Med 95:2113, 1977

Hepp H: Diagnostics in hysteroscopy. Endoscopy 10:232, 1978

Hermstein A, Neustadt B: Über den intramuralen Tubenteil. Z Geburtschilfe Gynaekol 88:43, 1924

Higgs GW, Moawad AH: The effect of ovarianhormones on the contractility of the rabbit oviductal isthmus. Can J Physiol Pharmacol 52:74, 1974

Hilfrich HJ, Almendral AC, Flaskamp D, et al: Untersuchungen über die diagnostiche Bedeutung der Hysterographie beim Korpuskarzinom. Geburtshilfe Frauenheilkd 29:346, 1969

Hindenburg HJ: Die Hysterokopie als klinische Routinemethode. III. Presented at the Europäischer Kongress f. Endoskopie (EECO), Berlin, June 14–17, 1981

Hoffken W, Junghans R, Zylka W: Die Grundlagen der Pneumoradiographie des rechten Herzens mit Kohlendioxyd. ROFO 86:292, 1957

Horwitz RC, Morton PC, Shaff MI, et al: A radiological approach to infertility—hysterosalpingography. Br J Radiol 52:255, 1979

Hosseinian AH, Lucero S, Kim MH: Hysteroscopic implantation of uterotubal junction blocking devices. In Sciarra JJ, Droegemueller W, Speidel JJ (eds): Advances in Female Sterilization Techniques, p 169. Hagerstown, Harper & Row, 1976

Huber SC, Piotow P, Orlans B, et al: IUDs reassessed—a decade of experience. Pop Rep Series B/2, 21, 1975

Hulf JA, Corall I, Strunin L, et al: Possible hazard of nitrous oxide for hysteroscopy. Br Med J 1:511, 1975

Hulf JA, Knights KM, Corall IM, et al: Proceedings: Arterialized venous pCO_2 changes during hysteroscopy. Br J Anaesth 48:273, 1976

Hulf JA, Corall IM, Knights KM, et al: Blood carbon dioxide tension changes during hysteroscopy. Fertil Steril 32:193, 1979

Hulka JF, Omran KF: Cauterization for tubal sterilization. In Richart RM, Prager DJ (eds): Human Sterilization, p 313. Springfield, IL, Charles C Thomas, 1972

Hyams MN: Sterilization of the female by coagulation of the uterine cornu. Am J Obstet Gynecol 28:96, 1934

Hysteroscopic sterilization. IPPF Med Bull 7:4, 1973

Iliesh AP, Kukute BG, Chuvasheva VI: Importance of hysteroscopy in diagnosing endometrial cancer. Akush Ginekol 2:52, 1981

Israel R: Current concepts in female sterilization. Clin Obstet Gynecol 17:139, 1974

Israngkun CH, Phaosavasdi S: Hysteroscopic sterilization: Complications in 269 cases. In Sciarra JJ, Droegemueller W, Speidel JJ (eds): Advances in Female Sterilization Techniques, p 148. Hagerstown, Harper & Row, 1976

Jewelewicz R, Khalaf S, Neuwirth RS, et al: Obstetric complications after treatment of intrauterine synechiae (Asherman's syndrome). Obstet Gynecol 47:701, 1976

Joelsson I, Levine RU, Moberger G: Hysteroscopy as an adjunct in determining the extent of carcinoma of the endometrium. Am J Obstet Gynecol 111:696, 1971

Johns A, Chiumecky J, Paton DM: Role of adrenergic nerves in ovulation and ovum transport. Lancet 2:1079, 1974

Johnsson JE: Hysterography and diagnostic curettage in carcinoma of the uterine body. Acta Radiol (Suppl) 326:1, 1973

Karacz B, Lindemann HJ: Hysteroskopie als Diagnostikum bei gynäkologischen Erkrankungen. Die Schwester 6, 1971

Karacz B, Lindemann HJ: Ergebnisse nach 230 transuterinen Tubensterilisationen per Hysteroskop. Fortschr Endosc 6:153, 1975

Kasby CB: Hysterosalpingography: An appraisal of current indications. Br J Radiol 53:279, 1980

Kennedy WH, Pilcher JF: Interior of uterus: Observed by hysteroscopic examination with findings in study of 25 cases. J Indiana Med Assoc 25:341, 1932

Klein SM, Garcia CR: Asherman's syndrome: A critique and current review. Fertil Steril 24:722, 1973

Kliment V, Stefanovic J, Kovancova L: Nase skuzenosti hysteroskopiose. Cesk Gynekol 39:29, 1974

Knudtson ML, Taylor PJ: Überempfindlichtkeitsreaktion auf Dextran 70 (Hyskon) während einer Hysteroskopie. Geburtshilfe Frauenheilkd 36:263, 1976

Koch UJ: International Meeting on Fertility Control, Genoa, 1980

Kocks J: Eine neue Methode der Sterilisation der Frauen. Zentralbl Gynaekol 2:617, 1878

Kohen M, Mattikov M, Middelton C Jr, et al: A study of three untoward reactions to dextran. J Allergy Clin Immunol 46:309, 1970

Kottmeier HL, Joelsson I: Hysteroskopi i diagnostiken av korpuskancer. Nord Med 86:990, 1971

Králová A: Hysteroskopie n gynekologické praxi. Cesk Gynekol 40:467, 1975

Kratochwil A: Ultraschalldiagnostik in der Gynäkologie. Gynaekol 9:166, 1976

Krebs HB, Petres RE, Dunn LJ, et al: Intrapartum fetal heart rate monitoring. III. Association of meconium with abnormal fetal heart rate patterns. Am J Obstet Gynecol 137:936, 1980

Kullander S, Sandahl B: Fetal chromosome analysis after transcervical placental biopsies during early pregnancy. Acta Obstet Gynecol Scand 52:355, 1973

Labwsetwar AP: Evidence for the involvement of a catecholaminergic pathway in gonadotrophin secretion for implantation in rats. J Reprod Fertil 33:545, 1973

Lee RS: Hysteroscopy. J Am Obstet Assoc 77:118, 1977

Leidenheimer H Jr: Office gynecology hysteroscopy. J Louisiana Med Soc 121:319, 1969

Levine RU, Neuwirth RS: Evaluation of a method of hysteroscopy with the use of 30% dextran. Am J Obstet Gynecol 113:696, 1972

Levine RU, Neuwirth RS: Simultaneous laparoscopy and hysteroscopy for intrauterine adhesions. Obstet Gynecol 42:441, 1973

Levine RU: A symposium on advances in fiberoptic hysteroscopy. Contemp Obstet Gynecol 3:115, 1974

Levy B, Lindner HR: The effects of adrenergic drugs on the rabbit oviduct. Eur J Pharmacol 18:15, 1972

Lindblom B, Hamberger L: Copper and contractility of the human fallopian tube. Am J Obstet Gynecol 141:398, 1981

Lindemann HJ: Eine neue Untersuchungsmethode für die Hysteroskopie. Endoscopy 4:194, 1971

Lindemann HJ: Hysteroscopy for the diagnosis of intrauterine causes of sterility. Presented at the VII World Congress on Fertility and Sterility, Tokyo/Kyoto, October 17–23, 1971

Lindemann HJ: Hysteroskopi v súvise s plánovanim rodićvstva. (Hysteroscopy in connection with planned parenthood.) Cesk Gynekol 37:522, 1972

Lindemann HJ: The use of CO_2 in the uterine cavity for hysteroscopy. Int J Fertil 17:221, 1972

Lindemann HJ: Transuterine Tubensterilisation per Hysteroskop. Geburtshilfe Frauenheilkd 33:709, 1973

Lindemann HJ: Utéroscopie. Med Hyg 31:1927, 1973

Lindemann HJ: Pneumometra für die Hysteroskopie. Geburtshilfe Frauenheilkd 33:18, 1973

Lindemann HJ: Eine neue Methode für die Hysteroskopie. Fortschr Endosc 4:185, 1973

Lindemann HJ: Historical aspects of hysteroscopy. Fertil Steril 24:230, 1973

Lindemann HJ: Die Hysteroskopie. Arch Gynaekol 214:241, 1973

Lindemann HJ: Mohr J: Tubensterilisation per Hysteroskop. Sexualmedizin 3:122, 1974

Lindemann HJ, Mohr J: Die Hysteroskopie als Untersuchungsmethode Infertilität der Frau. Fortschr Sterilitat 3:102, 1974

Lindemann HJ: Transuterine tubal sterilization by CO_2 hysteroscopy. In Sciarra JJ, Butler JC, Speidel JJ (eds): Hysteroscopic Sterilization, p 61. New York, Intercontinental Medical Book Corporation, 1974

Lindemann HJ: Transuterine tubal sterilization by hysteroscopy. J Reprod Med 13:21, 1974

Lindemann HJ, Mohr J: Ergebnisse von 274 transuterinen Tubensterilisationen per Hysteroskop. Geburtshilfe Frauenheilkd 34:775, 1974

Lindemann HJ: Fortschritte, Risiken und Grenzen der Endoskopie in der Gynäkologie. Fortschr Endosc 5:147, 1974

Lindemann HJ: A symposium on advances in fiberoptic hysteroscopy. Contemp Obstet Gynecol 3:115, 1974

Lindemann HJ: Die Wertigkeit der gynäkologischen Endoskopie gegenüber der Histologie und Zytologie. Fortschr Endosc 6:63, 1975

Lindemann HJ: Komplikationen bei der CO_2-Hysteroskopie. Arch Gynaekol 219:257, 1975

Lindemann HJ, Mohr J, Gallinat A, et al: Der Einfluss von CO_2-Gas während der Hysteroskopie. Geburtshilfe Frauenheilkd 36:153, 1976

Lindemann HJ, Mohr J: CO_2 hysteroscopy: Diagnosis and treatment. Am J Obstet Gynecol 124:129, 1976

Lindemann HJ, Siegler AM, Mohr J: The Hysteroflator 1000S. J Reprod Med 16:145, 1976

Lindemann HJ, Gallinat A: Physikalische und physiologische Grundlagen der CO_2-Hysteroskopie. Geburtshilfe Frauenheilkd 36:729, 1976

Lindemann HJ: Die Sterilisationsmethoden bei der Frau. Möglichkeiten der hysteroskopischen Sterilisation. Münch Med Wochenschr 118:903, 1976

Lindemann HJ: Hysteroskopie. In Frangenheim H (ed): Die Laparoskopie in der Gynäkologie, Chiurgie und Pädiatrie. Stuttgart, George Thieme Verlag, 1977

Lindemann HJ, Lueken RP: Transcervical amniocentesis via hysteroscopy within the first three months of pregnancy. In Phillips JM (ed): Endoscopy in Gynecology. St. Louis, Christian Board Publication, 1978

Lindemann HJ, Lueken RP: Development of the blastocyst as seen by hysteroscopy and the transcervical extraamniotic embryoscopy. Presented at the Ninth World Congress of Gynecology and Obstetrics, Tokyo, 1979

Lindemann HJ: CO_2 hysteroscopy today. Endoscopy 11:94, 1979

Lindemann HJ, Gallinat A, Lueken RP: Metromat. A new instrument for producing pneumometra. J Reprod Med 23:73, 1979

Lindemann HJ: Das fadenlose IUD. Helsinki-Keil-Grafenberg Symp 19:26, 1980

Lindemann HJ: Atlas der Hysteroskopie. Stuttgart, Gustav Fischer, 1980

Lindemann HJ, Gallinat A, Lueken RP: Intrauterinpessare in Situ. Coloratlas. Oberschleissheim, Germany, Nourypharma, 1980

Litwak B, Wiktorowskaja E: Regeneration der Uterusschleimhaut nach künstlichem Abort und hysteroskopisches Studium derselben. Monatschr Geburtsh Gynaekol 101:55, 1935

Liukko P, Grönroos M, Punnonen R, et al: Methods for evaluating the intrauterine location of carcinoma. Acta Obstet Gynecol Scand 58:275, 1979

Loffer FD, Pent D: Pregnancy after laparoscopic sterilization. Obstet Gynecol 55:643, 1980

Loffer FD, Pent D: Risks of laparoscopic fulguration and transection of the fallopian tubes. Obstet Gynecol 49:218, 1977

Lübke F: Erste Erfahrungen mit der Hysteroskopie. Geburtshilfe Frauenheilkd 34:387, 1974

Lübke F: The diagnostic value of intrauterine causes for sterility and infertility, using hysteroscopy. Presented at the VIII World Congress on Fertility and Sterility, Buenos Aires, Nov. 3–9, 1974

Lübke F: Hysteroskopie und Colpocoeliotomie. Arch Gynaekol 219:255, 1975

Lübke F: Kritische Bemerkungen zur Hysteroskopie. II. Presented at the Europaischer Kongress fur Endoskopie (EECO), Konstanz, April 16–19, 1975

Lueken RP, Gallinat A, Lindemann HJ: Hysteroskopische Untersuchungen nach Aspiration und instrumenteller Kürettage für den Schwangerschaftsabbruch. Geburtshilfe Frauenheilkd 37:776, 1977

Lueken RP, Lindemann HJ: Diagnosis and treatment of lost IUDs using CO_2-hysteroscopy. Endoscopy 9:119, 1977

Lueken RP, Lindemann HJ: Therapeutic possibilities with hysteroscopy. Endoscopy 10:232, 1978

Lucken RP, Krieg M: Transcervical amniocentesis for quantitative determination of fetoprotein. In Weitzel HK, Schneider J (eds): Alpha-Fetoprotein in Clinical Medicine. Sutttgart, Georg Thieme Verlag, 1979

Lueken RP, Lindemann HJ: Problems with IUDs use of hysteroscopy. In Proceedings of the First National Congress on Gynaecological Endoscopy, Bombay, 1979

Lueken RP: Position und Kinetik von Intrauterinpessaren. Keitumer Kreis 2:4, 1980

Lueken RP: Hysteroskopische Operationen. III. Presented at the Europäische Kongress für Endoscopie, West Berlin, 1981

Luys G: De l'hystéroscopie. Bull Mem Soc Med Paris 138:32, 1934

Lyon FA: Intrauterine visualization by means of a hysteroscope. Am J Obstet Gynecol 90:443, 1964

L'yvonnet M: De l'hystéroscopie. Thèse n° 176, Besançon 1973

Maathuis JB, Horbach JGM, van Hall EV: A comparison of the results of hysterosalpingography and laparoscopy in the diagnosis of fallopian tube dysfunction. Fertil Steril 23:428, 1972

MacDonald EJ, Airaksinen MM: The effect of 6-hydroxy dopamine on the oestrous cycle and fertility of rats. J Pharm Pharmacol 26:518, 1974

Mack TM, Pike MC, Henderson BE, et al: Estrogens and endometrial cancer in a retirement community. N Engl J Med 294:1262, 1976

Maddi VI, Wyso EM, Zinner EN: Dextran anaphylaxis. Angiology 20:243, 1969

March CM, Israel R: A critical reappraisal of hysteroscopic tubal fulguration for sterilization. Contraception 11:261, 1975

March CM, Israel R: Intrauterine adhesions secondary to elective abortion: Hysteroscopic diagnosis and management. Obstet Gynecol 48:422, 1976

March CM, Israel R: A comparison of steerable and rigid hysteroscopy for uterine visualization and cannulation of tubal ostia. Contraception 14:269, 1976

March CM, Israel R, March AD: Hysteroscopic management of intrauterine adhesions. Am J Obstet Gynecol 130:653, 1978

March CM, Israel R: Gestational outcome following hysteroscopic lysis of adhesions. Fertil Steril 36:455, 1980

Marchetti M, Valente S, Murari G: La cervicoisteroscopia a contatto nel follow-up della contraccezione meccanica. Ginecol Clin 2:1, 1981

Marleschki V: Ein weiterer Schritt in der Frühdiagnose des Intracervikal und Korpuskarzinomes. Krebsarzt 21:159, 1966

Marleschki V: Moderne Cerviscoscopie und Hysteroscopie; Abhandlungen der deutschen Akademie der Wissenschaften zu Berlin. Akad Verlag Berlin, 3:421, 1966

Marleschki V: Die moderne Zervikoskopie und Hysteroskopie. Zentralbl Gynaekol 88:637, 1966

Marleschki V: Hysteroskopische Feststellung der spontanen Perfusionsschwankungen am menschlichen Endometrium. Zentralbl Gynaekol 90:1094, 1968

Marleschki V: Das Universal Hysteroskop nach Marleschki. Urania 6:34, 1971

Marleschki V: Geburtserleichterung unter Kontrolle. Urania 11:34, 1971

Marleschki V: The hysteroscopic method of Marleschki. Amsterdam, Excerpta Medica, 1973

Marleschki V: Hysteroscopy in Gynaecological and Obstetric Emergencies: Urgent Endoscopy of Digestive and Abdominal Diseases, p 248. Basel, Karger, 1972

Marleschki V: Hysteroscopic study of uterine circulation in normal labor and in labor involving the use of abdominal decompression. Amsterdam, Excerpta Medica, 1973

Marshall JM: Effects of catecholamines on the smooth muscle of the female reproductive tract. Ann Rev Pharmacol 13:19, 1973

Masubuchi K, Tenzin M: Abstract of the 14th Japanese Congress of Obstet Gynecol, 1962

Masubuchi K, Tenzin M: Colpomicroscope. Clin Obstet Gynecol, 13:1705, 1959

Mather EC, Refsal KR, Gustafsson BK, et al: The use of fibre-optic techniques in clinical diagnosis and visual assessment of experimental intrauterine therapy in mares. J Reprod Fertil (Suppl) 27:293, 1979

Mattingly RF: TeLinde's Operative Gynecology, p 420. Philadelphia, JB Lippincott, 1977

McCrea LE: Clinical Cystoscopy, Vol 1, p 5. Philadelphia, FA Davis, 1945

Mencaglia L, Scarselli G, Marchionni M, et al: Aspetti microcolpoisteroscopici del canale cervicale. In Cittadini E, Gasparri F, Maneschi M, et al (eds): Fertilita e Sterilita. Palermo, Co Fe Se, 1981

Menken FC: L'endocervicoscopie. Bull Soc Sci Med Grand Duche Luxemb 104:97, 1967

Menken FC: Fortschritte der gynäkologischen Endoskopie. In Demling L, Allenjann R, (eds): Fortschritte der Endoskopie. Stuttgart, FK Schattauer, 1969

Menken FC: Hysteroskopie: Methode praxisreif. Selecta 25:2459, 1972

Menken FC: Ein neues Verfahren mit Vorrichtung zur Hysteroskopie. Endoscopy 3:200, 1971

Menken FC: Un nouveau système d'hystéroscopie. Soc Gynecol 4:1, 1972

Menken FC: Micro-endoscopy of the uterine cervix. Geburtshilfe Frauenheilkd 41:192, 1981

Merrill JA: Dissemination of cancer cells during surgical curettage. Am Surg 29:206, 1963

Mettler L, Semm K, Rimkus V: Conclusions d'une experimentation sur la sterilisation thermique transutérine. Gynaecologia 27:383, 1976

Metzler R, Habighorst LV, Diethelm L: Komplikationen des Retropneumoperitoneum unter Verwendung von Kohlendioxyd als Insufflationsgas. Radiologie 12:367, 1972

Meyenburg M: Anwendung der Ultraschall-Schnittbildtechnik zur Darstellung von Intrauterinpessaren. Geburtshilfe Frauenheilkd 38:950, 1978

Michlewitz H: Hysteroscopy: Its role in detection of endometrial cancer. Clin Obstet Gynecol 22:737, 1979

Mikulicz-Radecki F von, Freund A: Ein neues Hysteroskop und seine praktische Anwendung in der Gynäkologie. Geburtshilfe Gynaekol 92:13, 1927

Mikulicz-Radecki F von, Freund A: Das Tubenhysteroskop und seine diagnostiche Verwendung bei Sterilität, Sterilisierung und Tubenerkrankungen. Arch Gynaekol 123:68, 1927

Mickulicz-Radecki F von: Experimentelle Untersuchungen über Tubensterilization durch Electrokoagulation. Z Geburtshilfe Gynaekol 94:318, 1928

Mickulicz-Radecki F von: Weitere Erfahrungen mit der Hysteroskopie, insbesonders beim Studium des Endometriums. Zentralbl Gynaekol 53:258, 1929

Miyazawa K: Hyskon hysteroscopy: A preliminary report. Hawaii Med J 37:169, 1978

Mocquot P, Palmer R: Diagnostic et traitement des polypes intracavitaires de l'uterus. Paris Med 2:462, 1936

Mohr J, Lindemann HJ: Hysteroscopy as a diagnostic method in female sterility. Fortschr Androl 3:102, 1974

Mohr J, Lindemann HJ: Vergleichende Resultate zwischen CO_2 Hysteroskopie, Hysterosalpingographie und Histologie. Arch Gynaekol 219:256, 1975

Mohr J, Lindemann HJ: Hysteroscopy in the infertile patient. J Reprod Med 19:161, 1977

Mohr J: Hysteroscopy as a diagnostic tool in postmenopausal bleeding. In Phillips JM (ed): Endoscopy in Gynecology, p 347. Downey, CA, American Association of Gynecologic Laparoscopists, 1978

Mohr J, Lindemann HJ: CO_2-Hysteroskopie, eine Methode zur Entfernung okkulter Intrauterinpessare. Arch Gynaekol 224:31, 1977

Mohr J: Idealform des Intrauterinpessars. Keitumer Kreis 2:4, 1980

Mohri C: A study of the intrauterine selfmovement of early human fetus by hysteroscopy and its recording on the film. J Jpn Obstet Gynecol Soc 3:374, 1956

Mohri T, Mohri C: Hysteroscopy. World Gynecol Obstet 6:48, 1954

Mohri T, Mohri C, Yamadori F: The original production of the glassfibre hysteroscope and a study of the intrauterine observation of the human fetus, things attached to the fetus and inner side of the uterus wall in late pregnancy and the beginning of delivery by means of hysteroscopy and its recording on the film. J Jpn Obstet Gynecol Soc 15:87, 1968

Mohri T, Mohri C, Yamadori F: Tubuloscope: Flexible glass fiber endoscope for intratubal observation. Endoscopy 2:226, 1970

Mohri T, Mohri C: Anomalies uterines decelées par un nouvel hystéroscope. Med Trib 23:5, 1970

Mohri T: Our 25 Years' Experience with Endoscopes. Tokyo, Jinmu Shobo, 1975

Mohri T: L'hystéroscope à fibres optiques. Med Trib 13:4, 1971

Moore DC: Regional Block. Springfield IL, Charles C Thomas, 1957

Morris RT: Endoscopic tubes for direct inspection of the interior of the bladder and uterus. Trans Am Assoc Obstet Gynecol 6:275, 1893

Morrow CP, Townsend DE: Synopsis of Gynecologic Oncology, p 153. New York, John Wiley & Sons, 1981

Muller P, Keller B: Hystéroscopie cinematographique. Technique, premiers résultats, possibilités futures. Rev Fr Gynecol Obstet 53:329, 1958

Muller P, Colette C, Gillet JY Jr, et al: L'hystéroscopie en 1973. Gaz Med Fr 80:4979, 1973

Muller P, Beller B: Hysteroscopie. Encycl Med Chirurgie 10:1, 1960

Munde PF: Minor Surgical Gynecology, p 99. New York, W Wood, 1880

Nakanishi H, Wood C: Effects of adrenergic blocking

agents on human fallopian tube motility in vitro. J Reprod Fertil 16:21, 1968

Neil JR: "Oscopy" in obstetrics and gynaecology. Aust Fam Physician 8:841, 1979

Neubueser D, Vahrson H: Zur Diagnostik und Entfernung okkulter Intrauterinpessaren. Geburtshilfe Frauenheilkd 37:277, 1977

Neubueser D, Bailer P, Bosselmann K: Erfahrungen über die hysteroskopischen Tubensterilisation mit der Hochfrequenz- und der Thermomethode. Geburtshilfe Frauenheilkd 37:809, 1977

Neuwirth RS, Richart RM, Taylor HC Jr: Chemical induction of tubal blockade in the monkey. Obstet Gynecol 38:51, 1971

Neuwirth RS, Levine RU, Richart RM: Hysteroscopic tubal sterilization. I. A preliminary report. AM J Obstet Gynecol 116:82, 1973

Neuwirth RS: Hysteroscopy. Philadelphia, WB Saunders, 1975

Neuwirth RS: Tubal sterilization via laparoscopy and hysteroscopy. Acta Eur Fertil 6:265, 1975

Neuwirth RS: Hysteroscopy. In Major Problems in Obstetrics and Gynecology, Vol 8. Philadelphia, WB Saunders, 1975

Neuwirth RS, Amin HK: Excision of submucous fibroids with hysteroscopic control. Am J Obstet Gynecol 126:95, 1976

Neuwirth RS: A new technique for and additional experience with hysteroscopic resection of submucous fibroids. Am J Obstet Gynecol 131:91, 1978

Neuwirth RS: A new way to manage submucous fibroids. Contemp Obstet Gynecol 12:101, 1978

Neuwirth RS, Richart RM, Bolduc LR, et al: Sterilizzazione femminile con metilciano acrilato in ambulatorio. Co Fe Se 8:247, 1981

Neuwirth RS: Operative hysteroscopy. In Albano J, Cittidini E (eds): Endoscopia Ginecologica. Palermo, Co Fe Se 1981

Newell JW: Comparative study of various hysteroscopes. In Sclarra JJ, Butler JC, Speidel JJ (eds): Hysteroscopic Sterilization, p 27. New York, Intercontinental Medical Book Corporation, 1974

Ng AY, Chen C, Ratnam SS: Hysteroscopic sterilization with quinacrine sulphate and electrocoagulation. Aust NZ J Obstet Gynaecol 16:38, 1976

Nitze M: Eine neue Beobachtungs- und Untersuchungsmethode für Harnrohre, Harnblase und Rectum. Wien Med Wochenschr 29:650, 1879

Nitze M: Über eine neue Beleuchtungsmethode der Höhlen des menschlichen Körpers. Wien Med Presse 20:851, 1879

Noda S: Colpomicroscopy. J Osaka City Med Center 11:179, 1962

Noda S: Studies on colpomicroscopy especially on the visible depth of stained epithelia of the vaginal portion of the uterus. J Osaka City Med Center 11:179, 1962

Nolte H: Indikationen und Methoden der Regionalanästhesie in der Geburtshilfe. Klin Anasthesiol Intensivther 4:189, 1974

Norman O: Hysterography in cancer of the corpus of the uterus. Acta Radiol (Suppl) 79, 1950

Norman O: Hysterography in cancer of the uterus. Semin Roentgenol 4:244, 1969

Norment WB: A study of the uterine canal by direct observation and uterogram. Am J Surg 60:56, 1943

Norment WB: Method of study of uterine canal. South Surg 13:885, 1947

Norment WB: Visualization and photography of uterine canal in patients. North Carolina Med J 9:619, 1948

Norment WB: Improved instrument for diagnosis of pelvic lesions by hysterogram and water hysteroscope. North Carolina Med J 10:646, 1949

Norment WB: A diagnostic test for tumors of the uterine canal. Am J Surg 82:240, 1951

Norment WB: Hysteroscopy in diagnosis of pathological conditions of uterine canal. JAMA 148:917, 1952

Norment WB: Hysteroscopic examination in older women. Geriatrics 11:13, 1956

Norment WB: The hysteroscope. Am J Obstet Gynecol 71:426, 1956

Norment WB, Sikes CH: Photographing tumors of the uterine canal in patients. JAMA 160:101, 1956

Norment WB, Sikes CH, Berry FX, et al: Hysteroscopy. Surg Clin North Am 37:1377, 1957

Norment WB, Sikes CH: Fiber-optic hysteroscopy: an improved method for viewing the interior of the uterus. North Carol Med J 31:251, 1970.

Norment WB: Hysteroscopy. J South Carol Med Assoc 71:118, 1975

Novak ER, Woodruff JD: Novak's Gynecologic & Obstetric Pathology, p. 140. Philadelphia, WB Saunders, 1979

Obstetrician convicted in sterilization death is placed on probation. Ob Gyn News 9:4, 1974

Oelsner G, Amnon D, Insler V, et al: Outcome of pregnancy after treatment of intrauterine adhesions. Obstet Gynecol 44:341, 1974

Ohkawa K, Ohkawa R: Panendomicroscope and its clinical use. The Colposcopist, 1980

Ohkawa K, Ohkawa R: Early detection and prevention of cancer development from dysplasia of uterine cervix. In Nieburgs HE (ed): Prevention and Detection of Cancer, Vol 1, p 829. New York, Marcel Dekker, 1978

Ohkawa K, Ohkawa R: Panendomicroscope and its clinical use. Scientific Exhibition Monograph, IX World Congress of Gynecology and Obstetrics, 34:86, 1980

Onetto E, Saavedra R, Crisosto G, et al: The treatment of uterine synechiae with the help of iatrogenic pseudopregnancy. Int J Fertil 10:217, 1965

Orley, J, Kallay F: Vaginoskop für Säuglinge und Kinder. Zentralbl Gynaekol 95:411, 1973

Orozdanov G: Preparation and technic for contact hysteroscopy. Akush Ginekol (Sofua) 19:249, 1980

Palmer R: Endoscopic sterilization and transuterine blind routes. Gynecologie 27:271, 1976

Palmer R: L'hystéroscopie cervicale. Rev Fr Gynecol 40:88, 1945

Palmer R: Un nouvel hystéroscope. Bull Fed Soc Gynecol Obstet Fr 9:300, 1957

Palmer R, Michon R: L'hystéroscopie cervicale. Gynecol Obstet 42:134, 1942

Pantaleoni D: On endoscopic examination of the cavity of the womb. Med Press Circ 8:26, 1869

Parent B, Toubas C, Doerler B: L'hystéroscopie de contact. J Gynecol Obstet Biol Reprod 3:511, 1974

Parent B, et al: Hystéroscopie de Contact. Paris, D.E.P., 1976

Parent B, Barbot J, Doeufleu B, et al: Hystéroscopie de contact. Documentation scientifique. Paris, Laboratories Roland Marie S.A., 1976

Parent B, Doerler B, Barbot J, et al: Metrorragies postmenopausiques: Diagnostic par l'hystéroscope de contact. Acta Endoscopy 8:13, 1978

Pauerstein CJ: The Fallopian Tube: A Reappraisal. Philadelphia, Lea & Febiger, 1974

Pauerstein CJ, Fremming BD, Hodgson BJ, et al: The promise of pharmacologic modifications of ovum transport in contraceptive development. Am J Obstet Gynecol 116:161, 1973

Pederson H: Hysteroskopien plad i den gynaecologiske diagnostik. Ugeskr Laeger 142:1022, 1980

Perez CA, Zivnuska F, Askin F, et al: Prognostic significance of endometrical extension from primary carcinoma of the uterinecervix. Cancer 35:1493, 1975

Perino A, Quartararo P, Sajeva F, et al: Ruolo della microcolpoisteroscopia nello studio della patologia cervicale. I Protocollo di studio. Co Fe Se 8: 149, 1981

Persinaninov LS, Pobedinskii NM, Abramova MN, et al: Primeneni gisteroskopii ginekologischeskoi klinika. Akush Ginekol (Mosk) 46:3, 1970

Phillips, JM, Keith L: Gynecological Laparoscopy: Principles and Techniques. Miami, Symposium Specialists, 1974

Phillips JM: Hysteroscopy: An overview and history of intrauterine gas insufflation. J Reprod Med 16:329, 1976

Phillips JM: The impact of laparoscopy, hysteroscopy, fetoscopy and culdoscopy on gynecologic practice. J Reprod Med 16:187, 1976

Phillips JM: Endoscopy in Gynecology. Downey, CA, American Association of Gynecologists and Laparoscopists, 1978

Pineda RL, Tozzini RI: Histeroscopiá en esterilidad e infertilida. Obstet Ginecol Latino Am 38:139, 1980

Pineda RL, Tozzini RI: Estado actual de la histeroscopía en esterilidad. Obstet Ginecol Latino Am 39:169, 1981

Pobedinskii NM, Volobuev AI: Primeneni gisteroskopii v ginekologicheskoi klinike. Akush Ginekol (Mosk) 9:65, 1976

Poma PA, Diaz A: Hysteroscopy in the diagnosis of endometrial carcinoma: Case report. J Am Geriatr Soc 28:130, 1980

Popp LW: Deutsches Patentamt, Offenlegungsschrift 25 37 620: Tuben-Ballon-Pessar (TBP), 1975

Popp LW: Contraception by means of reversible tubal occlusion (film). Presented at the VIII World Congress of Gynecology and Obstetrics. Mexico, 1976

Popp LW: Deutsches Patentamt, Offenlegungsschrift 29 13 036: Krallenpessar zur temporären Infertilisierung der Frau durch den reversiblen Verschluss der Eileiterlumina, 1979

Popp LW, Lueken RP, Lindemann HJ: Hysterosonographie. Diagn Intensiv Ther 4:69, 1982

Porto R, Gaujoux J, Serment H: Premiers resultats d'une nouvelle méthode d'hystéroscopie: Communication à la Société Nationale de Gynécologie et d'Obstétrique de France (groupement de Marseille), June 20, 1972

Porto R: Une nouvelle méthode d'hystéroscopie. Marseille, Thèse, 1972

Porto R, Gaujoux J: Progrès récents en hystéroscopie. J Gynecol Obstet Biol Reprod (Supp 2) 1:406, 1972

Porto, R, Gaujoux J: Une nouvelle méthode d'hystéroscopie, instrumentation et technique. J Gynecol Obstet Biol Reprod 1:691, 1972

Porto R, Gaujoux J: Une nouvelle méthode d'hystéroscopie. Note préliminaire. CR Soc Fr Gynecol 42:89, 1972

Porto R, Serment H: Pneumo-hystéroscopie. Gaz Med Fr 80:4985, 1973

Porto R, Gaujoux J: Hystéroscopie: Technique et résultats. In Les Entretiens de Bichat (Chirurgie et Spécialités), pp 453–456. Paris, L'Expansion, 1973

Porto R: Rapport de l'hystéroscopie en pratique gynécologique. Gynaekologie 24:301, 1973

Porto R: La pneumo-hystéroscopie. Acta Endoscopy 3:84, 1973

Porto R: Pneumohysteroscopy: Instrumentation and technique. In Sciarra JJ, Butler JC, Speidel JJ (eds): Hysteroscopic Sterilization, p 51. New York, Intercontinental Medical Book Corporation, 1974

Porto R: Corrélation hystérographiques et hystéroscopiques. Presented at the Faculté de Médecine Broussais, Paris, June 15, 1974

Porto R: Hystéroscopie. In Encyclopédie Médico-Chirurgicale, Paris, 1974

Porto R: Hystéroscopie. Presented Travail de la Clinique Obstétricale et Gynécologique de la Faculté de Medicine de Marseille, Paris, 1975

Pous-Ivern LC: La histeroscopía con CO_2. Técnica, indicaciones y contraindicaciones. Reproduccion 3:295, 1971

Prudnikoff YV: Artificial sterilization of women by means of electrocoagulation. Thesis, Imperial Academy of Medicine, St. Petersburg, 1912

Pye A: Ambulatory hysteroscopy and intrauterine devices. Gynaekologie 27:75, 1976

Pye A: Pourquoi l'hystéroscopie en ambulatoire. Gynécologie 25:321, 1974

Pye A: L'endoscopie de contact en gynécologie. Gynaékologie, 25:317, 1974

Quakernack K, Schmidt EH, Lieder B, et al: The identification of IUDs by ultrasound in the uterine cavity. Eur J Obstet Gynecol Reprod Biol 4:203, 1975

Quiñones RG, Alvarado DA, Esperanza AR: Histeroscopía. Reporte preliminar. Ginecol Obstet Mex 27:683, 1970

Quiñones RG, Alvarado DA, Aznar RR: Histeroscopía. Una nueva téchnica. Ginecol Obstet Mex 32:237, 1972

Quiñones RG, Alvarado DA, Aznar RR: Tubal catheterization: Applications of a new technique. Am J Obstet Gynecol 114:674, 1972

Quiñones RG, Alvarado DA, Ramos RA: Histeroscopía. Una nueva téchnica. Ginecol Obstet Mex 32:237, 1972

Quiñones RG, Aznar RR, Alvarado DA: Tubal electrocauterization under hysteroscopic control. Contraception 7:195, 1973

Quiñones RG, Alvarado DA, Aznar RR: Tubal occlusion by electrocoagulation under hysteroscopy: A preliminary report. Int J Fertil 18:167, 1973

Quiñones RG: A symposium on advances in fiberoptic hysteroscopy. Contemp Obstet Gynecol 3:115, 1974

Quiñones RG, Alvarado DA, Ley E: Tubal electrocoagulation under hysteroscopic control (three hundred and fifty cases). Am J Obstet Gynecol 121:1111, 1975

Quiñones RG, Alvarado DA, Ley E: Hysteroscopic sterilization. Int J Gynaecol Obstet 14:27, 1976

Raabe N, Edström K, Frankman O: Hysteroscopic study of early pregnancy with an intrauterine device in situ. Presented at the Third International Conference on Intrauterine Contraception, 1974, p 64

Rakshit B: Intratubal blocking device for sterilization without laparotomy. Calcutta Med J 65:90, 1968

Rakshit B: Attempts at chemical blocking of the fallopian tube for female sterilization. J Obstet Gynaecol India 20:618, 1970

Rakshit B: The scope of liquid plastics and other chemicals for blocking the fallopian tube. In Richart RM, Prager DJ (eds): Human Sterilization, p 213. Springfield, IL, Charles C Thomas, 1972

Rao RP: Lost intrauterine devices and their localization. J Reprod Med 20:195, 1978

Reed TP, Erb RA: Hysteroscopic oviductal blocking with formed-in-place silicone rubber plugs. II. Clinical studies. J Reprod Med 23:69, 1979

Reed TP, Erb RA: Tubal occlusion with silicone rubber: An update. J Reprod Med 25:25, 1980

Reed TP, Erb RA, Cooper JM: Methods for improving tubal ostial observation, obturation, and perfusion with the hysteroscope. In Siegler AM, Lindemann HJ (eds): Hysteroscopy: Principles and Practice. Philadelphia, JB Lippincott, 1983

Reed TP, Erb RA, DeMaeyer JFDE: Tubal occlusion with silicone rubber: An update 1980. J Reprod Med 26:534, 1981

Reinermann T: Die Kontrolle des Heilungsverlaufes des Korpuskarzinoms durch Hysterographie. Fortschr Rontgen 102:292, 1965

Richart RM, Najar AJG, Neuwirth RS: Transvaginal human sterilization: A preliminary report. Am J Obstet Gynecol 111:108, 1971

Richart RM, Prager DJ: Human Sterilization, Springfield, IL, Charles C Thomas, 1972

Richart RM, Neuwirth RS, Taylor HC Jr: Experimental studies of fallopian tube occlusion. In Richart RM, Prager DJ (eds): Human Sterilization, p 360. Springfield, IL, Charles C Thomas, 1972

Richart RM, Neuwirth RS, Israngkun C, et al: Female ster-

ilization by electrocoagulation of tubal ostia using hysteroscopy. Am J Obstet Gynecol 117:801, 1973

Richart RM, Neuwirth RS, Bolduc LR: Single-application fertility regulating device: Description of a new instrument. Am J Obstet Gynecol 127:86, 1977

Riedel HH, Semm K: Das postpelviskopische (laparoskopische) subphrenische Schmerzsyndrom. Arch Gynaekol 20:228, 1979

Rimkus V, Semm K: Sterilization by carbon dioxide hysteroscopy. In Sciarra JJ, Butler JC, Spiedel JJ (eds): Hysteroscopic Sterilization, p 75. New York, Intercontinental Medical Book Corporation, 1974

Rimkus V, Semm K: Die Schwachstromkoagulation als Methode der Sterilisation unter hysteroskopischer Kontrolle. Arch Gynaekol 219:40, 1975

Rimkus V, Semm K: Hysteroscopic sterilization, a routine method? Int J Fertil 22:121, 1977

Ringrose C: Office tubal sterilization. Obstet Gynecol 42:151, 1973

Rioux JE: Sterilization of women: Benefits vs risks. Int J Gynaecol Obstet 16:48, 1978

Rioux JE, Yuzpe AA: Gynecologic endoscopic equipment. In Current Problems in Obstetrics and Gynecology. Chicago, Year Book Medical Publishers, 1981

Roberts S, Long L, Janasson O, et al: The isolation of cancer cells from the blood stream during uterine curettage. Surg Gynecol Obstet 111:3, 1960

Robertson JR: Ambulatory gynecologic urology. Clin Obstet Gynecol 17:255, 1974

Robertson JR: Letter: missing strings. Obstet Gynecol 45:601, 1975

Rochet Y, Dargent D, Bremond A, et al: Le devenir obstetrical de femmes opérées de synéchies utérines. J Gynecol Obstet Biol Reprod 8:723, 1979

Rosenfeld DL: A study of hysteroscopy as an adjunct to laparoscopy in the evaluation of the infertile woman. In Phillips JM (ed): Endoscopy in Gynecology, p 337. Downey, CA, American Association of Gynecologic Laparoscopists, 1978

Rubin IC: The nonoperative determination of patency of fallopian tubes. JAMA 74:1017, 1920

Rubin IC: Uterine endoscopy, endometroscopy with the aid of uterine insufflation. Am J Obstet Gynecol 10:313, 1925

Rubin IC: Uterotubal Insufflation. St. Louis, CV Mosby, 1947

Saidl J: Hysteroscopy. Casop Lek Cesk 68:905, 1929

Salat-Baroux J, Hamou J: Microhystéroscopie. Une nouvelle méthode, son application en gynécologie. Med Hyg 1377:1696, 1980

Salat-Baroux J, Hamou JE: Complications from microhysteroscopy. In Siegler AM, Lindemann HJ (eds): Hysteroscopy: Principles and Practice. Philadelphia, JB Lippincott, 1983

Salat-Baroux J, Hamou JE, Uzan S, et al: Postabortal hysteroscopy. In Siegler AM, Lindemann HJ (eds): Hysteroscopy: Principles and Practice. Philadelphia, JB Lippincott, 1983

Salgado C: Esterilizacão provocada pela injecão intrauterina de cáusticos. An Acad Bras Ginecol 11:503, 1941

Saling E: Die Amnioskopie. Ein neues Verfahren zum Erkennen von Gefahrenzustanden des Feten bei noch stehender Fruchtblase. Geburtshilfe Frauenheilkd 22:830, 1962

Saling E, Dudenhusen JW: The present situation of clinical monitoring of the fetus during labor. J Perinat Med 1:75, 1973

Sampson JA: Heterotopic or misplaced endometrial tissue. Am J Obstet Gynecol 10:649, 1925

Saveljeva GM, Breusenko VG: Die Bedeutung von zusätzlichen Üntersuchungsmethoden bei Kranken mit intrauteriner Pathologie. Zentralbl Gynaekol 101:976, 1979

Scarselli G, Marchionni M, Verni A: Hysteroscopy of contact and submucous myomas: Differential diagnosis between various benign and clinical patterns. Acta Eur Fertil 10:181, 1979

Scarselli G, Verni A, Marchionni M: Isteroscopia a contatto. In Maneschi M, Cittadini E, Quartararo P (eds): Fertilità e Sterilità. Palermo, Co Fe Se, 1979

Scarselli G, Mencaglia L, Hamou J: Atlante di Microisteroscopia. Palermo, Co Fe Se, 1981

Scarselli G, Mencaglia L, Pieroni G: Microcolpositeroscopia. Co Fe Se 8:251, 1981

Scarselli G, Mencaglia L, Pieroni G, et al: Microcolpoisteroscopia: Aspetti normali e patologici in vivo degli epiteli cervicali. Co Fe Se 8:255, 1981

Scarselli G, Mencaglia L, Branconi F, et al: Immagini dall'endometrio: L'iperplasia. Co Fe Se 8:265, 1981

Scarselli G, Mencaglia L: La microcolposcopia secondo Hamou. Notiz Assoc Ital Citolog 7:4, 1981

Scarselli G, Mencaglia L, Bruni V, et al: Salpingoscopia: Studio dell'orizio uterino-tubarico. In Fertility & Sterility. (Cittadini E, Gasparri F, Maneschi M, Quartararo P, Scarselli G, Eds.) Co Fe Se, Palermo 1981

Scarselli G, Mencaglia L, Colafranceschi M, et al: Microhysteroscopy: The reliability of a new hysteroscopic technique in the diagnosis of endometrial hyperplasia. Presented at the Tenth Annual Meeting of the American Association of Gynecologic Laparoscopists, Phoenix, November 4–8, 1981

Scarselli G, Mencaglia L, Hamou J: Atlante di Microcolposteroscopia. Palermo, Co Fe Se, 1981

Scarselli G, Mencaglia L, Branconi F, et al: Utilità della microisteroscopia panoramica nella diagnosi differenziale tra polipi endometriali, fibromiomi sottomucosi e iperplasie endometriali. In Cittadini E, Gasparri F, Maneschi M, Quartararo P, Scarselli G, (eds): Fertilità e sterilità. Palermo, Co Fe Se, 1981

Scarselli G, Mencaglia L, Colafranceschi M, et al: Microisteroscopia: Affidabilità di una nuova tecnica isteroscopica nella diagnosi della iperplasia endometriale. Oncol Ginecol 1:23, 1982

Scarselli G, Mencaglia L, Tantini C, et al: Intraoperative microsalpingoscopy of the ampullar fallopian tube. Act Eur Fertil 13:35, 1982

Schack L: Unsere Erfahrungen mit der Hysteroskopie. Zentralbl Gynaekol 60:1810, 1936

Schenker JG, Polishuk WZ: Regeneration of rabbit endometrium after cryosurgery. Obstet Gynecol 40:638, 1972

Schenker JG, Polishuk WZ: Regeneration of rabbit endometrium following intrauterine instillation of chemical agents. Gynecol Invest 4:1, 1973

Schmidt-Matthiesen H: Die Hysteroskopie als klinische Routinemethode. Geburtshilfe Frauenheilkd 26:1498, 1966

Schmidt EH, Wagner H, Quakernack K: Ergebnisse der Lageüberwachung von Intrauterinpessaren durch Ultraschall. Geburtshilfe Frauenheilkd 39:134, 1979

Schroeder C: Über den Ausbau und die Leistungen der Hysteroskopie. Arch Gynaekol 156:407, 1934

Schwartz PE, Goldstein HM, Wallace S, et al: Control of arterial hemorrhage using percutaneous arterial catheter techniques in patients with gynecologic malignancies. Gynecol Oncol 3:276, 1975

Schüller V, Walther G, Staehler G, et al: Beurteilung von Blasenwandveränderungen mit der intravesikalen Ultraschalltomographie. Urology 20:204, 1981

Schweppe KW, Wagner H, Beller FK: Schwangerschaftsunterbrechung durch Saugkürettage im Vergleich zur konventionellen Metallkürette. Med Welt 31:479, 1980

Sciarra JJ: Research and development programs to achieve practical outpatient sterilization. In Duncan CW, Falb RD, Speidel JJ (eds): Female Sterilization, p 159. New York, Academic Press, 1972

Sciarra JJ, Butler JC, Speidel JJ (eds): Hysteroscopic Sterilization. New York, Intercontinental Medical Book Corporation, 1974

Sciarra JJ, Droegemueller W, Speidel JJ (eds): Advances in Female Sterilization Techniques. Hagerstown, Harper & Row, 1976

Sciarra JJ, Valle RF: Hysteroscopy: A clinical experience with 320 patients. Am J Obstet Gynecol 127:340, 1977

Sciarra JJ: Hysteroscopic approaches for tubal closure. In Zatuchni GI, Labbok MH, Sciarra JJ (eds): Research Frontiers in Fertility Regulation, p 270. Hagerstown, Harper & Row, 1980

Segond R: Hystéroscopie. Bull Soc Obstet Gynecol 23:709, 1934

Segond R: L'hystéroscopie. Gaz Med Fr 42:285, 1935

Segond R: Le diagnostic des métrorragies par l'hystéroscopie. Gaz Med Fr 43:1031, 1936

Segond R: L'hystéroscopie, déscription des images critiques. Gaz Med Fr 44:271, 1937

Segond R: L'hystéroscopie. Etat actuel de sa technique et son emploi clinique. Sem Hop Paris 19:215, 1943

Seki M, Riedel HH, Viehweg G, et al: Ein Vergleich der Flüssigkeits- und CO_2-Hg Hysteroskopie bei Blutungsanomalien im reproduktiven Alter. Arch Gynaekologie 232:741, 1981

Semm K: Die Laparoskopie in der Gynäkologie. Geburtshilfe Frauenheilkd 27:1029, 1967

Semm K: Transabdominale oder transvaginale Eileiter-sterilisation mit einer neuen Koagulationszange. Endoscopy 6:40, 1970

Semm K: Sterilisierung durch Tubenkoagulation der pars intramuralis tubae per Hysteroskopiam. Endoscopy 5:218, 1973

Semm K, Rimkus V: Technische Bemerkungen zur CO_2 Hysteroskopie. Geburtshilfe Frauenheilkd 34:392, 1974

Semm K: Pelviskopie und Hysteroskopie. Farbatlas und Lehrbuch. Stuttgart, FK Schattauer, 1976

Semm K: Atlas of Gynecologic Laparoscopy and Hysteroscopy. Rice AL (trans): Philadelphia, Saunders, 1977

Semm K: Kontakt hysteroskopische Fetoskopie. Gynaekol Prax 2:369, 1978

Seymour HF: A method of endoscopic examination of the uterus with its indications. Proc R Soc Med 19:74, 1926

Seymour HF: Endoscopy of the uterus with a description of a hysteroscope. J Obstet Gynaecol Br Emp 33:52, 1926

Sheares BH: Sterilization of women by intra-uterine electro-cautery of the uterine cornu. J Obstet Gynaecol Br Emp 65:419, 1958

Shephard DA, Vandam LD: Anaphylaxis associated with the use of dextran. Anesthesiology 25:244, 1964

Shiu-Chiu C, Sugimoto O: Diagnostic hysteroscopy for postmenopausal uterine bleeding. Acta Obstet Gynecol Jap 30:1737, 1978

Siegler AM: Hysterosalpingography, 2d ed, New York, Medcom Press, 1974

Siegler AM: A symposium on advances in fiberoptic hysteroscopy. Contemp Obstet Gynecol 3:115, 1974

Siegler AM, Kemmann EK: Hysteroscopy. Obstet Gynecol Surv 30:567, 1975

Siegler AM: A comparison of gas and liquid for hysteroscopy. J Reprod Med 15:73, 1975

Siegler AM, Kemmann EK: Hysteroscopic removal of occult intrauterine contraceptive devices. Obstet Gynecol 46:604, 1975

Siegler AM, Kemmann EK, Gentile GP: Hysteroscopic procedures in 257 patients. Fertil Steril 27:1267, 1976

Siegler AM, Kemmann EK: Location and removal of misplaced or embedded intrauterine devices by hysteroscopy. J Reprod Med 16:139, 1976

Siegler AM: Hysterography and hysteroscopy in the infertile patient. J Reprod Med 18:143, 1977

Siegler AM, Lindemann HJ: Hysteroscopy. New York, Medcom Press, 1977

Siegler AM, Kontopoulos VG: Lysis of intrauterine adhesions under hysteroscopic control. A report of 25 operations. J Reprod Med 26:372, 1981

Siegler AM, Kemmann EK: Hysteroscopy. Obstet Gynecol Surv 30:567, 1975

Silander T: Hysteroscopy through a transparent rubber balloon. Surg Gynecol Obstet 114:125, 1962

Silander T: Hysteroscopy through a transparent rubber balloon in patients with carcinoma of the uterine endometrium. Acta Obstet Gynecol Scand 42:284, 1963

Silander T: Hysteroscopy through a transparent rubber balloon in patients with uterine bleeding. Acta Obstet Gynecol Scand 42:300, 1963

Simpson JL, Elias S, Malinak LR, et al: Heritable aspects of endometriosis. I. Genetic studies. Am J Obstet Gynecol 137:327, 1980

Smith DC, Prentice R, Thompson DJ, et al: Association of exogenous estrogens and endometrial carcinoma. N Engl J Med 293:1164, 1975

Speroff L, Glass RH, Kase NG: Clinical Gynecologic Endocrinology and Infertility, 2d ed, p 161. Baltimore, Williams & Wilkins, 1978

Starks GC: Correlation of meconium-stained amniotic fluid, early intrapartum fetal pH, and Apgar scores as predictors of perinatal outcome. Obstet Gynecol 56:604, 1980

Stauffer HM, Durant TM, Oppenheimer MJ: Gas embolism; roentgenologic considerations, including the experimental use of carbon dioxide as an intracardiac contrast material. Radiology 66:686, 1956

Stelmachow J: Place and role of hysteroscopy in gynecologic practice. Ginecol Pol 52:521, 1981

Stevenson TC, Taylor DS: The effect of methyl cyanoacrylate tissue adhesive on the human fallopian tube and endometrium. J Obstet Gynaecol Br Emp 79:1028, 1972

Stillman RJ, Schinfeld J, Schiff I: Use of the operating hysteroscope in the treatment of infertility caused by a cervical foreign body. Fertil Steril 33:335, 1980

Stjärne L, Brundin JO: Frequency–dependence of ^{3}H-noradrenaline secretion from human vasoconstrictor nerves: Modification by factors interfering with alpha or beta adrenoceptor or prostaglandin E_2 mediated control. Acta Physiol Scand 101:199, 1977

Stock RJ, Kanbour A: Prehysterectomy curettage. Obstet Gynecol 45:537, 1975

Sudmeyer W, Schilling K: Klinische Erfahrungen mit der intravenösen Applikation der Beta-Rezeptoren-Blockers Propranolol in der Anästhesie und Intensivpflege. Z Prakt Anasth Wiederbeleb 5:104, 1970

Sugimoto O: Obstetrical application of hysteroscopy. Sanfujinka Jissai 15:494, 1966

Sugimoto O: Hysteroscopy. I. Hysteroscope. Obstet Gynecol Ther Jpn 23:468, 1971

Sugimoto O: Hysteroscopy. II. Normal endometrial findings. Obstet Gynecol Ther Jpn 23:585, 1971

Sugimoto O: Hysteroscopy. III. Endometrial carcinoma. Obstet Gynecol Ther Jpn 23:693, 1971

Sugimoto O: Hysteroscopy. IV. Submucous myoma. Obstet Gynecol Ther Jpn 24:102, 1972

Sugimoto O: Hysteroscopy. V. Endometrial polyps. Obstet Gynecol Ther Jpn 24:217, 1972

Sugimoto O, Oshima M: Current and future status of hysteroscopy. Sanfujinka Jissai 21:377, 1972

Sugimoto O: Hysteroscopic sterilization by electrocoagulation. In Sciarra JJ, Butler JC, Speidel JJ (eds): Hysteroscopic Sterilization, p 107. New York. Intercontinental Medical Book Corporation, 1974

Sugimoto O: Hysteroscopic diagnosis of endometrial carcinoma. A report of fifty-three cases examined at the Woman's Clinic of Kyoto University Hospital. Am J Obstet Gynecol 121:105, 1975

Sugimoto O: Diagnostic and therapeutic hysteroscopy for traumatic intrauterine adhesions. Am J Obstet Gynecol 131:539, 1978

Sugimoto O: Hysteroscopic reversible sterilization. In Diagnostic and Therapeutic Hysteroscopy, p 208. Tokyo, Igaku–Shoin, 1978

Sweeney WJ: Accuracy of preoperative hysterosalpingograms. Obstet Gynecol 11:640, 1958

Sweeney WJ: The interstitial portion of the uterine tube. Its gross anatomy, course, and length. Obstet Gynecol 19:3, 1962

Swolin K, Rosencrantz M: Laparoscopy vs. hysterosalpingography in sterility investigation. A comparative study. Fertil Steril 23:270, 1972

Tatum HJ, Schmidt FH, Jain AK: Management and outcome of pregnancies associated with the copper intrauterine device. Am J Obstet Gynecol 126:869, 1976

Taylor PJ: Correlations in infertility: Symptomatology, hysterosalpingography, laparoscopy and hysteroscopy. J Reprod Med 18:339, 1977

Taylor PJ, Cumming DC: Hysteroscopy in 100 patients. Fertil Steril 31:301, 1979

Taylor PJ, Cumming DC: Laparoscopy in the infertile female. Curr Probl Obstet Gynecol 2:3, 1979

Taylor PJ, Graham G: Is diagnostic currettage harmful to women with unexplained infertility? Br J Obstet Gynaecol 89:296, 1982

Taylor PJ, Cumming DC, Hill PJ: Significance of intrauterine adhesions detected hysteroscopically in eumenorrheic infertile women and role of antecedent curettage in their formation. Am J Obstet Gynecol 139:239, 1981

Templeton AA, Kerr MG: An assessment of laparoscopy as the primary investigation in the subfertile female. Br J Obstet Gynaecol 84:760, 1977

Terruhn V: Die Ektopie in der Neugeborenenperiode. Eine vaginoskopische Studie. Geburtshilfe Frauenheilkd 39:568, 1979

Thom MH, White PJ, Williams RM, et al: Prevention and treatment of endometrial disease in climacteric women receiving estrogen therapy. Lancet 2:455, 1979

Thompson HE, Dafoe CA, Moulding TS, et al: Evaluation of experimental methods of occluding the uterotubal junction. In Duncan GW, Falb RD, Speidel JJ, (eds): Female Sterilization, p 107. New York, Academic Press, 1972

Tietze C: Therapeutic abortion in the United States. Am J Obstet Gynecol 101:784, 1968

Toaff R, Ballas S: Traumatic hypomenorrhea–amenorrhea (Asherman's syndrome). Fertil Steril 30:379, 1978

Tomaselli F, Donfrancesco E, Romao S: La sindrome di Asherman. Aspetti clinici e terapeutici. Minerva Ginecol 12:885, 1979

Townsend DE, Ostergard DR, Mischell D Jr, et al: Abnormal Papanicolaou smears. Am J Obstet Gynecol 108:429, 1970

Tozzini RI, Pineda RL: La histeroscopía como método diagnóstico en ginecología. Presented at the Actas de la Reunión Anual Nacional de FASCO, Resistencia, Argentina, September 1975

Tozzini RI, Pineda RL: El síndrome de amenorrea postraspado uterino y tratamiento de 50 casos. Obstet Ginecol Latino Am 36:114, 1978

Tozzini RI, Pineda RL: Histeroscopía en esterilidad. Presented at the Actas del IX Congreso Latinoamericano de Obstetricía y Ginecología, Lima, Peru, October 1978

Treisser A, Colau JC: Causes, diagnostic et traitement des perforations utérines. J Gynecol Obstet Biol Reprod 7:837, 1978

Vagner Z: Some comments on hysteroscopic technique. Cesk Gynekol 41:679, 1976

Valente S: Diagnostic significance of hysteroscopy in gynecologic pathology. Acta Medico 6:81, 1979

Valente S, Marcolin D, Labi L: Hysteroscopy in pre-treatment staging of endometrial cancer. Cancer Treat Rep 63, 358, 1979

Valente S, Marcolin D: L'isteroscopia Nella Pratica Clinica. S.E.M.E.S. s.r.l. Ed. Padua, 1980

Valente S, Marcolin D, Maggino T, Pollon S: Ruolo della isteroscopia da contatto nella patologia ginecologica. Ginecol Clin 2:104, 1980

Valente S, Marchetti M, Murari G: Contact hysteroscopy in the diagnosis of endometrial carcinoma. Eur J Ginecol Oncol 1:22, 1981

Valle RF, Sciarra JJ: Diagnostic and operative hysteroscopy. Minn Med 57:892, 1974

Valle RF, Freeman DW: Hysteroscopy in the management of the "lost" intrauterine device. Adv Plann Parent 10:164, 1975

Valle RF, Sciarra JJ: Hysteroscopy: A useful diagnostic adjunct in gynecology. Am J Obstet Gynecol 122:230, 1975

Valle RF, Freeman DW: Hysteroscopy in the localization and removal of intrauterine devices with "missing strings." Contraception 11:161, 1975

Valle RF, Sciarra JJ, Freeman DW: Hysteroscopic removal of intrauterine devices with missing filaments. Obstet Gynecol 49:55, 1977

Valle RF: Hysteroskopie: Methode und klinische Anwendung. Extr Gynaecologia 2:9, 1978

Valle RF: Clinical application of hysteroscopy. In Phillips JM (ed): Endoscopy in Gynecology, p 327. Downey, CA, American Association of Gynecologic Laparoscopists, 1978

Valle RF: Hysteroscopy. Obstet Gynecol Annu 7:245, 1978

Valle RF: Hysteroscopy: Diagnostic and therapeutic applications. J Reprod Med 20:115, 1978

Valle RF, Sciarra JJ: Current status of hysteroscopy in gynecologic practice. Fertil Steril 32:619, 1979

Valle RF: Hysteroscopy in the evaluation of female infertility. Am J Obstet Gynecol 137:425, 1980

Valle RF, Sabbagha RE: Management of first trimester pregnancy termination failures. Obstet Gynecol 55:625, 1980

Valle RF: Hysteroscopic evaluation of patients with abnormal uterine bleeding. Surg Gynecol Obstet 153:521, 1981

Van der Pas H: Die ambulante Hysteroskopie als Untersuchungsmethode in der Gynäkologie. Keitum/Sylt, Keitumer Kreis, 1980

Van der Pas H, Van Herendael BJ: Atlas on Hysteroscopy. (in press)

Varangot J, Parent B, Barbot J, et al: Hystéroscopie de contact. Nouv Presse Med 6:113, 1977

Virutamasen P, Hickok RL, Wallach EE: Local ovarian effects of catecholamines on human chorionic gonadotropin-induced ovulation in the rabbit. Fertil Steril 22:235, 1971

Vodianik ND, Zhilkin GV, El'tsova-Strelkova VM, et al: Diagnostic importance of hysteroscopy. Akush Ginekol (Mosk) 6:23, 1978

Volobuev AI: Use of hysteroscopy in gynecological clinical practice. Akush Ginekol (Mosk) 46:3, 1970

Volobuev AI: Hysteroscopy. Med Sestra 31:17, 1972

Volobuev AI: Comparative evaluation of hysteroscopy and hysterography for the diagnosis of intrauterine pathology. Akush Ginekol (Mosk) 49:20, 1973

Wagner H: Derzeitiger Stand der Intrauterinpessaranwendung. In Beller FK (ed): Fortschritte in der Geburtshilfe und Gynakologie. Karlsruhe, G. Braun, 1979

Wagner H: Lost IUD. Keitum/Sylt, Keitumer Kreis, 1980

Wagner H, Schweppe KW, Kronholz HL, et al: Möglichkeiten der Extraktion von Intrauterinpessaren bei eingetretener Schwangerschaft. Med Welt 31:1317, 1980

Wallach EE: Evaluation and management of uterine causes of infertility. Clin Obstet Gynecol 22:43, 1979

Wallach EE: What uterine factors limit fertility? A symposium. Contemp Obstet Gynecol 18:126, 1981

Wamsteker K: Hysteroscopie. Thesis, University of Leiden, Holland. 1977

Welch WR, Scully RE: Precancerous lesions of the endometrium. Hum Pathol 8:503, 1977

Weseley AC: A new study of intrauterine synechiae. Diagn Gynecol Obstet 3:127, 1981

Williams PP: Endoscopic contraception: A look at three methods. Med Times 104:67, 1976

Word B, Gravlee LC, Wideman GL: The fallacy of simple uterine curettage. Obstet Gynecol 12:642, 1958

Wulfsohn NL: A hysteroscope. J Obstet Gynaecol Br Emp 65:657, 1958

Yoonessi M, Antowiak JM, Mariano EJ: Hysteroscopy—past and present: A review of 72 cases. Diagn Gynecol Obstet 2:179, 1980

Zakrojczyk S: Contribution à l'étude de l'hystéroscopie. Thèse Médecine Paris n° 519, Libr. Rodstein, 1937

Zampi G, Colafranceschi M, Taddei G: Morfologia delle lesioni preneoplastiche dell 'endometrio. In Apporto alla ricerca di base al controllo della crescita neoplastica, p 429. Napoli, Idelson, 1981

Ziel HK, Finkle WD: Increased risk of endometrial carcinoma among users of conjugated estrogens. N Engl J Med 293:1167, 1975

Zielske F, Becker K, Knauf P: Schwangerschaften bei Intrauterinpessaren. Geburtshilfe Frauenheilkd 37:473, 1977

Zipkin B, Rosenfeld DL: Hysteroscopic removal of a Heyman radium capsule. J Reprod Med 22:133, 1979

Zipper J, Medel M, Prager R: Alterations in fertility induced by unilateral intrauterine instillation of cytotoxic compounds in rats. Am J Obstet Gynecol 101:971, 1968

Zipper J, Medel M, Pastene L, et al: Intrauterine instillation of chemical cytotoxic agents for tubal sterilization and treatment of functional metrorrhagias. Int J Fertil 14:280, 1969

Zipper JA, Stachetti E, Medel M: Human fertility control by transvaginal application quinacrine on the fallopian tube. Fertil Steril 21:581, 1970

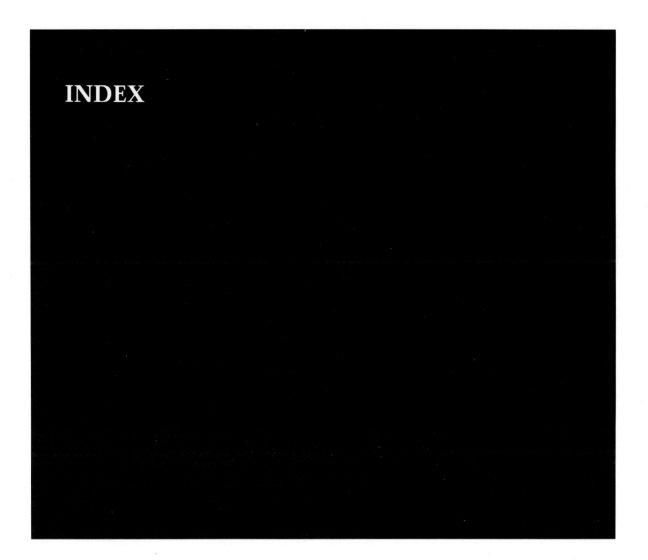

INDEX

An *f* following a page number indicates a figure; a *t* indicates tabular material.